Clinical Andrology

Clinical Andrology

Edited by Maisie Ellis

hayle
medical

New York

Hayle Medical,
750 Third Avenue, 9th Floor,
New York, NY 10017, USA

Visit us on the World Wide Web at:
www.haylemedical.com

ISBN: 978-1-63241-915-6

Cataloging-in-Publication Data

Clinical andrology / edited by Maisie Ellis.
    p. cm.
Includes bibliographical references and index.
ISBN 978-1-63241-915-6
1. Andrology. 2. Generative organs, Male. 3. Human reproduction--Endocrine aspects.
4. Men--Diseases. 5. Urology. I. Ellis, Maisie.
RC875 .C55 2020
612.6--dc23

Table of Contents

Preface

The world is advancing at a fast pace like never before. Therefore, the need is to keep up with the latest developments. This book was an idea that came to fruition when the specialists in the area realized the need to coordinate together and document essential themes in the subject. That's when I was requested to be the editor. Editing this book has been an honour as it brings together diverse authors researching on different streams of the field. The book collates essential materials contributed by veterans in the area which can be utilized by students and researchers alike.

Andrology is the medical specialty concerned with male reproductive and urological health. Anomalies of the genitalia, including the disorders of the connective tissues and alterations in the volume of cells such as in genital hypertrophy or macrogenitosomia, are under the scope of this discipline. Certain surgical procedures in men such as circumcision, vasectomy, vasovasostomy and orchidopexy are routine procedures in andrology. There are unique treatment strategies for the management of male genitourinary disorders such as erectile dysfunction, infertility, penile fracture, prostate cancer, testicular torsion, varicocele, etc. This book discusses the fundamentals as well as modern approaches of clinical andrology. It unfolds the innovative aspects of male reproductive and urological health which will be crucial for the progress of this field in the future. The extensive content of this book provides the readers with a thorough understanding of the subject.

Each chapter is a sole-standing publication that reflects each author's interpretation. Thus, the book displays a multi-facetted picture of our current understanding of application, resources and aspects of the field. I would like to thank the contributors of this book and my family for their endless support.

Editor

Targeting CXCR4 with CTCE-9908 inhibits prostate tumor metastasis

Donald Wong[4], Pridvi Kandagatla[1], Walter Korz[4] and Sreenivasa R Chinni[1,2,3*]

Abstract

Background: CXCL12/CXCR4 transactivation of epidermal growth factor family receptors in lipid raft membrane microdomains on cell surface is thought to mediate tumor growth and subsequent development of metastatic disease. CTCE-9908 is a known inhibitor of CXCR4. Herein, we tested the efficacy of CTCE-9908 in inhibiting prostate cancer cell growth, invasion, and metastasis.

Methods: We used a panel of *in vitro* assays utilizing human prostate cancer cell lines and an *in vivo* orthotopic prostate cancer model to assess the anti-tumoral activity of CTCE-9908.

Results: We demonstrated that (a) CTCE-9908 treatment resulted in no significant change in the growth of PC-3 and C4-2B cells; (b) 50 μg/ml of CTCE-9908 inhibited the invasive properties of PC-3 cells; (c) 25 mg/kg of CTCE-9908 did not alter primary tumor growth but it did significantly reduce total tumor burden in the animal including the growth of prostate and soft tissue metastases to lymph node and distant organ tissues. Histological analysis showed that CTCE-9908 treatment resulted in tumor necrosis in primary prostate tumors and no significant change in proliferation of tumor cells as measured by Ki-67 staining; (d) CTCE-9908 inhibited the tumor angiogenesis as measured by CD34 positive vessels in tumors.

Conclusions: These data suggest that CXCR4 inhibition by CTCE-9908 decreases the invasion potential *in vitro*, which then translated to a reduction of tumor spread with associated reduction in angiogenesis. Hence, CTCE-9908 may prove to be an efficacious novel agent to prevent and treat the spread of metastatic prostate cancer.

Keywords: CTCE-9908, CXCR4, CXCL12, Chemoinvasion and prostate cancer progression

Background

CXCR4 activation contributes to site-specific metastasis in several types of tumors, where circulating epithelial tumor cells express CXCR4 and common metastasis sites express abundant ligand, and ligand/receptor interaction has been shown to promote metastasis (reviewed in [1]). In prostate cancer patients, CXCR4 expression is upregulated during cancer progression [2] and aggressive cancer development [3,4]. We and others have previously shown that the CXCL12/CXCR4 axis plays an important role in PC cell proliferation, migration, and invasion [2,5-13]. Furthermore, we demonstrated that CXCL12/CXCR4 signals through the PI3 kinase/Akt pathway to induce matrix metalloproteinase

(MMP) expression and secretion, ultimately leading to migration and invasion of PC cells [5]. MMPs have been shown to be involved in the metastatic growth of prostate tumors in the bone and also appear to be activated at earlier time periods of tumor growth [14]; therefore, these data provide a mechanistic connection between "homing" of cancer cells to distant sites mediated by CXCL12/CXCR4 axis and followed by expression of MMPs which mediate invasion and proliferation. Similarly, our recent data demonstrate that CXCL12 binding to CXCR4 transactivates HER2 in PC cells to initiate chemo-invasive signaling and promotion of bone tumor growth, suggesting that this pathway is not only involved in initial seeding of bone metastases but also plays a key role in subsequent osseous expansion of metastases [10]. Furthermore, neutralization of CXCR4 in prostate cancer cells with anti-CXCR4 antibodies significantly reduced metastatic burden of experimental bone metastasis [13].

* Correspondence: schinni@med.wayne.edu
[1]Department of Urology, Wayne State University School of Medicine, 9200 Scott Hall 540 E. Canfield Avenue, Detroit, MI 48201, USA
[2]Department of Pathology, Wayne State University School of Medicine, 9200 Scott Hall 540 E. Canfield Avenue, Detroit, MI 48201, USA
Full list of author information is available at the end of the article

Targeting CXCR4 can have dual effects on inhibiting primary tumor growth and metastasis or mono effect on inhibiting either tumor growth or metastasis. Among CXCR4 inhibitors, AMD3100 is in clinical use for leukemia [15,16], and CTCE-9908 was granted approval by the FDA for osteosarcoma [17] based on its potent inhibitory activity in preclinical models of osteosarcoma [18]. AMD3100 is a bicyclam CXCR4 inhibitor that has been shown to be effective in reducing tumor growth in glioblastoma [19] and peritoneal metastasis in ovarian carcinoma [20]. CTCE-9908 is a peptide antagonist for CXCR4 and has shown to inhibit both primary tumor growth and metastases in osteosarcoma [18] and breast cancer models [21]. In a prostate cancer model, CTCE-9908 caused a reduction in tumor growth in a subcutaneous xenograft model via inhibiting angiogenesis by reducing the recruitment of pro-angiogenic myeloid precursor cells [22]. The current study assessed the efficacy of CTCE-9908 in an orthotopic prostate cancer model of primary tumor growth and metastases. The results show that CTCE-9908 is effective in reducing total tumor burden without significantly affecting the primary tumor growth.

Methods
Cell culture
PC-3 cells were obtained from American Type Culture Collection (Manassas, VA) and cultured in RPMI 1640 (Invitrogen Life Technologies, Carlsbad, CA) supplemented with 10% FBS and 1% Penicillin and Streptomycin. C4-2B cells were obtained from Dr. Leeland Chung and cultured in T media (Invitrogen Life Technologies, Carlsbad, CA) supplemented with 10% FBS and 1% Penicillin and Streptomycin.

Cell proliferation assay
1×10^4 PC-3 and C4-2B cells were seeded in a 96 well plate; the following day, cells were treated with varying concentrations (0–100 µg/ml) of CTCE-9908 dissolved in sterile dH_2O. After 24, 48, and 72 hours, cells were washed with PBS and exposed to 1X dye binding solution from CyQUANT® NF cell proliferation assay kit (Molecular Probes, Eugene, OR) for 60 min. Dye DNA-bound complexes were measured at 485 nm excitation and 530 nm emission.

Chemoinvasion assay
PC-3 cells were serum-starved for 4 hours. A total of 1.5-2.0×10^5 cells were seeded onto inserts in the upper chamber of trans-well culture plates (Becton Dickenson, San Diego, CA). Prior to seeding, the inserts were pre-coated with Matrigel. Untreated control and CTCE-9908 (1 and 50 µg/ml) pretreated PC-3 cells were seeded in Matrigel coated inserts. CXCL12 was placed in the bottom chamber to induce CXCR4-mediated chemoinvasion. After 24 hours,

the upper chambers were cleaned with cotton swabs to remove non-migrated/invaded cells, and the inserts were stained with Diff-Quik stain set (Dade Behring Inc., Newark, DE). The total number of migrated cells in a high power field was counted under a microscope, and the data presented is based on three independent experiments.

Orthotopic tumor growth and CTCE-9908 treatment
PC-3-GFP cells were grown subcutaneously as a tumor stock. The animal experiments were performed at Anti Cancer Inc., (San Diego, CA) in accordance with the principles and procedures outlined in the NIH Guide for the Care and Use of Laboratory Animals under assurance number A3873-1. Subcutaneous PC3-GFP tumor was excised, the necrotic areas removed, and 1 mm³ of tumor piece was implanted in the mouse ventral lobe of the prostate [23]. Animals were treated with 25 mg/kg/day CTCE-9908 daily, through subcutaneous injection at 3 days post-orthotopic tumor implantation for four weeks. Control animals were treated with water. The whole experiment was performed in three batches with six, four and ten animals in control group to a total of 20 mice and seven, four and ten animals in CTCE-9908 group to a total of 21 mice. Four weeks post tumor implantation, caliper measurements were made to determine the orthotpic prostate tumor volume by measuring perpendicular minor dimension (W) and major dimension (L) and volume was calculated by the $W^2 \times L \times 1/2$ formula. Whole body fluorescence measurements were made using Leica stereo fluorescence microscope (model LZ12) equipped with ST-133 Micromax high speed CCD camera (Princeton Instruments, Trenton, NJ) with anesthetized intact animals to determine total tumor burden including metastases. Starting two weeks after implantation whole body imaging was performed once a week. At the end of the study (four weeks) animals were euthanized and an open imaging was conducted to accurately document and quantitate tumor burden (primary tumors and metastatic tumor). Signals from individual organ metastasis were quantitated from control animals and CTCE-9908 treated animals.

Immunohistochemistry
Prostate tumors and lymph node metastases were paraffin embedded, and 4 µm thick sections were cut using microtome. Tissue sections were immunostained with anti-cytokeratin antibody, anti-Ki-67 antibody and anti-CD34 antibody. Vectastain Elite ABC kit was used to stain secondary antibody, and DAB chromogen was used to develop color. Images were captured with Axiovision software. For determining angiogenesis clusters of CD34 positive vessels (hot spots) were counted in 400× field in tumors and lymph node metastasis.

Statistical analysis

In vitro studies, statistical significance was determined by Student t-test and non-parametric ANOVA test, while in vivo assays were analyzed by Student t-test using GraphPad Prism software version 3.0 (GraphPad, San Diego, CA). $p \leq 0.05$ was considered to be statistically significant.

Results

CXCR4 inhibition by CTCE-9908 does not inhibit cell proliferation

In an effort to determine the effect of CTCE-9908 on proliferation, PC-3 and C4-2B cells were treated with increasing concentrations of CTCE-9908 ranging from 10 ng/ml to 100 µg/ml for 24 to 72 hours. CTCE-9908 treatment did not significantly affect the PC-3 cell proliferation (Figure 1). Similar trend was observed with C4-2B cells up to 48 treatment of CTCE-9908, but at 72 hours a modest inhibition of growth observed at higher concentrations of CTCE-9908.

CTCE-9908 inhibits CXCL12-induced cell invasion

Our previous reports demonstrate that CXCL12/CXCR4 activation induces protease expression and chemoinvasion of PC-3 cells. Herein, the effect of CTCE-9908 on CXCL12-induced chemoinvasion was tested in PC-3 cells as the drug have no growth inhibitory effect. As

expected, CXCL12 induced chemoinvasion of PC-3 cells; treatment with 50 µg/ml CTCE-9908 significantly reduced CXCL12-induced chemoinvasion of PC-3 cells (Figure 2). These results suggest that CTCE-9908 compound inhibits the CXCL12/CXCR4 axis and subsequent chemoinvasion of PC-3 cells.

CXCL12/CXCR4 inhibition by CTCE-9908 leads to inhibition of total tumor burden

To determine the efficacy of CTCE-9908 in inhibiting CXCL12/CXCR4-mediated tumor cell growth and dissemination, an orthotopic model of prostate cancer metastasis was utilized. GFP-transfected PC-3 tumor cells were implanted into the ventral lobes of murine prostate. GFP stable transfection did not affect CXCR4 expression (data not shown). Mice were treated with a daily dose of 25 mg CTCE-9908/kg mouse body weight for four weeks. Caliper measurements of tumor volume at the end of four weeks show a decrease in mean tumor volume in CTCE-9908 treated animals (Figure 3B), although this decrease was not statistically significant. Proliferation index was determined in control and CTCE-9908 treated prostate tumors by immunostaining tumor sections for Ki-67 expression. There is no significant difference present between Ki-67 positive tumor cells between these groups suggesting that proliferation rate of tumor cells was not affected by the CTCE-9908

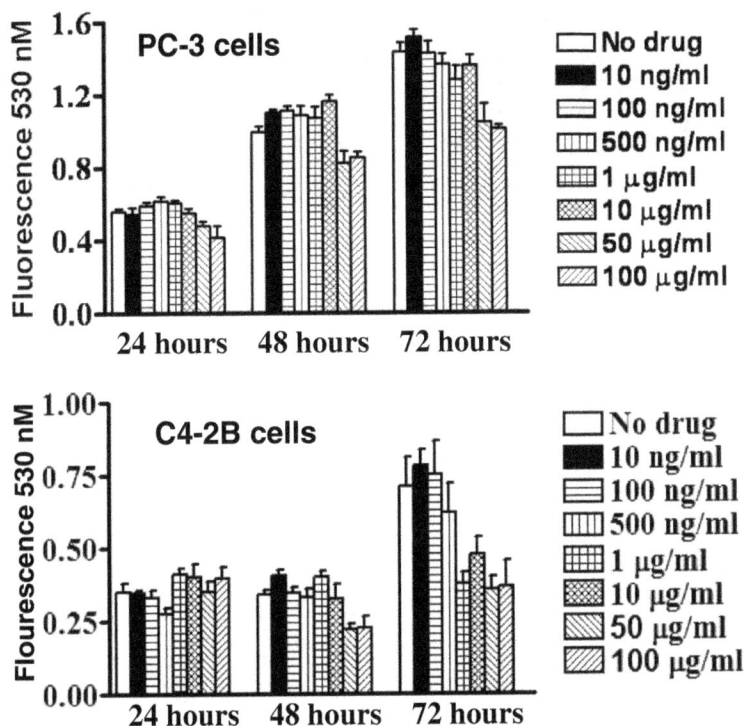

Figure 1 PC-3 cell proliferation in the presence of CTCE-9908. PC-3 and C4-2B cells were treated with 0, 10, 100, 500 ng/ml, 1, 10, 50 and 100 µg/ml concentrations of CTCE-9908 for 24 to 72 hours, and viable cells were determined with CyQUANT® NF cell proliferation assay.

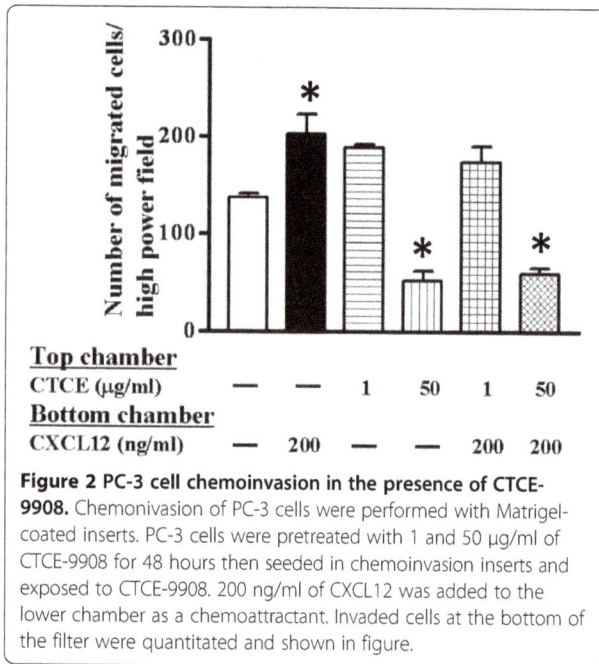

Figure 2 PC-3 cell chemoinvasion in the presence of CTCE-9908. Chemonivasion of PC-3 cells were performed with Matrigel-coated inserts. PC-3 cells were pretreated with 1 and 50 μg/ml of CTCE-9908 for 48 hours then seeded in chemoinvasion inserts and exposed to CTCE-9908. 200 ng/ml of CXCL12 was added to the lower chamber as a chemoattractant. Invaded cells at the bottom of the filter were quantitated and shown in figure.

(Additional file 1: Figure S1). The reduction in tumor growth may be due to increased necrosis of tumor cells as evidenced by low cytokeratin staining in CTCE-9908 treated mice (Additional file 2: Figure S2) which resulted in shrinkage of tumor.

CTCE-9908 treatment significantly reduced lymph node metastasis and distant metastases in orthotopic mouse model (Figure 3A), however significant reduction in primary tumor burden was not evident (Figure 3B). Total body fluorescence measurements show that CTCE-9908 treatment significantly inhibited total metastatic burden in mice (Figure 3C). Quantitation of site-specific metastases show that lymph node metastases were reduced by 40%, spleen metastasis by 75%, liver metastasis by 93%, and 95% reduction in distant metastases in CTCE-9908 treated mice (data not shown). Taken together, these data demonstrate that CTCE-9908 administration significantly inhibited dissemination of cancer cells to various sites in the mouse.

CTCE-9908 inhibits angiogenesis in prostate tumor tissues

Primary tumor tissue from control and CTCE-9908-treated mice were stained with anti-CD34 antibody to determine the effect of CTCE-9908 on tumor angiogenesis. As shown by immunohistochemistry, CTCE-9908

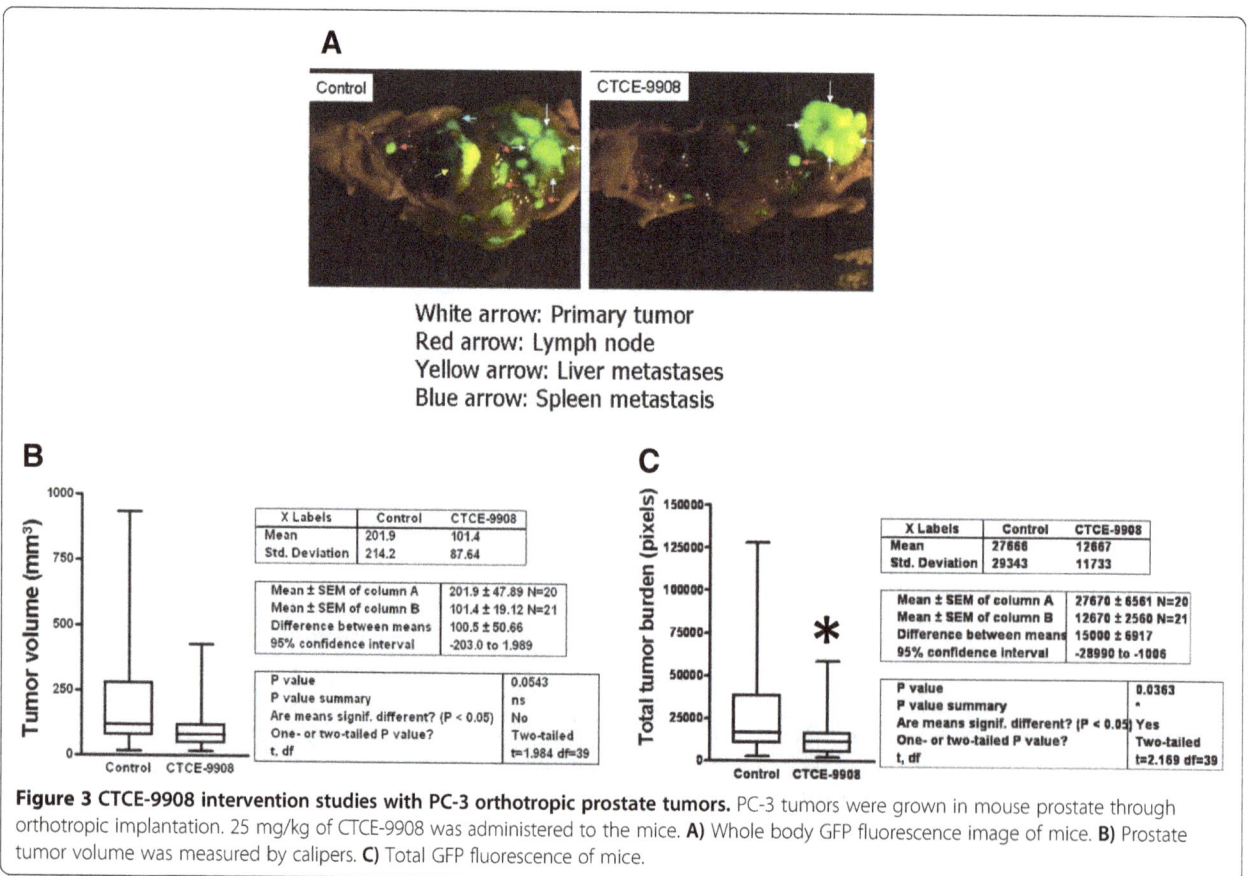

Figure 3 CTCE-9908 intervention studies with PC-3 orthotropic prostate tumors. PC-3 tumors were grown in mouse prostate through orthotropic implantation. 25 mg/kg of CTCE-9908 was administered to the mice. **A)** Whole body GFP fluorescence image of mice. **B)** Prostate tumor volume was measured by calipers. **C)** Total GFP fluorescence of mice.

treated tumors have fewer vessels, and these vessels are also smaller in size (Figure 4A). Quantitation of microvessel density in the hot spots of angiogenesis show a reduced CD34-positive vessel density in CTCE-9908 treated tumors (Figure 4B). Moreover, quantitation of CD34 positive vessel density in lymph node metastatic tissue shows a decrease in number in CTCE-9908 treated tumors (Additional file 3: Figure S3). These data suggest that CTCE-9908 treatment inhibited the angiogenesis of primary and lymph node metastatic tumors. The CTCE-9908-mediated inhibition of primary tumor angiogenesis lead to inhibition of metastasis.

Discussion

Previous studies demonstrate that tumor cells are capable of usurping immune cell chemoinvasive pathways for metastasis to secondary sites. Chemokines and chemokine receptors mediate physiological movement of immune cells in the body. Among the family of chemokine and chemokine receptors mediating tumor cell invasion and metastasis, CXCL12/CXCR4 has gained a central role in different types of tumors in mediating tumor growth, angiogenesis and metastasis. In prostate cancer cells, CXCL12 and CXCR4 play a key role in invasion and metastasis, leading to development and expansion of osseous metastasis. In this study we assessed the effect of inhibition of the CXCL12/CXCR4 pathway by a novel CXCR4 antagonist, CTCE-9908 on in vitro cell proliferation and invasion, and in vivo orthotopic tumor growth, metastasis, and angiogenesis of PC cells.

Previous studies report that CTCE-9908 compound inhibited cell proliferation in PC-3 cells at higher concentrations with no effect at lower concentrations [22]; our data is in line with these studies, as CTCE-9908 compound did not show significant inhibition in cell proliferation at 100 µM (which corresponds to 44 nM) concentration. This lack of inhibitory effect on PC-3 cells can be attributed to the fact that cultured PC-3 cells express low or no CXCL12 [5], and therefore CXCR4 activation could be low in these cells. Previous report by Provasnik et al. support this observation that CTCE-9908 administration do not inhibit the subcutaneous tumor growth [22]. As opposed to cultured cancer cells, in vivo bone tumors express CXCL12 in prostate cancer cells in addition to osteoblasts and endothelial cells. Primary tumors also express CXCL12 in epithelial cells. The CXCL12/CXCR4 axis has been shown to promote cell survival by inhibiting apoptosis in cancer cells; thus, CTCE-9908-mediated inhibition of the CXCL12/CXCR4 pathway leads to loss of protection from apoptosis and increased cell death. Our data support this notion, as CTCE-9908-treated tumors showed enhanced necrotic areas, suggesting that loss of the CXCL12/CXCR4 axis mediated cell survival leading to enhanced necrosis in tumor cells. But, we cannot rule out the role of growth inhibition of CTCE-9908 in our model as mean tumor growth is inhibited in CTCE-9908 treated group, though the data did not reach statistical significance.

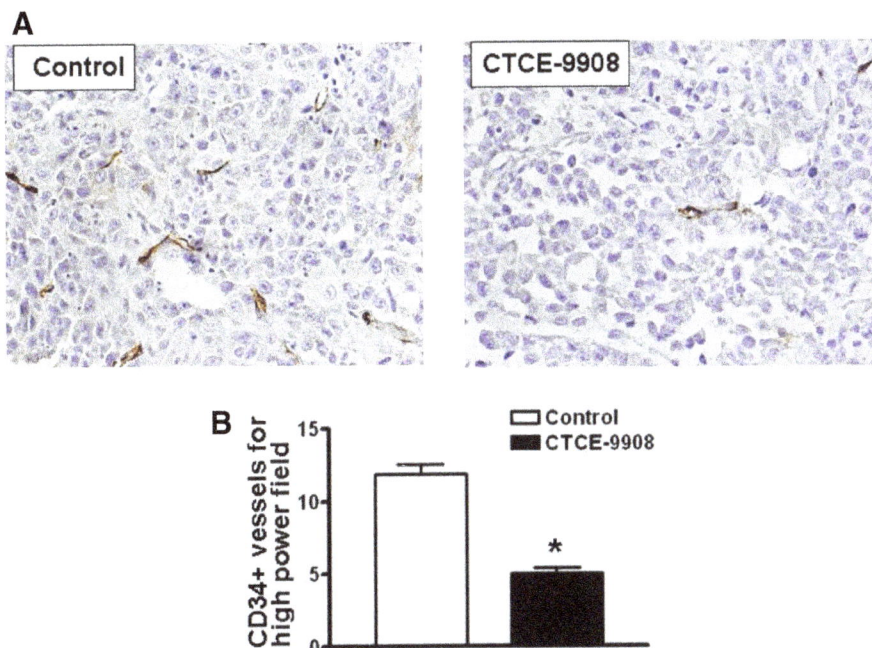

Figure 4 Microvessel density in CTCE-9908-treated PC-3 tumors. A) Prostate tumor tissues were stained with anti-CD 34 antibody. **B)** Quantitation of CD34+ vessels in control and CTCE-9908 treated prostate tumor tissue. *Represents statistically significant, where p = 0.0021.

We have previously shown that the CXCL12/CXCR4 axis in PC-3 cells induce MMP-9 expression via activation of PI3K and MAPK pathways, and this activation mediates *in vitro* cell invasion of PC-3 cells [24]. Bone colonizing PC-3 cells induce the expression of active MMP-9 at earlier time periods suggesting that CXCL12/CXCR4-mediated homing of PC cells to bone would functionally link with the expression of MMP-9 in local bone tumor microenvironment and induce invasive bone tumor growth [5]. To determine whether CTCE-9908 compound could inhibit invasion of PC-3 cells, we used the lower concentration of 50 µg/ml in cell invasion studies. Although this concentration of CTCE-9908 did not inhibit cell proliferation, our data suggest that 50 µg/ml CTCE-9908 potently inhibited the CXCL12-induced PC-3 cell invasion. To determine whether inhibition of invasion could translate into inhibition of metastasis formation, we treated mice implanted with orthotopic tumors with CTCE-9908. The whole body quantitation of fluorescence measurements shows that CTCE-9908 treatment significantly reduced total tumor burden as a measure of total body fluorescence. To our knowledge, this is the first report to document that targeting the CXCL12/CXCR4 axis through CTCE-9908 inhibited the metastatic burden in an orthotopic prostate cancer model system. Both lymph node and distant metastases were significantly inhibited in CTCE-9908 treated tumors, but distant metastases were strongly inhibited compared to lymph node metastases. Similar observations were found with CTCE-9908 in a breast cancer model where total metastatic burden was significantly inhibited upon CTCE-9908 administration [25]. CXCL12/CXCR4 mediated invasive function has implications in clinical management of patients as chemotherapy resistant tumors cells often express high levels of CXCR4 [26] and this may lead to the development of metastases in these patients via CXCL12/CXCR4 activation. In addtion, prostate cancer progenitor cells express CXCR4 [27] and often these cells are resistant to current chemo and radiation therapy practices, thus, combination therapy with anti-CXCR4 strategies consisting of CTCE-9908 may prevent the further spread of tumor in patients.

Tumor angiogenesis plays a key role in tumor growth and development of metastases. CXCL12/CXCR4 signaling has been shown to modulate the expression of angiogenic cytokines/chemokines in prostate cancer cells [28]. Expression of these proangiogenic factors can recruit endothelial precursor cells to the tumor sites to facilitate angiogenesis. To determine the effect of CXCR4 inhibition on tumor angiogenesis we measured hotspots of angiogenesis in primary and lymph node metastatic tumor tissues for CD34 positive blood vessels. CTCE-9908 treatment significantly inhibited angiogenesis in both primary and lymph node metastases. Porvasnik et al. reported that CTCE-9908 treatment reduced tumor angiogenesis by down regulating

VEGF production and myeloid derived suppressor cell (CD11b positive) recruitment into tumor tissues [22]. CD11b cells have been recently shown to express CXCR4 and migrate towards the CXCL12 expressing cells.

Our studies show that CTCE-9908 is efficacious in inhibiting total tumor burden without significantly reducing primary tumor burden suggesting that targeting CXCL12/CXCR4 axis may be therapeutically beneficial for the management of prostate cancer patients undergoing chemo or radiation therapy.

Conclusions
The data presented in the study demonstrate that CTCE-9908 is efficacious in preventing spread of tumor cells from primary site by inhibiting invasive and angiogenic functions of CXCL12/CXCR4 axis in primary tumor environment.

Additional files

Additional file 1: Figure S1. A) Immunohistochemical analysis of Ki-67 in PC-3 tumors. Control and CTCE-9908 treated prostate tumor tissues were stained for Ki-67 antigen. **B)** Quantitation of total Ki-67 positive cells in control and treated group. Statistical difference between groups is not significant, where $p = 0.0897$.

Additional file 2: Figure S2. Immunohistochemical analysis of cytokeratin in PC3 tumors. Control and CTCE-9908 treated prostate tumor tissues were stained for cytokeratin. Arrow represents low staining necrotic area.

Additional file 3: Figure S3. CD34 staining of lymph node metastasis in control (left) and CTCE-9908 treated mice (right). A representative hot spot of CD34+ vessels is shown. Graphical representation of microvessel densities between control and treated groups of metastatic tumor sections. *represents statistically significant, where $p = 0.0296$.

Competing interests
Dr. Donald Wong and Mr. Walter Korz are the employees of British Canadian BioScience Corporation.

Authors' contributions
DW and WK participated in study design and acquisition of animal experimental data. PK carried out immunohistochemical experiments and involved in preparation of figures. SRC is actively involved in all aspects of study and responsible for drafting manuscript. All authors read and approved the final manuscript.

Acknowledgements
We would like to thank Dr. Charles J. Rosser (MD Anderson Cancer Center Orlando, Orlando, FL, USA) for critically reading and editing the manuscript to improve intellectual content.
Supported by Fund for Cancer Research, U.S. Department of Defense, Idea Award W81XWH-09-1-0250 and NIH R01CA151557 to Sreenivasa R. Chinni.

Author details
[1]Department of Urology, Wayne State University School of Medicine, 9200 Scott Hall 540 E. Canfield Avenue, Detroit, MI 48201, USA. [2]Department of Pathology, Wayne State University School of Medicine, 9200 Scott Hall 540 E. Canfield Avenue, Detroit, MI 48201, USA. [3]The Barbara Ann Karmanos Cancer Institute, Detroit, MI 48201, USA. [4]British Canadian BioScience Corporation, Vancouver, Canada.

References

1. Balkwill F: Cancer and the chemokine network. *Nat Rev Cancer* 2004, 4(7):540–550.
2. Sun YX, Wang J, Shelburne CE, Lopatin DE, Chinnaiyan AM, Rubin MA, Pienta KJ, Taichman RS: Expression of CXCR4 and CXCL12 (SDF-1) in human prostate cancers (PCa) in vivo. *J Cell Biochem* 2003, 89(3):462–473.
3. Wallace TA, Prueitt RL, Yi M, Howe TM, Gillespie JW, Yfantis HG, Stephens RM, Caporaso NE, Loffredo CA, Ambs S: Tumor immunobiological differences in prostate cancer between African-American and European-American men. *Cancer Res* 2008, 68(3):927–936.
4. Akashi T, Koizumi K, Tsuneyama K, Saiki I, Takano Y, Fuse H: Chemokine receptor CXCR4 expression and prognosis in patients with metastatic prostate cancer. *Cancer Sci* 2008, 99(3):539–542.
5. Chinni SR, Sivalogan S, Dong Z, Filho JC, Deng X, Bonfil RD, Cher ML: CXCL12/CXCR4 signaling activates Akt-1 and MMP-9 expression in prostate cancer cells: the role of bone microenvironment-associated CXCL12. *Prostate* 2006, 66(1):32–48.
6. Taichman RS, Cooper C, Keller ET, Pienta KJ, Taichman NS, McCauley LK: Use of the stromal cell-derived factor-1/CXCR4 pathway in prostate cancer metastasis to bone. *Cancer Res* 2002, 62(6):1832–1837.
7. Arya M, Patel HR, McGurk C, Tatoud R, Klocker H, Masters J, Williamson M: The importance of the CXCL12-CXCR4 chemokine ligand-receptor interaction in prostate cancer metastasis. *J Exp Ther Oncol* 2004, 4(4):291–303.
8. Kukreja P, Abdel-Mageed AB, Mondal D, Liu K, Agrawal KC: Up-regulation of CXCR4 expression in PC-3 cells by stromal-derived factor-1alpha (CXCL12) increases endothelial adhesion and transendothelial migration: role of MEK/ERK signaling pathway-dependent NF-kappaB activation. *Cancer Res* 2005, 65(21):9891–9898.
9. Singh S, Singh UP, Grizzle WE, Lillard JW Jr: CXCL12-CXCR4 interactions modulate prostate cancer cell migration, metalloproteinase expression and invasion. *Lab Invest* 2004, 84(12):1666–1676.
10. Chinni SR, Yamamoto H, Dong Z, Sabbota A, Bonfil RD, Cher ML: CXCL12/CXCR4 Transactivates HER2 in Lipid Rafts of Prostate Cancer Cells and Promotes Growth of Metastatic Deposits in Bone. *Molecular cancer research: MCR* 2008, 6(3):446–457.
11. Darash-Yahana M, Pikarsky E, Abramovitch R, Zeira E, Pal B, Karplus R, Beider K, Avniel S, Kasem S, Galun E, et al: Role of high expression levels of CXCR4 in tumor growth, vascularization, and metastasis. *Faseb J* 2004, 18(11):1240–1242.
12. Vaday GG, Hua SB, Peehl DM, Pauling MH, Lin YH, Zhu L, Lawrence DM, Foda HD, Zucker S: CXCR4 and CXCL12 (SDF-1) in prostate cancer: inhibitory effects of human single chain Fv antibodies. *Clin Cancer Res* 2004, 10(16):5630–5639.
13. Sun YX, Schneider A, Jung Y, Wang J, Dai J, Cook K, Osman NI, Koh-Paige AJ, Shim H, Pienta KJ, et al: Skeletal localization and neutralization of the SDF-1(CXCL12)/CXCR4 axis blocks prostate cancer metastasis and growth in osseous sites in vivo. *J Bone Miner Res* 2005, 20(2):318–329.
14. Dong Z, Bonfil RD, Chinni S, Deng X, Trindade Filho JC, Bernardo M, Vaishampayan U, Che M, Sloane BF, Sheng S, et al: Matrix metalloproteinase activity and osteoclasts in experimental prostate cancer bone metastasis tissue. *Am J Pathol* 2005, 166(4):1173–1186.
15. Sun X, Cheng G, Hao M, Zheng J, Zhou X, Zhang J, Taichman RS, Pienta KJ, Wang J: CXCL12 / CXCR4 / CXCR7 chemokine axis and cancer progression. *Cancer Metastasis Rev* 2011, 29(4):709–722.
16. DiPersio JF, Micallef IN, Stiff PJ, Bolwell BJ, Maziarz RT, Jacobsen E, Nademanee A, McCarty J, Bridger G, Calandra G: Phase III prospective randomized double-blind placebo-controlled trial of plerixafor plus granulocyte colony-stimulating factor compared with placebo plus granulocyte colony-stimulating factor for autologous stem-cell mobilization and transplantation for patients with non-Hodgkin's lymphoma. *J Clin Oncol* 2009, 27(28):4767–4773.
17. Burger JA, Stewart DJ: CXCR4 chemokine receptor antagonists: perspectives in SCLC. *Expert Opin Investig Drugs* 2009, 18(4):481–490.
18. Kim SY, Lee CH, Midura BV, Yeung C, Mendoza A, Hong SH, Ren L, Wong D, Korz W, Merzouk A, et al: Inhibition of the CXCR4/CXCL12 chemokine pathway reduces the development of murine pulmonary metastases. *Clin Exp Metastasis* 2008, 25(3):201–211.
19. Rubin JB, Kung AL, Klein RS, Chan JA, Sun Y, Schmidt K, Kieran MW, Luster AD, Segal RA: A small-molecule antagonist of CXCR4 inhibits intracranial growth of primary brain tumors. *Proc Natl Acad Sci USA* 2003, 100(23):13513–13518.
20. Kajiyama H, Shibata K, Terauchi M, Ino K, Nawa A, Kikkawa F: Involvement of SDF-1alpha/CXCR4 axis in the enhanced peritoneal metastasis of epithelial ovarian carcinoma. *Int J Cancer* 2008, 122(1):91–99.
21. Huang EH, Singh B, Cristofanilli M, Gelovani J, Wei C, Vincent L, Cook KR, Lucci A: A CXCR4 antagonist CTCE-9908 inhibits primary tumor growth and metastasis of breast cancer. *J Surg Res* 2009, 155(2):231–236.
22. Porvasnik S, Sakamoto N, Kusmartsev S, Eruslanov E, Kim WJ, Cao W, Urbanek C, Wong D, Goodison S, Rosser CJ: Effects of CXCR4 antagonist CTCE-9908 on prostate tumor growth. *Prostate* 2009, 69(13):1460–1469.
23. Glinskii AB, Smith BA, Jiang P, Li XM, Yang M, Hoffman RM, Glinsky GV: Viable circulating metastatic cells produced in orthotopic but not ectopic prostate cancer models. *Cancer Res* 2003, 63(14):4239–4243.
24. Bonfil RD, Sabbota A, Nabha S, Bernardo MM, Dong Z, Meng H, Yamamoto H, Chinni SR, Lim IT, Chang M, et al: Inhibition of human prostate cancer growth, osteolysis and angiogenesis in a bone metastasis model by a novel mechanism-based selective gelatinase inhibitor. *Int J Cancer* 2006, 118(11):2721–2726.
25. Richert MM, Vaidya KS, Mills CN, Wong D, Korz W, Hurst DR, Welch DR: Inhibition of CXCR4 by CTCE-9908 inhibits breast cancer metastasis to lung and bone. *Oncol Rep* 2009, 21(3):761–767.
26. Hatano K, Yamaguchi S, Nimura K, Murakami K, Nagahara A, Fujita K, Uemura M, Nakai Y, Tsuchiya M, Nakayama M, et al: Residual prostate cancer cells after docetaxel therapy increase the tumorigenic potential via constitutive signaling of CXCR4, ERK1/2 and c-Myc. *Molecular cancer research: MCR* 2013, 11(9):1088–1100.
27. Dubrovska A, Elliott J, Salamone RJ, Telegeev GD, Stakhovsky AE, Schepotin IB, Yan F, Wang Y, Bouchez LC, Kularatne SA, et al: CXCR4 expression in prostate cancer progenitor cells. *PLoS One* 2012, 7(2):e31226.
28. Wang J, Sun Y, Song W, Nor JE, Wang CY, Taichman RS: Diverse signaling pathways through the SDF-1/CXCR4 chemokine axis in prostate cancer cell lines leads to altered patterns of cytokine secretion and angiogenesis. *Cell Signal* 2005, 17(12):1578–1592.

2

Factor V Leiden mutation triggering four major complications to standard dose cisplatin-chemotherapy for testicular seminoma

Klaus-Peter Dieckmann[1*], Petra Anheuser[1], Ralf Gehrckens[2], Sven Philip Aries[3], Raphael Ikogho[1] and Wiebke Hollburg[4]

Abstract

Background: Major life-threatening complications secondary to cisplatin-based chemotherapy are rare in patients with testicular germ cell tumour (GCT). The incidence of complications increases with dosage of chemotherapy and with a variety of patient-related as well as disease-related conditions. We here report the first case of GCT experiencing as many as four major complications most of which can be explained by the conjunction of several predispositions.

Case presentation: A 48 year old patient with testicular seminoma and bulky retroperitoneal and mediastinal metastases underwent cisplatin based chemotherapy. During the third cycle of chemotherapy, he developed thrombosis of the central venous port device, subtotal splenic infarction, and Bleomycin induced pneumonitis (BIP). Three months after completion of therapy, he was struck by thalamic infarction. Genetic testing then revealed heterozygote mutation of Factor V Leiden (FVL). He received full-dose warfarin anticoagulation treatment and steroid treatment for BIP. 18 months thereafter, the patient is still disease-free, oncologically. Neurological symptoms have disappeared, but pulmonary dysfunction persists with a vital capacity of 50%.

Conclusion: The unique co-incidence of four major complications occurring in this patient were obviously triggered by the genetically determined predisposition of the patient to thrombotic events (FVL). Additionally, several patient-related and disease-related conditions contributed to the unique pattern of complications, i.e. (1) the slightly advanced age (48 years), (2) the prothrombotic condition caused by the disease of cancer, (3) the central venous port device, (4) retroperitoneal bulky metastasis, and (5) cisplatin chemotherapy. Whether or not FVL contributed to the pulmonary fibrosis as well, remains elusive. Practically, in the case of one major vascular complication during cisplatin chemotherapy at standard dose, genetic testing for hereditary thrombophilia should be considered. Thus, precautions for preventing further complications could be initiated.

Keywords: Seminoma, Cisplatin chemotherapy, Thrombosis, Thrombophilia, Factor V Leiden, Bleomycin induced pneumonitis

* Correspondence: DieckmannKP@t-online.de
[1]Albertinen-Krankenhaus, Department of Urology, Suentelstrasse 11a, D-22457 Hamburg, Germany
Full list of author information is available at the end of the article

Background

Testicular germ cell tumours (GCTs) represent a paradigm for a curable neoplasm [1]. Combination chemotherapy with cisplatin, etoposide and bleomycin (PEB) can cure metastasized disease and even far advanced disease (i.e. poor prognosis according to the IGCCCG classification) can be salvaged in about 50% [2]. However, systemic treatment is quite toxic even by application of standard doses and it involves the potential of numerous adverse reactions arising acutely at the time of treatment and other sequels developing in the long term [3]. The most frequent untoward reactions occurring at the time of treatment or immediately thereafter encompass myelodepression with neutropenic fever, alopecia, gastrointestinal toxicity, peripheral neurotoxicity, and impairment of fertility. These side-effects are experienced by almost all of the patients with varying degrees of severity, and usually, these events can be managed successfully. However occasionally, more serious and even life threatening complications may ensue mainly involving vascular and pulmonary events. Deep venous thrombosis (DVT) is encountered in about 8% of GCT patients receiving cisplatin-based chemotherapy for metastatic disease [4]. Pulmonary embolism secondary to DVT may occur in up to 6% of cases [5,6]. Arterial complications e. g. peripheral arterial thrombotic occlusion, myocardial infarctions, and cerebral vascular events are reported in about 0.3% of GCT patients receiving chemotherapy [7]. Pulmonary fibrosis represents the most important complication involving the lungs. This complication is also called bleomycin induced pneumonitis (BIP) because it is clearly associated with bleomycin if given in cumulative dosages of more than 300 mg [8,9]. About 7% of chemotherapy cases will experience BIP with 1% being fatal [10].

Multiple complications occurring synchronously or metachronously in one patient have been reported [4,7]. But rarely, more than three serious complications will be encountered in one individual [11]. Here we report a case who experienced as many as four serious complications secondary to cisplatin-combination chemotherapy, three vascular events and one pulmonary.

Case presentation

This 48 years old patient with uneventful history presented with a left sided testicular seminoma. Beta Human chorionic gonadotropin (bHCG) was elevated to 247 U/l (normal range to 2 U/l) while Alpha fetoprotein and Lactate dehydrogenase were within normal limits. Computed tomography of chest and abdomen revealed a retroperitoneal mass of 6 cm in size (Figure 1) and another one of 2 cm size in the mediastinum corresponding to clinical stage III (Lugano Classification) and

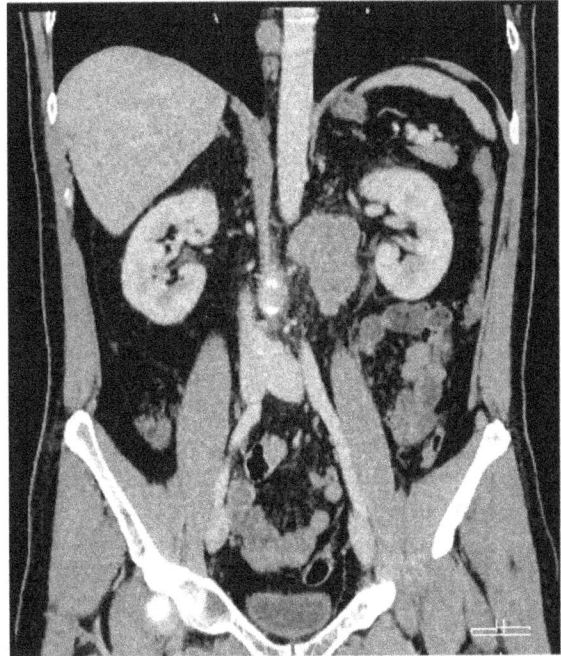

Figure 1 Abdominal computed tomography, coronary section view showing the large retroperitoneal metastasis of seminoma before initiation of chemotherapy.

to the good prognosis group according to IGCCCG classification [12].

The patient underwent inguinal orchiectomy and according to the patient´s wish, a centralvenous port system with access to the right subclavian vein was implanted at the same time. Low-dose anticoagulation treatment was instituted thereafter with low molecular weight heparin (Enoxiparin 40 mg daily). Three cycles of the cisplatin/etoposide/ bleomycin chemotherapy regimen (PEB) were administered without delay between the cycles. Acute side effects involved recurrent singultus during all cycles, complete alopecia after the third cycle. Routine laboratory examinations done weekly during chemotherapy revealed transient increase of gamma glutarate dehydrogenase, as well anemia with hemoglobin of 8.9 g/dl. Serum creatinine increased during the application of the third cycle of treatment to 1.5 mg/dl indicating a considerable impairment of renal function. Also during the third cycle, the patient reported of increasing dyspnea upon slight exercise. In addition, at the end of the third cycle, the patient experienced a sudden episode of left upper abdominal pain. Routine restaging with computed tomography of chest and abdomen after completion of the second cycle of chemotherapy revealed partial remission of the lymphadenopathy but no other significant findings. Final restaging after the third cycle documented complete remission of the mediastinal mass and subtotal remission of the retroperitoneal mass.

Accordingly, serum bHCG had returned to normal. Thus, cure had been achieved, oncologically. However, chest CT also revealed fibrotic changes bilaterally in the caudal parts of the lungs consistent with the typical findings in Bleomycin induced pneumonitis (Figure 2). Accordingly, pulmonary function testing revealed a decrease of vital capacity to 44%. Also, the chest CT revealed thrombosis of the centralvenous port system with extension of thrombotic material into the subclavian vein (Figure 3). In addition, the abdominal CT revealed splenic infarction involving approximately one third of the organ (Figure 3). Therapeutically, anticoagulation therapy was increased to 80 mg Enoxaparin daily and the venous port system was removed surgically. In addition, corticosteroid therapy with 50 mg Prednisolone p/o was applied for treatment of BIP resulting in some improvement of dyspnea, subsequently. Three months after completion of chemotherapy and despite ongoing full dose heparin-based anticoagulation therapy, the patient experienced a sudden loss of speech and amnesic aphasia. Magnetic resonance imaging of the brain disclosed infarction of the right-sided thalamic region (Figure 4) as well as several additional small older ischemic regions in the temporal and occipital cortex, respectively.

After all these complications genetic testing for inherited thrombophilia documented heterozygote mutation of factor V Leiden (FVL).

The patient was placed on life-long warfarin anticoagulation therapy. 18 months after completion of chemotherapy, follow-up examinations revealed ongoing complete remission, oncologically. The neurological symptoms had resolved totally. The corticosteroid therapy had been terminated 14 months after onset of BIP. Exertional dyspnea has improved meanwhile, however, vital capacity is still no more than 50%.

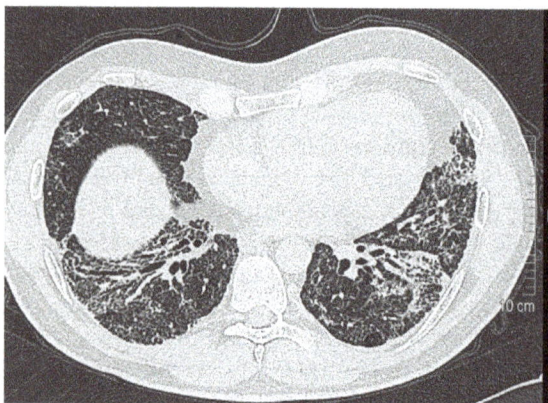

Figure 3 Computed tomography of chest and abdomen, coronary section, performed after third cycle of chemotherapy, showing the central venous port device with thrombosis (arrow) and subtotal splenic infarction (arrow).

Conclusion

Generally, the occurrence of complications secondary to a chemotherapeutic agent is dependent on both the applied dosage of the drug and the predisposition of the individual patient to acquire particular complications. Accordingly, high dose chemotherapy is associated with a much higher frequency of major complications. With respect to the susceptibility of the patient to acquire complications, older age is clearly one general predisposing factor as well as pre-existing chronic diseases e.g. Diabetes mellitus, renal insufficiency, chronic vascular disease. As most of the patients with testicular GCT are young and otherwise healthy, and as most of the metastasized cases only require standard dose chemotherapy, major complications are rather infrequent. Two or more critical events arising simultaneously or consecutively in one such patient are even more infrequent. Thus, the conjunction of four serious events as experienced by our patient is truly exceptional. O´Reilly reported a 26 year old patient with testicular seminoma and no significant comorbidity who sequentially experienced cerebral stroke, deep vein thrombosis and pulmonary embolism during PVB chemotherapy [11]. A 33 year old Dutch patient with GCT who was otherwise healthy developed cerebral stroke and myocardial infarction upon cisplatin-based therapy [13]. Likewise, in a German series, two

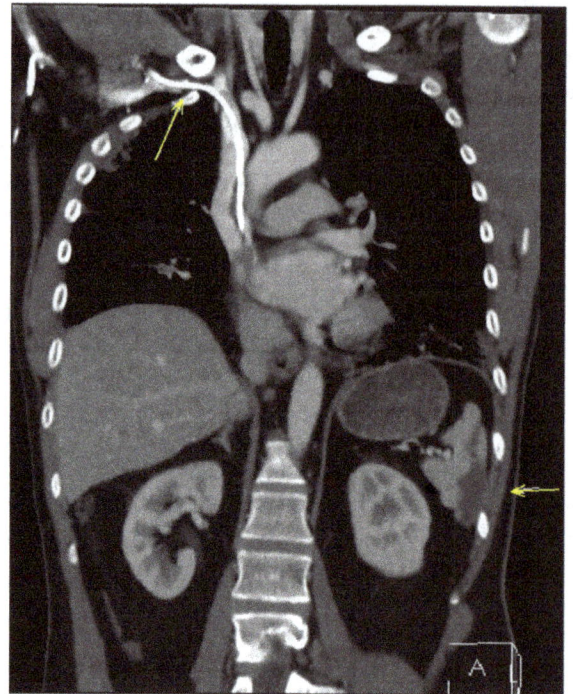

Figure 2 Chest Computed tomography performed after third cycle of chemotherapy showing diffuse interstitial infiltrates, bilaterally, consistent with Bleomycin induced pneumonitis.

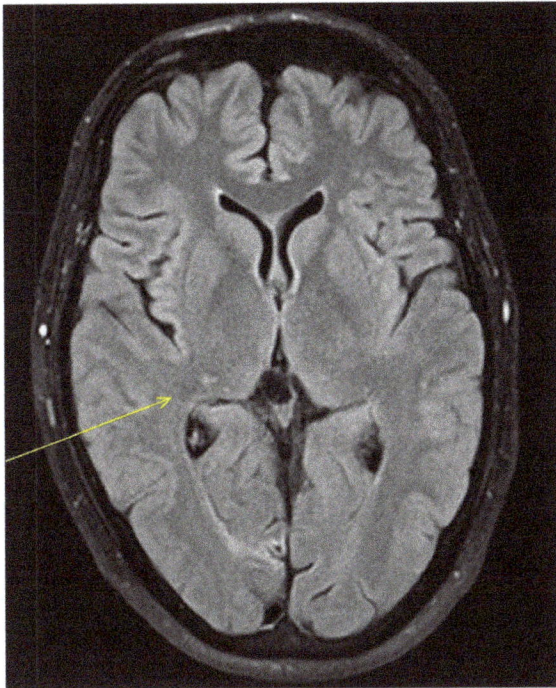

Figure 4 Axial Magnetic resonance Imaging (MRI) of the Brain with Fluid Attenuated Inversion Recovery (FLAIR sequence), three months after completion of chemotherapy: Hyperintense lesion in the right thalamic region (arrow) indicating thalamic infarction.

patients (36 and 44 years of age) with both, myocardial infarction and cerebral stroke were reported. Also in that report, five cases with multivessel myocardial infarction as well as two cases with pulmonary embolism occurring in conjunction with cerebral stroke and with peripheral arterial thrombosis, respectively, were documented [7].

With respect to the present patient, it is probably the unique combination of a number of particular conditions that instigated this extraordinary pattern of untoward events.

Undoubtedly, the thrombophilic predisposition of this patient documented by the mutation of Factor V Leiden (FVL) represents the paramount pathogenetic factor that triggered the major vascular complications. Heterozygote status of FVL mutation is prevalent in around 5% of the Caucasian population involving a seven-fold increase of the thrombogenic risk in afflicted subjects [14]. Evidently, FVL does also modestly increase the risk of arterial thrombosis [15-17], at least in the presence of additional prothrombotic conditions [18]. Even splenic infarction, one of the events of our patient, has been documented in a case with FVL mutation [19].

Thus, our patient was bearing a genetically determined significantly increased risk of thrombosis which was superimposed by at least four additional synergistic thrombogenic factors: age, cancer, central venous port

system, and cisplatin chemotherapy. (I) Firstly, the slightly advanced age of 48 years confers a minor increase of general thrombotic risk by comparison to the average GCT patient. (II) Cancer itself generally increases the risk of thrombosis [20,21]. Moreover, there is also clear evidence of further increased thrombotic risk in those individuals who have both, cancer and FVL mutation [14]. On top of that, our patient had a huge retroperitoneal mass that potentially might compromise venous backflow from the lower limbs thus predisposing to intravasal clotting [4]. (III) Central venous port devices generally involve a high potential of thrombosis due to contact and irritation of vascular walls with the synthetic port material [22]. In the presence of FVL mutation, an additional 3 – 6 fold thrombotic risk has been documented [23,24]. (IV) Cisplatin combination chemotherapy involves considerable thrombogenic risk [25] possibly caused by endothelial damage [6,26,27]. Whether or not anti-emetic steroid therapy and BIP-related corticoid administration may have advanced the thrombotic risk in our patient is at least conceivable [28]. In all, our patient experienced three thrombotic events during or immediately after cisplatin-based chemotherapy. Obviously these complications were initiated and promoted by the conjunction of the patient´s genetically determined increased risk of thrombosis on the one side, and several disease-related as well as treatment related synergistic prothrombotic factors on the other side.

With regard to the Bleomycin-related pulmonary fibrosis the patient used to be a non-smoker and he had no apparent predisposing pulmonary conditions. Yet, two minor precipitating factors could be noted, i.e. the slightly advanced age of 48 years and the impaired renal function developing during the third cycle of chemotherapy, both of these conditions are known to be associated with the occurrence of BIP [8]. At least on the experimental level there is some evidence that FVL mutation may promote pulmonary fibrosis, too [29]. Thus conceivably, the pulmonary and the vascular complications occurring in the present patient may share predisposing factors.

From a clinical point of view, it must be asked how and if at all these events could have been prevented. Probably, the pulmonary complication represents much of a chance event that had not been predictable at the time of treatment. Two of the three vascular complications were endo-arterial events. So, low dose heparin anticoagulation would probably not have been sufficient to prevent further vascular events. If acetylic salicylic acid (ASA) would have been beneficial in this case remains elusive. However, what should be learned from this extraordinary case is that genetic testing for hereditary clotting disorders should be considered in all those

GCT patients experiencing one major vascular complication. Then, life-threatening further complications could be prevented by full dose warfarin medication or other modern oral anticoagulation treatment.

Consent

Written informed consent was obtained from the patient for publication of this Case report and the accompanying images. A copy of the written consent is available for review by the Editor of this journal.

Abbreviations

GCT: Germ cell tumour; PEB: Cisplatin, Etoposide, Bleomycin (chemotherapy); IGCCCG: International germ cell cancer consensus group; BIP: Bleomycin induced peumonitis; CT: Computed tomography; FVL: Factor V leiden; DVT: Deep vein thrombosis; BHCG: Beta human chorionic gonadotropin; p/o: Per oral (medication).

Competing interests

The authors declare that they have no competing interests.

Authors' contributions

KPD conceived the study, wrote the manuscript. PA co-conceived the study, did most of the literature research. RG did most of the radiological examinations, assisted in drafting the manuscript. SPA did the pulmonary examinations, guided particular parts of the clinical management. RI guided particular parts of the clinical management, co-conceived the study. WH did most of the clinical management, assisted in drafting the manuscript. All authors have critically revised and finally approved the manuscript.

Acknowledgements

Dr. Saskia Kleier, Humangenetik at Gynaekologicum, Hamburg, gave valuable advice regarding the diagnosis of Factor V Leiden mutation. Dr. Hendrik Job, Department of Radiology, Albertinen-Krankenhaus Hamburg, assisted in selecting appropriate imaging material for publication.
The present study did not receive any funding.

Author details

[1]Albertinen-Krankenhaus, Department of Urology, Suentelstrasse 11a, D-22457 Hamburg, Germany. [2]Albertinen-Krankenhaus, Department of Diagnostic Radiology, Hamburg, Germany. [3]Elbpneumologie, Mörkenstrasse 47, D-22767 Hamburg, Germany. [4]Hämatologisch-onkologische Praxis Altona (HOPA), Mörkenstrasse 47, D-22767 Hamburg, Germany.

References

1. Hanna N, Einhorn LH. Testicular cancer: a reflection on 50 years of discovery. J Clin Oncol. 2014;32(28):3085–92.
2. Calabrò F, Albers P, Bokemeyer C, Martin C, Einhorn LH, Horwich A, et al. The contemporary role of chemotherapy for advanced testis cancer: a systematic review of the literature. Eur Urol. 2012;61:1212–21.
3. Abouassaly R, Fossa SD, Giwercman A, Kollmannsberger C, Motzer RJ, Schmoll HJ, et al. Sequelae of treatment in long-term survivors of testis cancer. Eur Urol. 2011;60(3):516–26.
4. Piketty AC, Flechon A, Laplanche A, Nouyrigat E, Droz JP, Theodore C, et al. The risk of thrombo-embolic events is increased in patients with germ-cell tumours and can be predicted by serum lactate dehydrogenase and body surface area. Br J Cancer. 2005;93:909–14.
5. Weijl NI, Rutten MF, Zwinderman AH, Keizer HJ, Nooy MA, Rosendaal FR, et al. Thromboembolic events during chemotherapy for germ cell cancer: a cohort study and review of the literature. J Clin Oncol. 2000;18:2169–78.
6. Nuver J, Smit AJ, van der Meer J, van den Berg MP, van der Graaf WT, Meinardi MT, et al. Acute chemotherapy-induced cardiovascular changes in patients with testicular cancer. J Clin Oncol. 2005;23:9130–7.
7. Dieckmann KP, Gerl A, Witt J, Hartmann JT, German Testicular Cancer Study Group. Myocardial infarction and other major vascular events during chemotherapy for testicular cancer. Ann Oncol. 2010;21:1607–11.
8. Sleijfer S. Bleomycin-induced pneumonitis. Chest. 2001;120:617–24.
9. O'Sullivan JM, Huddart RA, Norman AR, Nicholls J, Dearnaley DP, Horwich A. Predicting the risk of bleomycin lung toxicity in patients with germ-cell tumours. Ann Oncol. 2003;14:91–6.
10. Efstathiou E, Logothetis CJ. Review of late complications of treatment and late relapse in testicular cancer. J Natl Compr Canc Netw. 2006;4:1059–70.
11. O'Reilly A, Maceneaney P, Mayer N, O'Reilly SP, Power DG. Testicular cancer and platinum: a double-edged sword. J Clin Oncol. 2014;32(12):e46–8.
12. International Germ Cell Cancer Consensus Group. International germ cell consensus classification: a prognostic factor-based staging system for metastatic germ cell cancers. J Clin Oncol. 1997;15(2):594–603.
13. Brouha ME, Bloemendal HJ, Kappelle LJ, Winter JB. Cerebral infarction and myocardial infarction due to cisplatin-containing chemotherapy].[Article in Dutch. Ned Tijdschr Geneeskd. 2003;147:457–60.
14. Blom JW, Doggen CJ, Osanto S, Rosendaal FR. Malignancies, prothrombotic mutations, and the risk of venous thrombosis. JAMA. 2005;293(6):715–22.
15. Voetsch B, Loscalzo J. Genetic determinants of arterial thrombosis. Arterioscler Thromb Vasc Biol. 2004;24(2):216–29.
16. Page C, Rubin LE, Gusberg RJ, Dardik A. Arterial thrombosis associated with heterozygous factor V Leiden disorder, hyperhomocysteinemia, and peripheral arterial disease: importance of synergistic factors. J Vasc Surg. 2005;42(5):1014–48.
17. de Paula Sabino A, Ribeiro DD, Carvalho M, Cardoso J, Dusse LM, Fernandes AP. Factor V Leiden and increased risk for arterial thrombotic disease in young Brazilian patients. Blood Coagul Fibrinolysis. 2006;17(4):271–5.
18. Mandegar MH, Saidi B, Roshanali F. Extensive arterial thrombosis in a patient with factor V Leiden mutation. Interact Cardiovasc Thorac Surg. 2010;11(1):127–9.
19. Lopez F, Mega A, Schiffman F, Sweeney J. Splenic infarction from factor V Leiden mutation. Am J Hematol. 1999;62(1):62–3.
20. De Cicco M. The prothrombotic state in cancer: pathogenic mechanisms. Crit Rev Oncol Hematol. 2004;50:187–96.
21. Blann AD, Dunmore S. Arterial and venous thrombosis in cancer patients. Cardiol Res Pract. 2011;2011:394740.
22. Honecker F, Koychev D, Luhmann AD, Langer F, Dieckmann KP, Bokemeyer C, et al. Venous thromboembolic events in germ cell cancer patients undergoing platinum-based chemotherapy. Onkologie. 2013;36(11):663–8.
23. Mandalà M, Curigliano G, Bucciarelli P, Ferretti G, Mannucci PM, Colleoni M, et al. Factor V Leiden and G20210A prothrombin mutation and the risk of subclavian vein thrombosis in patients with breast cancer and a central venous catheter. Ann Oncol. 2004;15(4):590–3.
24. Van Rooden CJ, Rosendaal FR, Meinders AE, Van Oostayen JA, Van Der Meer FJ, Huisman MV. The contribution of factor V Leiden and prothrombin G20210A mutation to the risk of central venous catheter-related thrombosis. Haematologica. 2004;89(2):201–6.
25. Starling N, Rao S, Cunningham D, Iveson T, Nicolson M, Coxon F, et al. Thromboembolism in patients with advanced gastroesophageal cancer treated with anthracycline, platinum, and fluoropyrimidine combination chemotherapy: a report from the UK national cancer research institute upper gastrointestinal clinical studies group. J Clin Oncol. 2009;27(23):3786–93.
26. Dieckmann KP, Struss WJ, Budde U. Evidence for acute vascular toxicity of cisplatin-based chemotherapy in patients with germ cell tumour. Anticancer Res. 2011;31(12):4501–5.
27. Nuver J, De Haas EC, Van Zweeden M, Gietema JA, Meijer C. Vascular damage in testicular cancer patients: a study on endothelial activation by bleomycin and cisplatin in vitro. Oncol Rep. 2010;23(1):247–53.
28. Johannesdottir SA, Horváth-Puhó E, Dekkers OM, Cannegieter SC, Jørgensen JO, Ehrenstein V, et al. Use of glucocorticoids and risk of venous thromboembolism: a nationwide population-based case–control study. JAMA Intern Med. 2013;173(9):743–52.
29. Xu Z, Westrick RJ, Shen YC, Eitzman DT. Pulmonary fibrosis is increased in mice carrying the factor V Leiden mutation following bleomycin injury. Thromb Haemost. 2001;85(3):441–4.

3

Malignant acanthosis nigricans associated with prostate cancer

Joanna Kubicka-Wołkowska[1*], Sylwia Dębska-Szmich[1], Maja Lisik-Habib[1], Marcin Noweta[2] and Piotr Potemski[1]

Abstract

Background: Acanthosis nigricans is characterized by hyperpigmentation and hyperkeratosis of the skin or mucous membranes. Its malignant form is associated with internal neoplasms, especially gastric adenocarcinoma (55–61%). Coexistence with prostate cancer is uncommon. In the paraneoplastic type of this dermatosis, the skin and mucous lesions are characteristically of more sudden onset and more severe than those in the benign form. The efficacy of various treatment strategies remains disappointing.

Case presentation: We here report a case of 66-year-old Caucasian patient with metastatic prostate cancer and a mild form of acanthosis nigricans that preceded the diagnosis of malignancy and resolved with chemotherapy in parallel with the prostate cancer. The dermatosis recurred when the prostate cancer progressed.

Conclusion: Concurrent acanthosis nigricans and prostate cancer is rare, and few such cases have been reported. Anti-tumor therapy occasionally results in regression of this dermatosis. Underlying malignant disease should be suspected in individuals with elderly-onset of acanthosis nigricans.

Keywords: Acanthosis nigricans, Prostate cancer, Paraneoplastic syndrome

Background

Acanthosis nigricans (AN) manifests with hyperkeratotic areas with excessive pigmentation predominantly localized in the axillae, groin, on the nape of the neck or around the anus; the lesions less frequently affect oral mucous membranes. The diagnosis is based on the clinical characteristics of the lesions. AN can be classified into two forms: benign and malignant [1]. The first is more common and usually accompanies endocrinological disorders (type 2 diabetes, acromegaly, Cushing syndrome, hypothyroidism, and insulin resistance). It may also be congenital or produced by certain medications, including fusidic acid, nicotinic acid and certain hormones; in the latter, it characteristically regresses within 4–10 weeks of cessation of treatment [2]. A malignant form of AN (ANM) is associated with internal neoplasms, particularly gastric adenocarcinoma (55–61%) [3]; the associated neoplasms are less frequently located in the lungs, ovaries, breasts, kidneys, prostate or bladder [3-5]. The skin pathology may appear concurrently with the

cancer (61%), as well as many years before (18%) or after its detection [6]. A coexisting neoplasm should always be suspected in patients with sudden onset of AN. Some reports have cited the presence of malignancy in almost 100% of cases of AN in elderly subjects [4]. Thus, a thorough evaluation for presence of malignancy is strongly recommended when AN is diagnosed in an elderly person.

The pathogenesis of AN is still widely debated; several possibilities are under consideration. Currently, it is presumed that certain cytokines, such as transforming growth factor-α (TGF-α), insulin-like growth factor 1 and fibroblast growth factor participate in the development of typical AN skin lesions. These tumor-produced substances stimulate keratinocytes, melanocytes and fibroblasts to proliferate. Many reports indicate that TGF-α plays a pivotal role in the development and progression of ANM [7-10]. In pathological conditions, excess TGF-α is produced and acts through epidermal growth factor receptors to induce hyperstimulation of keratinocytes. Ellis *et al.* and Koyama *et al.* independently reported resolution of skin lesions and decrease in urine and serum concentrations of TGF-α following surgical removal of malignant tumors in two patients

* Correspondence: zuz.ka@interia.pl
[1]Department of Chemotherapy, Medical University of Lodz, Paderewskiego 4, 93-509 Lodz, Poland
Full list of author information is available at the end of the article

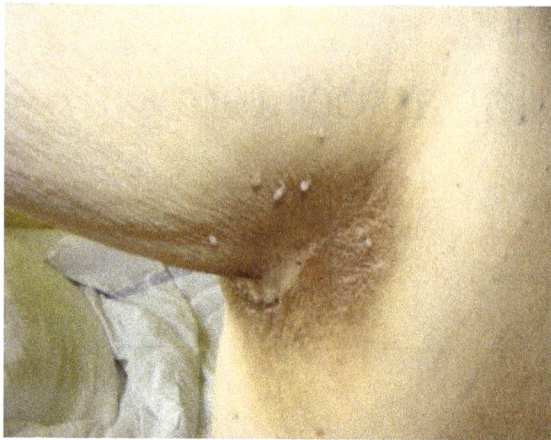

Figure 1 Acanthosis nigricans before starting chemotherapy.
Right axilla

[7,8]. The factors responsible for development of skin lesions in patients with benign AN associated with endocrinopathies, obesity or diabetes are hyperinsulinemia and insulin resistance. Excessive proliferation and growth are induced particularly by insulin-like growth factor 1 [9,11].

Herein we report a patient who developed ANM almost 1 year prior to the diagnosis of prostate cancer. Not only did complete remission of the skin lesions occur following administration of chemotherapy, progression of the underlying malignancy was accompanied by recurrence of AN.

Case presentation

In December 2012, a 66-year-old patient with castration-resistant prostate cancer with bone metastases was admitted to the Chemotherapy Department, Medical University of Lodz to begin anti-neoplastic therapy. The patient had developed otherwise asymptomatic symmetric brownish skin discoloration affecting mainly his armpits in 2009. Because he had no associated symptoms, the family doctor he consulted had not started any therapy or performed

any diagnostic tests. At the beginning of 2010, he was diagnosed as having type 2 diabetes and commenced oral antidiabetics, which were effective in controlling his diabetes. He had no history of other medical problems, endocrinopathies or dermatological disorders. Prostate cancer was diagnosed in February 2010 on biopsies taken because of a high prostate-specific antigen (PSA) serum concentration (13.56 ng/mL) and abnormal findings on digital rectal examination and trans-rectal ultrasonography. The neoplasm was classified as highly aggressive (Gleason score $4 + 4 = 8$) and categorized as T2cN0M0 (IIB). The patient accordingly underwent bilateral pelvic lymphadenectomy and prostatectomy in the Urological and Transplantation Ward of Pirogow Memorial Hospital in Lodz. The final pathological evaluation revealed T3bN0 disease, positive resection margins and Gleason score 9 $(4 + 5)$. In April 2011, bone scintigraphy revealed bone metastases and the patient began palliative hormonal therapy (luteinizing hormone-releasing hormone analog plus an antiandrogen). He is currently still receiving luteinizing hormone-releasing hormone analog injections. From June to October 2012, he received palliative radiation therapy to the pelvis, thoracic spine and right humerus for severe pain. Despite a good initial response to hormonal therapy, the patient's prostate cancer eventually progressed and he was considered to have developed castration-resistant disease. In December 2012 he was referred to our Department for cytotoxic treatment. On admission, he was in good general condition (Eastern Cooperative Oncology Group performance status 1/2), his main complaint being of generalized bone pain. Dermatological evaluation revealed focal hyperpigmentation of the skin localized symmetrically in his axillae (Figure 1). The brownish skin discoloration was accompanied by verrucous-like lesions and mild pruritus. Mucous membranes and other areas of the skin were not affected. A diagnosis of AN was made based on the typical clinical appearance of his lesions. Aside from moderate grade gynecomastia probably attributable to hormonal treatment, there were no other relevant abnormalities on physical examination. Laboratory tests showed a castrate

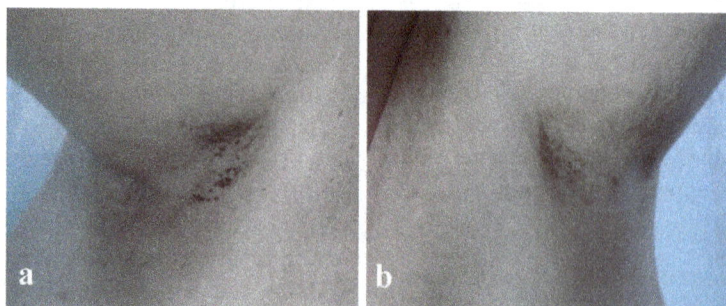

Figure 2 Regression of skin lesions after five cycles of chemotherapy. Right (a) and left (b) axilla.

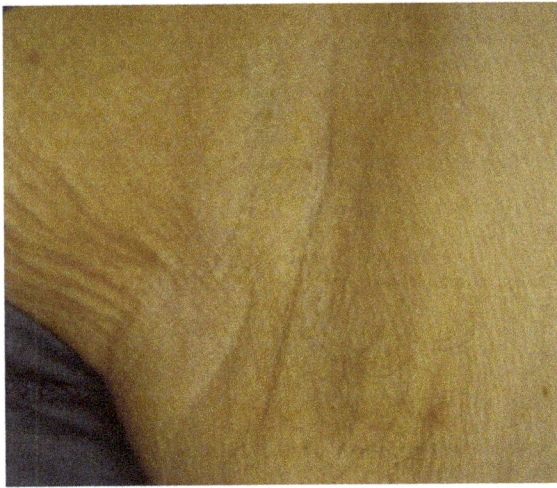

Figure 3 Complete regression of skin condition (right axilla).

serum concentration of testosterone (<0.03 ng/mL) and increased concentrations of alkaline phosphatase (382 U/L), lactate dehydrogenase (269 U/L) and PSA (1280 ng/mL). Complete blood count revealed slightly decreased white blood cell count (4.19 × 103/µL), hemoglobin 11.5 g/dL, and hematocrit (35.1%). Electrolytes and other biochemical tests were within normal limits. After all clinical data had been collected, the patient was deemed eligible to receive standard cytotoxic treatment and accordingly received eight cycles of prednisone with docetaxel (75 mg/m^2 every 3 weeks) from December 2012 to June 2013. Partial remission of skin lesions was apparent after five cycles of chemotherapy (Figure 2). After completion of the eight cycles, not only had his skin lesions completely regressed (Figure 3), but he also had reduced bone pain, a decrease in PSA serum concentration (162.6 ng/mL), improvement in his general well-being, and slight improvement in his bone metastases according to scintigraphy. In September 2013, recurrence of AN was noted in the form of non-itchy hyperpigmentation of the skin of the abdomen and areolae (Figure 4). There were no dermal lesions in the

axillae. At the beginning of October, there was a sudden deterioration in the patient's general condition with an increase in PSA concentration to 2852 ng/mL. Paraparesis caused by disease progression forced the patient to use a wheelchair. He has now received five cycles of second line chemotherapy with mitoxantrone and his prostate cancer is considered stable.

Discussion
The initial skin lesions of ANM appear as areas of excessive keratosis and pigmentation that with time evolve into verrucous-like lesions. Unlike the benign form of AN, ANM occurs in the elderly (>40 years), has a rapid onset and spreads quickly, typically involving the mucous membranes or perianal area. Lesions in the oral cavity may involve the lips, gums, tongue, and palate and reportedly occur in 53% of patients [12]. In extreme cases, almost all of the skin is involved or sudden outbreaks of multiple seborrheic keratoses occur (Leser–Trelat sign). ANM is mainly associated with intra-abdominal malignancies (70–90%), especially gastric adenocarcinoma [3]. An association with prostate cancer is uncommon; to our knowledge, only a few such cases have been reported [3,5,13,14]. Results of treatment aimed at relief of accompanying symptoms such as pruritus and pain in the oral cavity or anus, remain disappointing. However, the skin condition sometimes resolves with tumor-specific treatment (surgical resection, chemotherapy, radiotherapy), cyproheptadine, psoralen and ultraviolet A, or retinoids [15-19].

Conclusions
An association between AN and prostate cancer is unusual. Reported cases of paraneoplastic AN, including those without severe skin lesions, emphasize the importance of vigilance concerning possible associated neoplasms, especially when the dermatosis has developed in an elderly individual. Even when the skin condition is relatively asymptomatic and perceived only as a cosmetic problem, it is essential to thoroughly investigate the possibility of neoplastic disease. Cooperation between urologists, oncologists and family doctors is crucial.

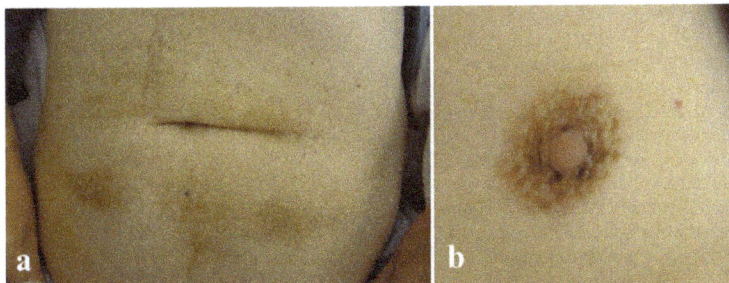

Figure 4 Skin hyperpigmentation on the abdomen (a) and areola (b). Recurrence of AN.

Consent

Written informed consent was obtained from the patient for publication of this manuscript and accompanying images. A copy of the written consent is available for review by the Editor-in-Chief of this journal; however, the patient wishes his personal data to remain confidential.

Abbreviations

AN: Acanthosis nigricans; ANM: Malignant acanthosis nigricans; TGF-α: Transforming growth factor alpha; PSA: Prostate-specific antigen.

Competing interests

The authors declare that they have no competing interests.

Authors' contributions

JKW was responsible for the concept and draft of this report. All authors were involved in revision and preparation of the final version of the manuscript and they all approved it.

Acknowledgement

This study was supported by a grant from the Chemotherapy Clinic of the Medical University of Lodz (UM 501/1-034-02/501-91-263).

Author details

¹Department of Chemotherapy, Medical University of Lodz, Paderewskiego 4, 93-509 Lodz, Poland. ²Department of Dermatology, Paediatric Dermatology and Dermatological Oncology, Medical University of Lodz, Lodz, Poland.

References

1. Yamada Y, Iwabuchi H, Yamada M, Kobayashi D, Uchiyama K, Fujibayashi T: A case of acanthosis nigricans identified by multiple oral papillomas with gastric adenocarcinoma. *Asian J Oral Maxillofac Surg* 2010, **22**:154–158.
2. Schwartz RA, Janniger EJ: Acanthosis nigricans – a common significant disorder usually unassociated with malignancy. *Przegl Dermatol* 2011, **98**:1–6. Article in Polish.
3. Rigel DS, Jacobs MI: Malignant acanthosis nigricans: a review. *J Dermatol Surg Oncol* 1980, **11**:923–927.
4. Kamińska-Winciorek G, Brzezińska-Wcisło L, Lis-Swiety A, Krauze E: Paraneoplastic type of acanthosis nigricans in patient with hepatocellular carcinoma. *Adv Med Sci* 2007, **52**:254–256.
5. Lenzner U, Ramsauer J, Petzoldt W, Meigel W: Acanthosis nigricans maligna. Case report and review of the literature. *Hautarzt* 1998, **49**:41–47. Article in German.
6. Krawczyk M, Mykała-Cieśla J, Kołodziej-Jaskuła A: Acanthosis nigricans as a paraneoplastic syndrome. Case reports and review of literature. *Pol Arch Med Wewn* 2009, **119**:180–183.
7. Ellis DL, Kafka SP, Chow JC, Nanney LB, Inman WH, McCadden ME, King LE Jr: Melanoma, growth factors, acanthosis nigricans, the sign of Leser-Trelat, and multiple acrochordons. A possible role for alpha-transforming growth factor in cutaneous paraneoplastic syndromes. *New Engl J Med* 1987, **317**:1582–1587.
8. Koyama S, Ikeda K, Sato M, Shibahara K, Yuhara K, Fukutomi H, Fukunaga K, Kanazawa N, Yuzawa K, Fukao K, Iijima T, Kikuchi M, Tomiya T, Fujiwara K: Transforming growth factor alpha (TGF-alpha)–producing gastric carcinoma with acanthosis nigricans: an endocrine effect of TGF-alpha in the pathogenesis of cutaneous paraneoplastic syndrome and epithelial hyperplasia of the esophagus. *J Gastroenterol* 1997, **32**:71–77.
9. Torley D, Bellus GA, Munro CS: Genes, growth factors and acanthosis nigricans. *Br J Dermatol* 2002, **147**:1096–1101.
10. Wilgenbus K, Lentner A, Kuckelkorn R, Handt S, Mittermayer C: Further evidence that acanthosis nigricans maligna is linked to enhanced secretion by the tumour of transforming growth factor alpha. *Arch Dermatol Res* 1992, **284**:266–270.
11. Higgins SP, Freemark M, Prose NS: Acanthosis nigricans: a practical approach to evaluation and management. *Dermatol Online J* 2008, **14**:2.
12. Petkowicz B, Berger M, Szeszko Ł, Piotrkowicz J: Acanthosis nigricans maligna in oral cavity as a symptom of malignant neoplasm of the gastrointestinal tract. *Gastroenterol Pol* 2011, **18**:41–44. Article in Polish.
13. Curth HO, Hilberg AW, Machacek GF: The site and histology of the cancer associated with malignant acanthosis nigricans. *Cancer* 1962, **15**:364–382.
14. Weger W, Ginter-Hanselmayer G, Hammer HF, Hödl S: Florid cutaneous papillomatosis with acanthosis nigricans in a patient with carcinomas of the lung and prostate. *J Am Acad Dermatol* 2007, **57**:907–908.
15. Anderson SH, Hudson-Peacock M, Muller AF: Malignant acanthosis nigricans: potential role of chemotherapy. *Br J Dermatol* 1999, **141**:714–716.
16. Bonnekoh B, Thiele B, Merk H, Mahrle G: Systemic photochemotherapy (PUVA) in acanthosis nigricans maligna: regression of keratosis, hyperpigmentation and pruritus. *Z Hautkr* 1989, **64**:1059–1062. Article in German.
17. Nomachi K, Mori M, Matsuda N: Improvement of oral lesions associated with malignant acanthosis nigricans after treatment of lung cancer. *Oral Surg Oral Med Oral Pathol* 1989, **68**:74–79.
18. Kebria MM, Belinson J, Kim R, Mekhail TM: Malignant acanthosis nigricans, tripe palms and the sign of Leser-Trélat, a hint to the diagnosis of early stage ovarian cancer: a case report and review of the literature. *Gynecol Oncol* 2006, **10**:353–355.
19. Mekhail TM, Markman M: Acanthosis nigricans with endometrial carcinoma: case report and review of the literature. *Gynecol Oncol* 2002, **84**:332–334.

4

The addition of a sagittal image fusion improves the prostate cancer detection in a sensor-based MRI /ultrasound fusion guided targeted biopsy

Karsten Günzel[1†], Hannes Cash[1*†], John Buckendahl[1], Maximilian Königbauer[1], Patrick Asbach[2], Matthias Haas[2], Jörg Neymeyer[1], Stefan Hinz[1], Kurt Miller[1] and Carsten Kempkensteffen[1]

Abstract

Background: To explore the diagnostic benefit of an additional image fusion of the sagittal plane in addition to the standard axial image fusion, using a sensor-based MRI/US fusion platform.

Methods: During July 2013 and September 2015, 251 patients with at least one suspicious lesion on mpMRI (rated by PI-RADS) were included into the analysis. All patients underwent MRI/US targeted biopsy (TB) in combination with a 10 core systematic prostate biopsy (SB). All biopsies were performed on a sensor-based fusion system. Group A included 162 men who received TB by an axial MRI/US image fusion. Group B comprised 89 men in whom the TB was performed with an additional sagittal image fusion.

Results: The median age in group A was 67 years (IQR 61–72) and in group B 68 years (IQR 60–71). The median PSA level in group A was 8.10 ng/ml (IQR 6.05–14) and in group B 8.59 ng/ml (IQR 5.65–12.32). In group A the proportion of patients with a suspicious digital rectal examination (DRE) (14 vs. 29%, $p = 0.007$) and the proportion of primary biopsies (33 vs 46%, $p = 0.046$) were significantly lower. The rate of PI-RADS 3 lesions were overrepresented in group A compared to group B (19 vs. 9%; $p = 0.044$). Classified according to PI-RADS 3, 4 and 5, the detection rates of TB were 42, 48, 75% in group A and 25, 74, 90% in group B. The rate of PCa with a Gleason score ≥ 7 missed by TB was 33% (18 cases) in group A and 9% (5 cases) in group B; p-value 0.072. An explorative multivariate binary logistic regression analysis revealed that PI-RADS, a suspicious DRE and performing an additional sagittal image fusion were significant predictors for PCa detection in TB. 9 PCa were only detected by TB with sagittal fusion (sTB) and sTB identified 10 additional clinically significant PCa (Gleason ≥ 7).

Conclusion: Performing an additional sagittal image fusion besides the standard axial fusion appears to improve the accuracy of the sensor-based MRI/US fusion platform.

Keywords: Multiparametric magnetic resonance imaging, Targeted biopsy, Prostate cancer detection, MRI/US fusion biopsy

* Correspondence: hannes.cash@charite.de
Karsten Günzel and Hannes Cash are co-first authors.
†Equal contributors
[1]Department of Urology, Charité — University Medicine Berlin,
Hindenburgdamm 30, 12203 Berlin, Germany
Full list of author information is available at the end of the article

Background

Prostate cancer (PCa) is the most common malignancy of men and the only tumour, which is diagnosed according to the guidelines by untargeted systematic biopsies of the entire organ [1, 2]. Because prostate cancer is often not visualized in conventional transrectal ultrasound, there is a risk to miss clinically significant PCa (Gleason ≥7) with a random systematic transrectal prostate biopsy (SB) [3, 4]. Due to a high soft-tissue contrast, a high resolution (T2-weighted anatomical sequences) and the registration of functional parameters (diffusion-weighted and dynamic contrast-enhanced sequences (DWI and DCE), MR spectroscopy imaging) a multiparametric magnetic resonance imaging (mpMRI) of the prostate provides a high sensitivity, specificity and negative predictive value in the detection and localization of clinically significant prostate cancers [5, 6]. For standardization of evaluation of the mpMRI the "European Society of Urogenital Radiology" (ESUR) established the "Prostate Imaging Reporting and Data System" (PI-RADS), which introduced a 5-point Likert scale for each region (peripheral and central glandular sections) with corresponding scores for each sequence (T2, DWI, DCE, and MR-Spectroscopy) [7, 8]. The correlation of the level of PI-RADS with the overall detection rate of PCa and the detection of significant PCa has been demonstrated in various studies [9–13]. The increasing utilization of mpMRI of the prostate and the consecutive MRI/ultrasound fusion guided targeted biopsy (TB) resulted in an improved detection of PCa compared to SB, the current standard of care [14–17]. A difficulty is the exact fusion of mpMRI with transrectal ultrasound for TB. Various possibilities of MRI/ultrasound (MRI/US) image fusion, such as cognitive fusion, sensor-based fusion or organ-based fusion are available to perform TB. Despite the technological progress of different fusion platforms, several studies have shown that clinically significant PCa can still be overlooked by TB [17–20]. For the sensor-bases TB we previously analyzed the possible pitfalls of TB, such as reader variability for mpMRI, an imprecise targeting of the suspicious lesion [21]. Traditionally sensor-based fusion of the MRI image and the real-time ultrasound image is performed by the operator in the axial plane according to anatomical landmarks (i.e. prostatic apex, periprostatic vessels, BPH nodes etc.). In order to further improve the targeting accuracy and reduce a possible image fusion error, this study evaluated the use of an additional image fusion in the sagittal plane according to a 3-point technique. In a cohort of 791 men, who underwent a MRI/US fusion biopsy with an organ-based fusion system, Hong et al. demonstrated that the combination of axial and sagittal approaches detected more clinically significant PCa [22]. For sensor-based fusion platforms there is currently no data on the effect of an added sagittal image fusion.

Methods

Study population

In the period of July 2013 to September 2015, 251 patients, who showed at least one suspicious lesion on mpMRI (PI-RADS ≥3) and underwent a consecutive TB in combination with a 10-core systematic prostate biopsy (SB), were consecutively included into the retrospective analysis. The indication for a mpMRI has largely been provided by attending outpatient urologists. Parts of the cohort were analysed in a previous study [13]. All patients were recorded regardless to the number of prior prostate biopsies. The data collection was based on the patients medical history, clinical findings and the physical patient files. Patient data was prospectively collected in a START conform database [23]. The analysis in regard to the axial and sagittal image fusion was performed retrospectively. All patients signed an informed consent for the intervention, data acquisition and data evaluation. The study was performed according to the declaration of Helsinki and the analysis was approved by the Institutional Review Board of the Charité University Medicine Berlin.

Multiparametric magnetic resonance imaging

A 3-Tesla mpMRI (Magnetom Skyra, Siemens Medical Systems, Erlangen, Germany) without an endorectal coil was performed for all patients before prostate biopsy. The MRI protocol contained high spatial resolution T2-weighted turbo spin-echo sequences in axial, sagittal and coronal orientation, axial turbo spin-echo T1 weighted images, axial diffusion weighted images (b-values 0.400 and 800 s/mm^2) and dynamic contrast-enhanced sequences. The evaluation of the mpMRI was performed by experienced radiologists according to the guidelines of the European Society of Urogenital Radiology (ESUR) [8]. From a PI-RADS score of 3, the indication for MRI/US fusion biopsy was made.

MRI-ultrasound fusion prostate biopsy and systematic biopsy

The prostate biopsies were performed under antibiotic prophylaxis with a fluoroquinolone according to the EAU guidelines [2], with a high-end ultrasound device HiVision Preirus (Hitachi Medical Systems, Tokyo, Japan) and an endocavity endfire probe (EUP V53W, Hitachi Medical Systems, Tokyo, Japan). All biopsies were taken in lithotomy position. At first TB were performed. T2 and DWI sequences of the axial planes in mpMRI were imported to the ultrasonic device. After that, the suspicious lesions were marked in axial orientation of the mpMRI sequences by the urologist experienced with mpMRI. The MRI/US image fusion was performed using sensor-based registration. The movement of the probe with an attached tracker was detected in a low magnetic field (0.1 Tesla), which was generated by a mini bird receiver. Until December 2014 only axial MRI/US image fusion was performed. For this purpose, the same plane in ultrasound and MRI was identified according to anatomical landmarks (prostatic apex, periprostatic vessels, BPH nodes, intraprostatic cysts) Depending on the anatomical conditions, the angle of axial plane in the MRI image was corrected to match the angulation of the ultrasound probe and image. The previously marked suspect lesions were transferred to the real-time ultrasound image by the platform's software, followed by a 2–5 targeted biopies in an axial orientation. After an analysis of possible reasons for targeted biopsy failure, as of December 2014 the targeted biopsies were performed after MRI/US image fusion in both the axial and sagittal plane [21]. The total number of targeted biopsies remained unchanged. For the sagittal image fusion, a T2-weighted sequence in sagittal orientation was used to mark the bladder neck, the apex of the prostate and the seminal vesicle angle. Based on these marks the MRI and the ultrasound image were fused by the software. Thereafter, TB was carried out in a sagittal orientation of the MRI and ultrasound image. For sampling, we used a long biopsy needle (18 g × 25 cm, Bard Magnum biopsy instrument, Tempe, United States). After performing TB, local anaesthesia with a bupivacaine was injected at the dorsal prostatic capsule and a 10-core SB was conducted without changing the examiner. The SB scheme included cores from: left/right apex, left/right lateral mid gland, left/right base, left/right ventral and left/right para-urethral. All tissue-samples were documented by their extraction location and shipped separately for histopathological evaluation by our experienced pathologists.

Group distribution
Group A included all patients who have received an MRI/US image fusion only in the axial plane. Group B, are included all patients who have received MRI/US image fusion in the axial and sagittal plane. Figure 1 shows a flow chart for the patient inclusion and the group distribution.

Statistical analysis
PASW Version 22 (SPSS Inc. 1998–2010, Chicago, Illinois 60606, USA) was used for statistical analyses. Categorical data were presented by absolute and relative frequencies.

Continuous variables were measured by means and standard deviation when normal distributed or by medians and quartiles. Continuous variables were evaluated with the Kolmogorov-Smirnov-test for normal distribution. We used chi-square test, Student's t-test and Mann-Whitney U test to calculate statistical differences between numerical and categorical variables. Univariate and multivariate binary regression analysis were performed to evaluate significant parameters in the descriptive analysis as predictors for PCa detection. A p-value of $p < 0.05$ was considered statistical significant.

Results
Demographic data, clinical characteristics and MRI findings are presented in Table 1 divided in group A (patients without additional sagittal image fusion) and group B (patients with additional sagittal image fusion). The median age in group A was 67 years (IQR 61–72) and in group B 68 years (IQR 60–71). Both groups showed statistically similar prostate volumes (48 vs. 50 ml). The median PSA level in group A was 8.10 ng/ml (IQR 6.05–14.00) and in group B 8.59 ng/ml (IQR 5.65–12.32). The proportion of patients with a suspicious digital rectal examination (DRE) (14 vs. 29%, $p = 0.007$) and the proportion of patients with primary biopsies (33 vs 46%, $p = 0.041$) were significantly lower in group A. The rate of PI-RADS 3 lesions were overrepresented in group A (19 vs. 9%; $p = 0.044$). With 43% compared to 30% in group A PI-RADS 5 lesions were more frequently represented in group B ($p = 0.051$). No significant differences were observed for lesion positions, number of suspicious lesions in mpMRI and lesion sizes. The mean number of cores taken per patient and the mean number of TB per patient were significant higher in Group A (13.7 vs. 13.2 and 3.8 vs. 3.4; $p = 0.009$ and 0.031). The analysis showed a significant higher overall cancer detection rate (CDR) (85 vs. 72%; $p = 0.019$) and a significant higher detection rate in TB (76 vs. 55%; $p = 0.001$) in group B, please see Table 2. Furthermore there was a significant lower number of patients diagnosed with a clinically significant PCa in group A (61 vs. 78%; $p = 0.025$). Classified according to

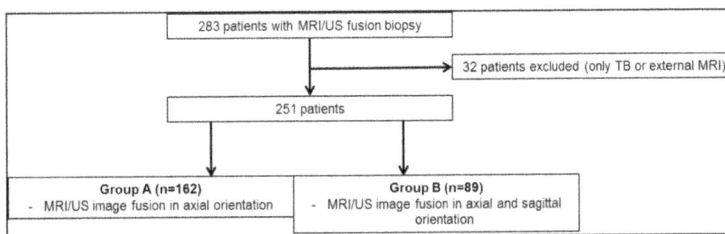

Fig. 1 Patient inclusion and group distribution. Group A included patients between July 2013 and December 2014 where an axial targeted biopsy was the standard Group B included patients between December 2014 and September 2015 where and axial and sagittal targeted biopsy was performed without increasing the total number of targeted biopsy cores

Table 1 Patient demographics and magnetic resonance imaging findings (n = 251)

	Group A (n = 162)	Group B (N = 89)	p-value
Median (IQR) age, years	67 (61–72)	68 (60–71)	0.846
Median (IQR) PSA. ng/ml	8.10 (6.05–14.00)	8.59 (5.65–12.32)	0.997
Median IQR f/t PSA-ratio,%	12 (9–17)	13 (9–19)	0.309
Median (IQR) prostate volume, ml	48 (35–60)	50 (37–70)	0.087
Suspicous DRE, n (%)	23 (14%)	26 (29%)	0.007
No. of prior biopsies, n (%)			
Primary biopsy	53 (33%)	41 (46%)	0.041
1	59 (36%)	28 (32%)	0.489
2	33 (20%)	13 (15%)	0.308
≥3	17 (10%)	7 (8%)	0.655
Localization of lesions with maximum PI-RADS on mpMRI, n (%)			
Apex	72 (44%)	35 (39%)	0.505
Midgland	43 (27%)	32 (36%)	0.149
Base	47 (29%)	22 (25%)	0.555
Anterior	45 (28%)	28 (32%)	0.563
Median (IQR) no. of lesions per patient	1 (1–2)	1 (1–2)	0.451
Maximum diameter of lesions (mm)	14 (10–17)	13 (10–18)	0.885
Mean (SD) of cores taken per patient	13.7 (±1.6)	13.2 (±1.2)	0.009
Mean (SD) TBs per patient	3.8 (±1.5)	3.4 (±0.9)	0.031
Maximum mpMRI Score, n (%)[a]			
PI-RADS 3	31 (19%)	8 (9%)	0.044
PI-RADS 4	83 (51%)	43 (48%)	0.693
PI-RADS 5	48 (30%)	38 (43%)	0.051

PSA prostate-specific antigen, IQR interquartile range, SD standard deviation, DRE digital rectal examination, mpMRI multiparametric magnetic resonance imaging, PI-RADS Prostate Imaging Reporting and Data System, TB targeted biopsy
[a]For patients with multiple lesions the highest PI-RADS score is stated

Table 2 Cancer Detection Rate and Gleason pattern

	Group A (n = 162)	Group B (N = 89)	p-value
Overall CDR	117 (72%)	76 (85%)	0.019
SB	108 (67%)	68 (76%)	0.115
TB	89 (55%)	68 (76%)	0.001
PI-RADS 3 (n = 39)			
Overall CDR	17 (55%)	5 (63%)	>0.999
SB	15 (48%)	3 (38%)	0.702
TB	13 (42%)	2 (25%)	0.450
PI-RADS 4 (n = 126)			
Overall CDR	55 (66%)	36 (84%)	0.058
SB	48 (58%)	33 (77%)	0.049
TB	40 (48%)	32 (74%)	0.007
PI-RADS 5 (n = 86)			
Overall CDR	45 (94%)	35 (92%)	>0.999
SB	45 (94%)	32 (84%)	0.175
TB	36 (75%)	34 (90%)	0.102
Detected GS ≥7 in TB	54 (61%)	53 (78%)	0.025
Missed PCa (GS ≥7) in TB	18 (33%*)	5 (9%*)	0.072

CDR = Cancer Dection Rate; GS = Gleason Score; SB = Random Biopsy; TB = Target biopsy; * % of GS ≥7 detected by TB

Table 3. Table 4 shows the comparison of the biopsy results of the axial (aTB) and sagittal (sTB) MRI/US fusion biopsy. Depending on PI-RADS, lesion diameter and lesion localization, PCa detection rates of aTB and sTB were statistically equivalent except a higher detection of PCa by aTB for PI-RADS 4 lesions (70 vs. 44%, *p* = 0.007). Furthermore, Table 4 shows the additional detection of PCa in total and of PCa with a Gleason score ≥7 due sTB depending on PI-RADS, lesion diameter and lesion localization. Overall, nine PCas were only detected by sTB and sTB identified 10 additional clinically significant PCa (Gleason ≥7).

Discussion

Since the introduction of MRI/US fusion biopsy of the prostate, several studies have demonstrated an improvement in prostate cancer detection rates as well as the identification of clinically relevant tumours [14, 15, 24–26]. Due to this increasing value of MRI/US fusion biopsy for

PI-RADS 3, 4 and 5, the detection rates of TB were 42, 48, 75% in group A and 25, 74, 90% in group B. The rate of PCa with a Gleason score ≥7 missed by TB was **33%** (18 cases) in group A and **9%** (5 cases) in group B (*p* = 0.072). The overall cancer detection rates and the PI-RADS based analyses for SB and TB for men without suspicious DRE and prior negative biopsy are shown in Additional file 1 Table S1 and Additional file 2 Table S2. An explorative multivariate binary logistic regression analysis revealed that PI-RADS, a suspicious DRE and performing an additional sagittal image fusion were significant predictors for PCa detection in TB, please see

Table 3 Predictors for prostate cancer detection in the Targeted Biopsy

	Univariate analysis		Multivariate analysis	
	OR	p-value	OR	p-value
Suspicious DRE	4.539	<0.001	2.777	0.024
Primary biopsy	1.175	0.553		
PI-RADS	2.712	<0.001	2.240	<0.001
Sagittal image fusion	2.656	0.001	2.105	0.017

Table 4 Cancer Detection Rate of the Targeted Biopsy in relation to an axial and sagittal image fusion

Group B n = 89	Overall CDR in TB (sTB + aTB)	CDR in aTB	CDR in sTB	Additional PCa detected only by sTB*	Additional GS ≥7 in sTB#
Overall	68 (76%)	59 (66%)	50 (56%)	9 (13%)	10 (19%)
PI-RADS					
3 (n = 8)	2 (25%)	2 (25%)	2 (25%)	0	0
4 (n = 43)	32 (74%)	30 (70%)	19 (44%)	2 (5%)	4 (9%)
5 (n = 38)	34 (90%)	27 (71%)	29 (76%)	7 (18%)	6 (16%)
Maximum diameter of lesion					
1–10 (n = 27)	18 (67%)	15 (56%)	10 (37%)	3 (11%)	3 (11%)
11–20 (n = 50)	38 (76%)	33 (66%)	29 (58%)	5 (10%)	5 (10%)
>20 (n = 12)	12 (100%)	11 (92%)	11 (92%)	1 (8%)	2 (17%)
Localization of lesion					
Apex (n = 35)	26 (74%)	23 (66%)	19 (54%)	3 (9%)	3 (9%)
Midgland (n = 32)	23 (72%)	18 (56%)	15 (47%)	5 (16%)	5 (16%)
Base (n = 22)	19 (86%)	18 (82%)	16 (73%)	1 (5%)	2 (9%)
Anterior (n = 28)	26 (93%)	22 (79%)	22 (79%)	4 (14%)	5 (18%)

aTB = axial fusion TB; sTB = sagittal fusion TB; * compared to overall CDR or TB (aTB + sTB);
#Either detection of GS ≥7 only by sTB or Gleason upgrade in the sTB biopsy core compared to the aTB core; percentage of GS ≥7 detected by TB (aTB + sTB) n = 53

primary diagnosis and monitoring of prostate cancer various fusion systems have been established. A variety fusion systems (UroNav, BiopSee, Urostation, Artemis, HiVison-Preirus, etc.) have been reported in the current literature [13, 14, 22, 24, 26, 27]. Uniform treatment regimens for the implementation of MRI/US fusion biopsies do not exist. In a large patient cohort Hong et al. demonstrated for organ based MRI/US fusion biopsies that the combination of sagittal and axial biopsy approaches identified additional clinically significant prostate cancers [22]. It can be assumed that the correctness of the image fusion of MRI and transrectal ultrasound has an important influence on the accuracy of targeted sampling. Our study showed a significant increase in prostate cancer detection rate of TB by 55% in the group without sagittal fusion to 76% in the group with additional sagittal fusion and the improvement remained even when men with a positive DRE and a primary biopsy were excluded. In addition, the proportion of detected clinically significant PCa (Gleason-score ≥7) increased from 61% in group A to 78% in group B. The sole analysis of the detection rates of axial TB results in an increase of 56 to 66% in group B. The observed increase in detection rates might be related to various factors. In the sensor-based MRI/US image fusion, the same layers in the T2-weighted MRI sequence and the transrectal ultrasound image in axial or sagittal orientation are fused. Identifying the same layers in MRI and US are the basis of fusion accuracy. Angular deviations of the display plane in transrectal ultrasound and MRI lead to inaccuracies of image fusion. In our study, the angle correction for axial image fusion was carried out manually by the urologist. In the sagittal image fusion, the angular offset is software-based by three identical points,

which are simultaneously marked in MRI and ultrasound in two different layers. Gaziev et al. showed an increase in the detection rate of prostate cancer by performing perineal MRI/US fusion biopsies of the prostate with increasing experience of the examiner [28]. It is tempting to speculate, that in our study the learning curve of the examiner has likewise lead to an increase in the detection rate in the TB after implementation of additional sagittal image fusion. Another important factor influencing the detection rate of TB is the PI-RADS score [12, 13]. Our study cohort showed a significant decrease of percentage of PI-RADS 3 lesions and a non-significant increase in the proportion of PI-RADS 5 lesions in the patient group with additional sagittal fusion. Also in the univariate and multivariate regression analysis the level of PI-RADS was identified as a significant predictor for PCa detection. This may have occurred to an increased PCa detection in group B, but the sagittal image fusion remained an independent predictor for cancer detection by TB. A suspicious digital rectal examination as described by Radtke et al. and Potter et al. presents a further risk factor for the detection of PCa in TB and SB [18, 29]. Similar to the previously published studies, our univariate and multivariate regression analyses of the whole cohort revealed a significant correlation of a suspicious DRE with PCa detection rate. The higher TB detection rate in group B, that included more men with a suspicious DRE, may therefore have been influenced, but the higher detection rate in group B compared to group A persisted when the analysis excluded men with a suspicious DRE. In our regression analysis, the proportion of biopsy naive men was not a significant predictor for PCa detection, although two large studies showed an influence on cancer detection

[12, 22]. Therefore, the significantly higher proportion of primary biopsies in group B may have affected the detection rate of the TB. Again, the improved detection rate in group B remained when men with a positive DRE and a primary biopsy were excluded from the analysis.

The additional implementation of the sagittal image fusion resulted in an increase in the detection rate of 10% for TB. By sagittal fusion, nine (13%) additional prostate cancers were detected and ten (19%) additional clinically significant tumors were identified. The improvement of the axial TB, when adding a sagittal TB was independent of the lesion size or localization of the lesions. Moreover, performing a sagittal image fusion was a significant predictor in univariate and multivariate regression analysis for the detection of prostate cancer in the TB. In the group of patients with sagittal fusion, the proportion of overlooked clinically significant tumors by TB dropped to 9% compared to 33% in the group of patients without sagittal fusion. The reduced rate of missed PCa after the introduction of the sagittal image fusion was not accompanied with an increase of the number of targeted biopsies.

Adding the sagittal image fusion when performing TB on a sensor-based platform may reduce the targeting error that may be inevitable in some cases [21]. In our institution we have therefore established the additional sagittal image fusion firmly in our MRI/US fusion biopsy protocol.

Because of the retrospective study design the investigation has several limitations. Unconsidered confounders may have also influenced the study results, e.g. a selection bias of patients by referring outpatient urologist. The inhomogeneity of the two study groups in terms of baseline characteristics may have affected the study results. To ensure the data consistency, we performed logistic regression analyses for the evaluation of predictors of PCa detection by targeted biopsy. In order to clearly demonstrate the impact of an additional sagittal image fusion on the detection rate of TB would require prospective randomized studies.

Conclusion
Performing a sagittal image fusion in addition to the standard the axial fusion improves the accuracy to detect PCa by targeted biopsies performed with a sensor-based MRI/US fusion platform.

Additional files

Additional file 1: Table S1. Cancer Detection Rates in Group A and B excluding men with abnormal DRE.

Additional file 2: Table S2. Cancer Detection Rate and Gleason pattern in Group A and B excluding men with abnormal DRE and including only men with prior negative biopsy.

Abbreviations
DCE: Dynamic contrast-enhanced sequences; DWI: Diffusion-weighted; ESUR: European society of urogenital radiology; mpMRI: Multiparametric magnetic resonance imaging; MRI/US: MRI/ultrasound; PCa: Prostate cancer; SB: Systematic transrectal prostate biopsy; TB: MRI/ultrasound fusion guided targeted biopsy

Acknowledgements
None.

Funding
None.

Authors' contributions
KG, HC, CK: Protocol/project development. KG, HC, JB, MK, PA, MH: Data collection or management. KG, HC, CK: Data analysis. KG, HC, CK: Manuscript writing/editing. PA, JN, SH, KM: Critical manuscript revision. JN, SH, KM, CK: Supervision.

Competing interests
H. Cash reports receiving honoraria as a speaker on national conferences for Hitachi Medical Systems. All other authors have no competing interests.

Author details
Department of Urology, Charité — University Medicine Berlin, Hindenburgdamm 30, 12203 Berlin, Germany. 2Departement of Radiology, Charité — University Medicine Berlin, Hindenburgdamm 30, 12203 Berlin, Germany.

References
1. Siegel RL, Miller KD, Jemal A. Cancer statistics, 2015. CA Cancer J Clin. 2015; 65(1):5–29.
2. Heidenreich A, Bastian PJ, Bellmunt J, Bolla M, Joniau S, van der Kwast T, et al. EAU guidelines on prostate cancer. part 1: screening, diagnosis, and local treatment with curative intent-update 2013. Eur Urol. 2014;65(1):124–37.
3. Rodriguez-Covarrubias F, Gonzalez-Ramirez A, Aguilar-Davidov B, Castillejos-Molina R, Sotomayor M, Feria-Bernal G. Extended sampling at first biopsy improves cancer detection rate: results of a prospective, randomized trial comparing 12 versus 18-core prostate biopsy. J Urol. 2011;185(6):2132–6.
4. Campos-Fernandes JL, Bastien L, Nicolaiew N, Robert G, Terry S, Vacherot F, et al. Prostate cancer detection rate in patients with repeated extended 21-sample needle biopsy. Eur Urol. 2009;55(3):600–6.
5. Futterer JJ, Briganti A, De Visschere P, Emberton M, Giannarini G, Kirkham A, et al. Can clinically significant prostate cancer Be detected with multiparametric magnetic resonance imaging? a systematic review of the literature. Eur Urol. 2015;68(6):1045–53.
6. Arumainayagam N, Ahmed HU, Moore CM, Freeman A, Allen C, Sohaib SA, et al. Multiparametric MR imaging for detection of clinically significant prostate cancer: a validation cohort study with transperineal template prostate mapping as the reference standard. Radiology. 2013;268(3):761–9.
7. Hamoen EH, de Rooij M, Witjes JA, Barentsz JO, Rovers MM. Use of the prostate imaging reporting and data system (PI-RADS) for prostate cancer detection with multiparametric magnetic resonance imaging: a diagnostic meta-analysis. Eur Urol. 2015;67(6):1112–21.
8. Barentsz JO, Richenberg J, Clements R, Choyke P, Verma S, Villeirs G, et al. ESUR prostate MR guidelines 2012. Eur Radiol. 2012;22(4):746–57.
9. Arsov C, Rabenalt R, Blondin D, Quentin M, Hiester A, Godehardt E, et al. Prospective randomized trial comparing magnetic resonance imaging (MRI)-guided in-bore biopsy to MRI-ultrasound fusion and transrectal ultrasound-guided prostate biopsy in patients with prior negative biopsies. Eur Urol. 2015;68(4):713–20.

10. Baco E, Rud E, Eri LM, Moen G, Vlatkovic L, Svindland A, et al. A Randomized Controlled Trial To Assess and Compare the Outcomes of Two-core Prostate Biopsy Guided by Fused Magnetic Resonance and Transrectal Ultrasound Images and Traditional 12-core Systematic Biopsy. Eur Urol. 2016;69(1):149–56.

11. Borkowetz A, Platzek I, Toma M, Laniado M, Baretton G, Froehner M, et al. Comparison of systematic transrectal biopsy to transperineal magnetic resonance imaging/ultrasound-fusion biopsy for the diagnosis of prostate cancer. BJU Int. 2015;116(6):873–9.

12. Filson CP, Natarajan S, Margolis DJ, Huang J, Lieu P, Dorey FJ, et al. Prostate cancer detection with magnetic resonance-ultrasound fusion biopsy: The role of systematic and targeted biopsies. Cancer. 2016;122(6):884–92.

13. Cash H, Maxeiner A, Stephan C, Fischer T, Durmus T, Holzmann J, et al. The detection of significant prostate cancer is correlated with the Prostate Imaging Reporting and Data System (PI-RADS) in MRI/transrectal ultrasound fusion biopsy. World J Urol. 2016;34(4):525–32.

14. Siddiqui MM, Rais-Bahrami S, Turkbey B, George AK, Rothwax J, Shakir N, et al. Comparison of MR/ultrasound fusion-guided biopsy with ultrasound-guided biopsy for the diagnosis of prostate cancer. JAMA. 2015;313(4):390–7.

15. Siddiqui MM, Rais-Bahrami S, Truong H, Stamatakis L, Vourganti S, Nix J, et al. Magnetic resonance imaging/ultrasound-fusion biopsy significantly upgrades prostate cancer versus systematic 12-core transrectal ultrasound biopsy. Eur Urol. 2013;64(5):713–9.

16. Pokorny MR, de Rooij M, Duncan E, Schroder FH, Parkinson R, Barentsz JO, et al. Prospective study of diagnostic accuracy comparing prostate cancer detection by transrectal ultrasound-guided biopsy versus magnetic resonance (MR) imaging with subsequent MR-guided biopsy in men without previous prostate biopsies. Eur Urol. 2014;66(1):22–9.

17. Salami SS, Ben-Levi E, Yaskiv O, Ryniker L, Turkbey B, Kavoussi LR, et al. In patients with a previous negative prostate biopsy and a suspicious lesion on magnetic resonance imaging, is a 12-core biopsy still necessary in addition to a targeted biopsy? BJU Int. 2015;115(4):562–70.

18. Radtke JP, Kuru TH, Boxler S, Alt CD, Popeneciu IV, Huettenbrink C, et al. Comparative analysis of transperineal template saturation prostate biopsy versus magnetic resonance imaging targeted biopsy with magnetic resonance imaging-ultrasound fusion guidance. J Urol. 2015;193(1):87–94.

19. Distler F, Radtke JP, Kesch C, Roethke M, Schlemmer HP, Roth W, et al. [Value of MRI/ultrasound fusion in primary biopsy for the diagnosis of prostate cancer]. Urologe A. 2016;55(2):146–55.

20. Radtke JP, Schwab C, Wolf MB, Freitag MT, Alt CD, Kesch C, et al. Multiparametric Magnetic Resonance Imaging (MRI) and MRI-Transrectal Ultrasound Fusion Biopsy for Index Tumor Detection: Correlation with Radical Prostatectomy Specimen. Eur Urol. 2016;70(5):846–853.

21. Cash H, Gunzel K, Maxeiner A, Stephan C, Fischer T, Durmus T, et al. Prostate cancer detection on transrectal ultrasonography-guided random biopsy despite negative real-time magnetic resonance imaging/ultrasonography fusion-guided targeted biopsy: reasons for targeted biopsy failure. BJU Int. 2016;118(1):35–43.

22. Hong CW, Rais-Bahrami S, Walton-Diaz A, Shakir N, Su D, George AK, et al. Comparison of magnetic resonance imaging and ultrasound (MRI-US) fusion-guided prostate biopsies obtained from axial and sagittal approaches. BJU Int. 2015;115(5):772–9.

23. Moore CM, Kasivisvanathan V, Eggener S, Emberton M, Futterer JJ, Gill IS, et al. Standards of reporting for MRI-targeted biopsy studies (START) of the prostate: recommendations from an international working group. Eur Urol. 2013;64(4):544–52.

24. Sonn GA, Chang E, Natarajan S, Margolis DJ, Macairan M, Lieu P, et al. Value of targeted prostate biopsy using magnetic resonance-ultrasound fusion in men with prior negative biopsy and elevated prostate-specific antigen. Eur Urol. 2014;65(4):809–15.

25. Wysock JS, Rosenkrantz AB, Huang WC, Stifelman MD, Lepor H, Deng FM, et al. A prospective, blinded comparison of magnetic resonance (MR) imaging-ultrasound fusion and visual estimation in the performance of MR-targeted prostate biopsy: the PROFUS trial. Eur Urol. 2014;66(2):343–51.

26. Delongchamps NB, Peyromaure M, Schull A, Beuvon F, Bouazza N, Flam T, et al. Prebiopsy magnetic resonance imaging and prostate cancer detection: comparison of random and targeted biopsies. J Urol. 2013;189(2):493–9.

27. Kuru TH, Roethke MC, Seidenader J, Simpfendorfer T, Boxler S, Alammar K, et al. Critical evaluation of magnetic resonance imaging targeted, transrectal ultrasound guided transperineal fusion biopsy for detection of prostate cancer. J Urol. 2013;190(4):1380–6.

28. Gaziev G, Wadhwa K, Barrett T, Koo BC, Gallagher FA, Serrao E, et al. Defining the learning curve for multiparametric magnetic resonance imaging (MRI) of the prostate using MRI-transrectal ultrasonography (TRUS) fusion-guided transperineal prostate biopsies as a validation tool. BJU Int. 2016;117(1):80–6.

29. Potter SR, Horniger W, Tinzl M, Bartsch G, Partin AW. Age, prostate-specific antigen, and digital rectal examination as determinants of the probability of having prostate cancer. Urology. 2001;57(6):1100–4.

5

A discrepancy of penile hemodynamics during visual sexual stimulation observed by near-infrared spectroscopy

Evgenii Kim[1†], Songhyun Lee[2†], Zephaniah Phillips V[1] and Jae G Kim[1,2*]

Abstract

Background: In this paper, we observed a discrepancy of penile hemodynamics dependent on location by using near infrared spectroscopy (NIRS) sensor, and showcase NIRS as a potentially suitable sensor in supplementing the diagnosis and treatment of erectile dysfunction.

Methods: To observe the effect that location has on penile hemodynamics, the NIRS sensor was placed on the top and the side of genital organ, and oxy- (HbO), deoxy-(RHb), and total (HbT) hemoglobin concentration changes were acquired. Our results from 6 healthy subjects show that hemodynamic changes vary depending on where the probe was placed. To observe a statistical difference between the signals, a Wilcoxon signed-rank test was performed.

Results: The result shows a significant difference ($p < 0.05$) between concentration changes of RHb and HbT depending on the probes' location. Moreover, the sensor placed on the top of the organ shows a rise of HbO and HbT concentration while RHb concentration decreased. However, hemodynamics from the side of the organ showed that RHb concentration increased along with HbO.

Conclusions: The outcomes demonstrates an ability of NIRS to be sensitive enough to detect the different hemodynamic changes in various locations of a healthy male genital organ during visual sexual stimulation. The results also show the importance of sensor location on the genital organ for the resulting hemodynamic changes. We can foresee our results as a way for clinicians to obtain more accurate hemodynamic measurements from the penis, and also show the likelihood for NIRS enhanced diagnosis tool of male erectile dysfunction over the current standards.

Keywords: NIRS, Hemodynamic, Erectile dysfunction, Penile erection

Background

Male erectile dysfunction (ED) is a disease that affects a large group of men and can have a severe negative effect on the subject's life. ED has been found to affect 5-20% of the world's male population [1]. ED is defined as the inability to achieve and maintain a penile erection sufficient enough to achieve satisfactory sexual performance and can have tremendous psychological health effects for the patient [2]. The inability to maintain a penile erection is biologically marked by the lack of blood flow to the penis. A normal penile erection is a result of many different dynamic, neural, and vascular interactions [3], therefore accurate measurements of penile hemodynamics is crucial in the diagnosis of erectile dysfunction.

There are many ways to assess the vascular functionality during penile erection including: selective pudendal angiography [4,5], duplex ultrasonography [6-9], and cavernosometry [9-11]. The issues with these assessments are the expense of the equipment, system complexity, and the fact that these tests require complete relaxation of the cavernous muscle. A common procedure to achieve muscle relaxation is the injection of an

* Correspondence: jaekim@gist.ac.kr
†Equal contributors
[1]School of Information and Communications, Gwangju Institute of Science and Technology, Gwangju 500-712, Korea
[2]Department of Medical System Engineering, Gwangju Institute of Science and Technology, Gwangju 500-712, Korea

intracavernosal vasoactive agent [12,13]. This invasive procedure can be seen as a less than ideal approach of measuring ED due to the inconvenience for the subject. When conducting studies regarding erectile dysfunction and the genital organ in general, it is critical that the subject feels comfortable with the experiment's paradigm. Any uncertainness about the paradigm may temporarily induce psychological erectile dysfunction, and may affect the final result [14].

Near Infrared Spectroscopy (NIRS) has shown to be a suitable sensor to detect the hemodynamic changes in the body under certain conditions. NIRS has been applied to detect hemodynamic changes in subjects with diseases ranging from epilepsy, Alzheimer's, and including erectile dysfunction [15-19]. The compactness and convenience of NIRS systems make it an ideal sensor for observations of the genital organ hemodynamics during sexual stimulation. In the case of erectile dysfunction, the studies have largely been focused on the change in total blood volume and tissue oxygenation in the male genital organ [20,21]. However, to the best of our knowledge, there hasn't been a thorough study showing the specific oxy- (HbO) and deoxy- (RHb) hemoglobin concentration changes and the effect of sensor location on the penile hemodynamics.

The aim of our study is to show that NIRS is a convenient, portable, and most importantly, a sensitive enough system to detect HbO and RHb changes during an erection of the genital organ. We also demonstrate that penile hemodynamics varies depending on the probe location on the genital organ. The dependency of penile hemodynamics according to NIRS probe location can be used to improve the diagnosis, treatment and overall understanding of male erectile dysfunction.

Methods

NIRS system

Our in house-built continuous wave NIRS probe consisted of one light emitting diodes (LED) (Epitex Inc. L735/850-40D32) and one monolithic photodiodes (Texas Instruments Inc. OPT101). The light emitting diode and photodiode was fixed onto the probe with a separation of 1 cm by means of a polydimethylsiloxane (PDMS) probe holder. The LED sequenced between the two wavelengths of 735 and 850 nm in order to obtain relative concentration changes of HbO and RHb. The sampling rate of the system was 2 Hz.

Calculation of oxy-, deoxy-, and total hemoglobin concentration change

The detailed description of calculation of HbO, RHb, and HbT can be found in our previous report [22]. In the NIR range, we can assume that tissue background absorption is negligible and that HbO and RHb are the main chromophores in human tissue. Therefore, the change in optical density (ΔOD) at two wavelengths (735 and 850 nm) can be associated with the changes of HbO (ΔHbO) and RHb (ΔRHb) by

$$\begin{bmatrix} \Delta OD^{735} \\ \Delta OD^{850} \end{bmatrix} = \begin{bmatrix} \varepsilon_{RHb}^{735} & \varepsilon_{HbO}^{735} \\ \varepsilon_{RHb}^{850} & \varepsilon_{HbO}^{850} \end{bmatrix} \begin{bmatrix} \Delta RHb \\ \Delta HbO \end{bmatrix} L \qquad (1)$$

where $\Delta OD = OD_{Transient} - OD_{Baseline}$, ε_{HbO}^{750}, ε_{HbO}^{735}, ε_{RHb}^{850}, ε_{HbO}^{850} are extinction coefficients of RHb and HbO at wavelengths of 735 and 850 nm, L is an optical path length between the light source and detector.

In a scattering medium, L is not exactly equal to the source-detector separation, d, but rather approximated as $L = dDPF$ (*DPF*: differential path length factor) [22]. If the scattering property of tissue is constant during the measurements, ΔHbO, ΔRHb, and ΔHbT can be obtained by

$$\begin{bmatrix} \Delta RHb \\ \Delta HbO \end{bmatrix} = \frac{1}{d \cdot DPF} \begin{bmatrix} \varepsilon_{RHb}^{735} & \varepsilon_{HbO}^{735} \\ \varepsilon_{RHb}^{850} & \varepsilon_{HbO}^{850} \end{bmatrix}^{-1} \begin{bmatrix} \Delta OD^{735} \\ \Delta OD^{850} \end{bmatrix} \qquad (2)$$

$$\Delta HbT = \Delta RHb + \Delta HbO \qquad (3)$$

The raw data have been passed through Butterworth lowpass filter with cutoff frequency at 0.3 Hz, to eliminate physiological artifacts such as: heartbeat, respiration etc.

Experimental setup

Our study consisted of three different placements of the probes, for three different experiments: a single probe placed on the side of the genital organ, a single probe placed on the top of the genital organ, and two identical probes placed on the top and side of the genital organ (Figure 1). The subject was the sole determinant of the exact location to place a probe on the genital organ, however received training beforehand of proper placement of the probe. The probe was affixed to the genital organ using commercial medical tape. A stable signal was confirmed by the subject and also by experiment administrator before the experiment began. The ability of the subject to attach the system himself demonstrated the overall convenience of the NIRS probe.

Experiment paradigm

This study has been reviewed and approved by the Gwangju Institute of Science and Technology's institutional review board (IRB 20140319-HR-10-02-02). The first two experiments were run for 6 healthy male subjects, age ranging from 28 ± 3 years old, with no previous history of ED. The informed written consent was obtained from each subject before the experiments. Each subject was placed in a dark experiment room with a chair and monitor. Before the experiment began, the administrator instructed the subject how to attach the probe. After that, the experiment was administered

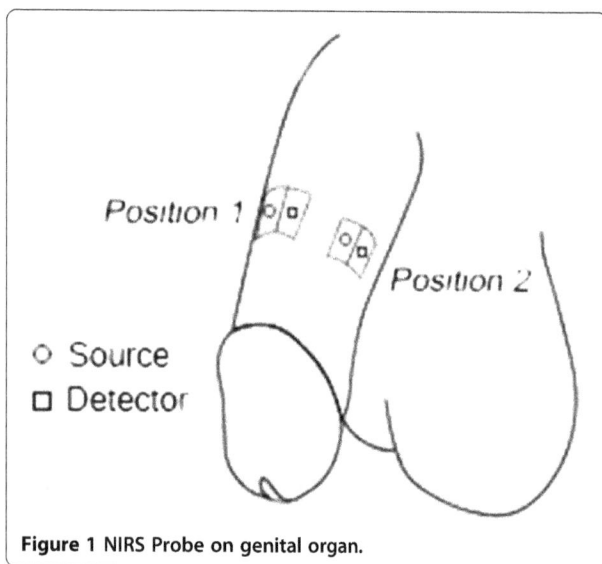

Figure 1 NIRS Probe on genital organ.

remotely by an experiment administrator in another room. A single probe was attached on the subject's left-middle of the genital organ for the first experiment and a single probe was attached on the top and middle of the genital organ for the second experiment. (Figure 1) The first and second experiment involved the same subjects, but occurred on different days. As mentioned previously, the subject attached the probe and a stable signal was confirmed remotely by the administrator. The subject sat down and was shown two types of videos: a still image of a cross for one minute (baseline), and adult video (sexual stimulation) for two minutes, for a total of 4 minutes. (Table 1) The preference for adult video was obtained via questionnaire prior to the start of the experiment.

Because of the intriguing results that was collected from the first two experiments, a third experiment was design to simultaneously measure hemodynamic changes from the top and left middle of the genital organ three times, using just one subject, utilizing the same sequencing of videos. Two exact probes were designed with the same specifications, and affixed by the subject with commercial medical tape. This experiment was designed to eliminate the variability of individualistic factors such as interest in stimulation video and the individual condition of each subject.

Results and discussion

The results section can be divided into two distinct sections. Our first set of results was acquired from six

Table 1 Sequence of videos

Type of video	Baseline	Sexual video	Baseline
Duration	1 minute	2 minutes	1 minute

healthy male subjects with a probe placed on the left side (from the viewpoint of the subject) of the genital organ for one trial and a probe placed on top of the genital organ for another trial. The trials were independent of each other with appropriate rest in between and different visual sexual stimulations as to create the same sensation in the subject. The collection and post processing of the data occurred in entirely by using Matlab software.

Figure 2 shows the averaged HbO, RHb, and HbT concentration changes acquired from six subjects from the first two experiments. When the NIRS probe placed on the side of the genital organ, we can see from Figure 2a that HbO, RHb, and HbT concentration rises during the sexual stimulation period. Then, when the probe is placed on the top of the genital organ, Figure 2b indicates that the RHb decreases while HbO and HbT increases. Compared to Figure 2b, Figure 2a shows a much higher relative concentration changes for total hemoglobin.

Figure 3 demonstrates the discrepancy of concentration changes of HbO, RHb, and HbT during penile erection between the top and the side of the genital organ simultaneously obtained from one subject. The resting stage after stimulation had been extended to one more additional minute due to subject's slow return back to a flaccid state. This proves the usefulness of NIRS as a real-time penile hemodynamic monitoring device. The figure shows the same pattern that has been observed from the two first experiments; an increase of HbO, RHb and HbT on the side of genital organ while the probe placed on the top showed not as substantial increase in HbO, a larger decrease in RHb concentration, and therefore a decrease in HbT.

In addition, the third experiment results show not only the different behavior of RHb but also the difference of response time between HbO and RHb occuring after the visual sexual stimulation. The probe placed on the side of genital organ showed that HbO change occurs before the change of RHb while the reversed response time between HbO and RHb was observed from the probe located on the top of the genital organ. (Figure 3c and d) This result implies the importance of multi-location measurement of penile hemodynamics in erectile dysfunction since it can provide distinct physiological process of penile hemodynamic from the genital organ during erection.

The changes of HbO, RHb and HbT concentration during the visual sexual stimulation are averaged from all three experiments and are compared between the top and the side of the genital organ. (Figure 4) HbO from the side probe showed greater increase than that from the top probe, and RHb from the side probe increased while it decreased from the top probe during the visual

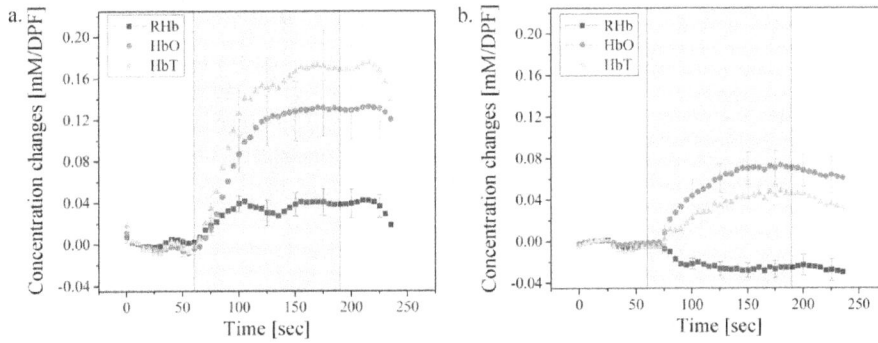

Figure 2 The average hemodynamic changes from all subjects during. (a) first experiment, a NIRS probe on the side; **(b)** second experiment, a NIRS probe on the top (error bars represents the standard errors from six subjects data).

sexual stimulation. While the probe located on the side shows greater increase of HbT, the probe on the top showed much smaller increase or decrease of HbT depending on the amplitude between HbO and RHb. A Wilcoxon rank-sum test was performed between signals from the top and side, and it showed that RHb and HbT concentration changes during erection are significantly different between the side and the top of the genital organ ($p < 0.05$) while HbO concentration change did not show the statistical difference ($p = 0.07$).

Thereby, the results from the three experiments demonstrate that the distinction of physiological process occurs at different location during penile erection. The penile hemodynamics from the side of genital organ is similar to the hemodynamics from venous occlusion of the arm, which shows an increase of both HbO and

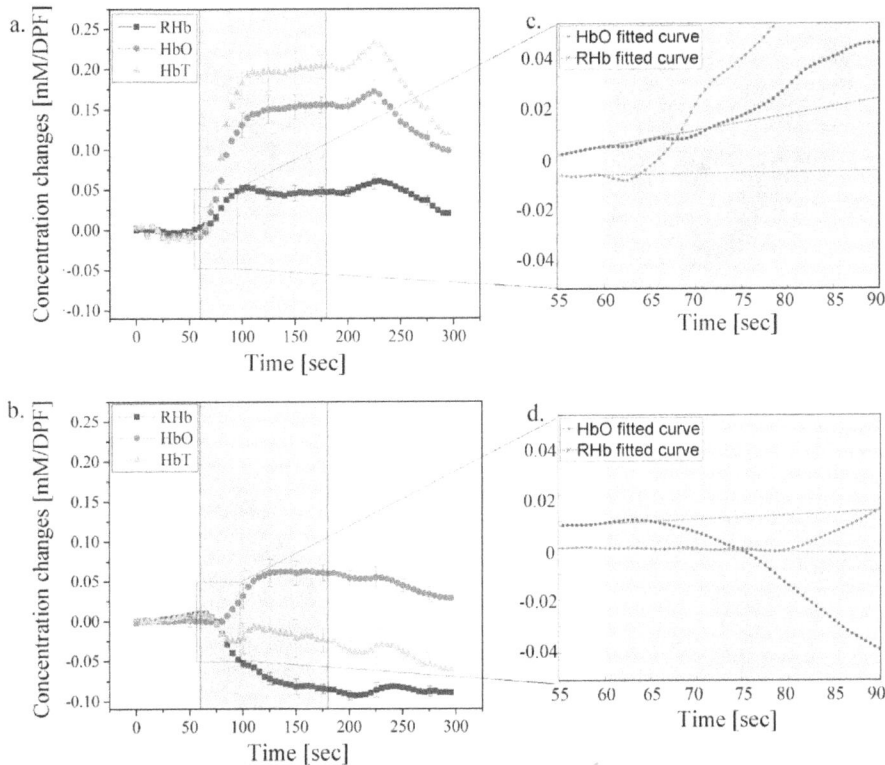

Figure 3 The simultaneous measurement of hemoglobin concentration changes from one subject (averaged from three trials).
(a) a probe on the side; **(b)** a probe on the top; **(c)** and **(d)** are enlarged part of the signal obtained from side and top during the first 30 sec of stimulation, respectively (error bars represents the standard errors from three trials).

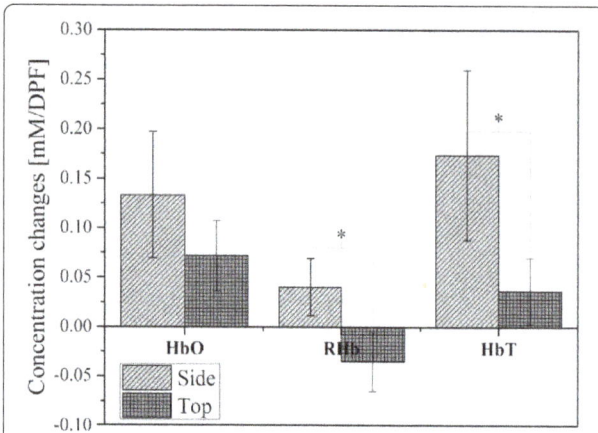

Figure 4 The level of concentration changes at the end of stimulus from the all experiments (error bars represents the standard errors from all three experiments) (* represents p < 0.05).

rapid increase of blood volume fills the corporal tissue. The increased blood volume in erectile chambers compresses the thin-walled penile venules which prevents the venous drainage of blood to maintain the erection. (Figure 5) Therefore, we see the increase of HbO due to the flow of arterial blood into corporal tissue while the compression to penile venules induces smaller increase of RHb.

Unlike the hemodynamics observed at the side of genital organ, the penile hemodynamics from the top of genital organ showed a decrease of RHb while HbO increased during visual sexual stimulation. The probe on the top of genital organ collects less signals from corporal cavernosa which is shown as a smaller increase of HbO than that from the side of genital organ. The decrease of RHb tells us that the expansion of corporal tissue caused less compression of dorsal vein due to its bigger diameter than the penile venules located on the side of genital organ so that there is less accumulation of venous blood but still with an increase of arterial blood on the top region of genital organ. All the results proved that NIRS is sensitive to monitor the penile hemodynamics during erection and multi-location measurements may tell us the details of erectile dysfunction and weaker erections.

RHb. This can be explained by understanding the process of erection as follows. Visual sexual stimulation causes a sexual arousal in brain which in turn releases the nitric oxide from nerve endings near blood vessels within the corpora cavernosa and spongiosum. This induces the dilation of penile arteries, and the resulting

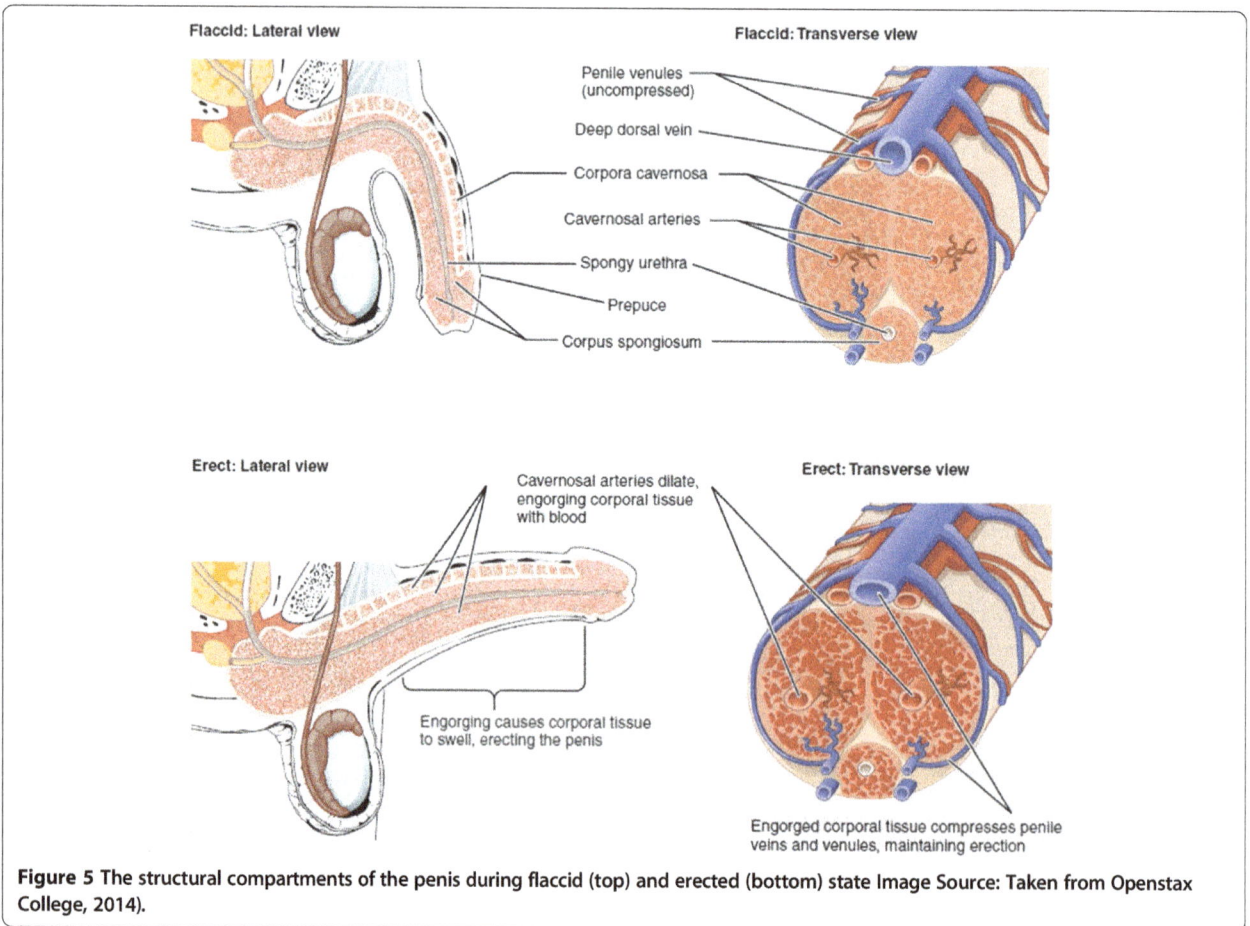

Figure 5 The structural compartments of the penis during flaccid (top) and erected (bottom) state Image Source: Taken from Openstax College, 2014).

Conclusions

This preliminary study has shown strong indication that NIRS can be a very important device for the understanding of erectile dysfunction due to its ability to detect different hemodynamic changes in various locations of a healthy male genital organ during visual sexual stimulation. Our data set shows that different locations of the genital organ may show a substantial increase in HbO, RHb and HbT, or a rise of HbO and HbT, but a decrease in RHb during visual sexual stimulation. Especially in the case of the studies of the genital organ and erectile dysfunction, it is vastly important that the measurement system should be comfortable for the subject, while at the same time, provide sufficient and high quality data for researchers and clinicians alike. We hope that the unique insight gained by applying NIRS can be useful in the diagnosis of male erectile dysfunction and weak erection.

For our future studies, we hope to expand upon our findings in this paper to understand what other physiological changes the body undergoes during sexual stimulation. Since a healthy penile erection is a result of many complex psychological and physiological reactions, and the impairments in any of these reactions may cause ED, it is important to develop a system to observe these reactions. NIRS presents a realistic solution to conveniently observe the psychological and physiological changes that the body undergoes during sexual stimulation by using a single system. In turn, we would like to apply our system to the cases of erectile dysfunction patient to see if NIRS can observe different hemodynamic changes in ED cases than from the healthy subjects we have shown in this study. As it can be seen, NIRS gives a promising outlook for a biosensor that can greatly enhance the diagnosis and treatment of erectile dysfunction and weak erection.

Abbreviations
ED: Erectile dysfunction; HbO: Oxy hemoglobin; HbT: Total hemoglobin; LED: Light emitting diodes; NIRS: Near infrared spectroscopy; PDMS: Polydimethylsiloxane; RHb: Deoxy hemoglobin.

Competing interests
The authors declare that they have no competing interests.

Authors' contributions
EK and SL were primarily responsible for experiment design, sensor design, data processing, and overall understanding of how to apply NIRS for the purpose of erectile dysfunction. This specific research was conducted with the assistance of ZPV and guidance of the corresponding author JGK. JGK has participated in many projects involving application of various biomedical optical imaging techniques toward diagnosis, rehabilitation, and critical care. All authors participated in the discussion about the proposal and contributed to the analysis of the results. All authors read and approved the final manuscript.

Acknowledgments
This work was partially supported by the National Research Foundation of Korea (NRF) Grants (NRF-2012K1A2B1A03000757, NRF-2013R1A1A2013625), Institute of Medical System Engineering (iMSE) in the GIST(Gwangju Institute of Science and Technology), and GIST and DGIST(Daegu Gyeongbuk Institute of Science and Technology), Korea, under the Practical Research and Development support program supervised by the GIST-DGIST.

References
1. Feldman HA, Goldstein I, Hatzichristou DG, Krane RJ, McKinlay JB. Impotence and its medical and psychosocial correlates: results of the Massachusetts Male Aging Study. J Urol. 1994;151:54–61.
2. Lue TF. Erectile dysfunction. N Engl J Med. 2000;342:1802.
3. Kaminetsky J. Epidemiology and pathophysiology of male sexual dysfunction. Int J Impot Res. 2008;20:S3–S10.
4. Rosen MP, Greenfield AJ, Walker TG, Grant P, Guben JK, Dubrow J, et al. Arteriogenic impotence: findings in 195 impotent men examined with selective internal pudendal angiography. Young Investigator's Award. Radiology. 1990;174:1043–8.
5. Polascik TJ, Walsh PC. Radical retropubic prostatectomy: the influence of accessory pudendal arteries on the recovery of sexual function. J Urol. 1995;154:150–2.
6. Kim SC, Moon YT, Oh CH. Non-visualization versus normal appearance of cavernous arteries on selective internal pudendal pharmaco-angiograms: comparison with Duplex scanning, cavernosal artery systolic occlusion pressure and penile brachial index. Br J Urol. 1994;73:185–9.
7. Meuleman E, Bemelmans B, Van Asten W, Doesburg W, Skotnicki S, Debruyne F. Assessment of penile blood flow by duplex ultrasonography in 44 men with normal erectile potency in different phases of erection. J Urol. 1992;147:51–6.
8. Shabsigh R, Fishman I, Shotland Y, Karacan I, Dunn J. Comparison of penile duplex ultrasonography with nocturnal penile tumescence monitoring for the evaluation of erectile impotence. J Urol. 1990;143:924–7.
9. Sattar AA, Wery D, Golzarian J, Raviv G, Schulman CC, Wespes E. Correlation of nocturnal penile tumescence monitoring, duplex ultrasonography and infusion cavernosometry for the diagnosis of erectile dysfunction. J Urol. 1996;155:1274–6.
10. Jasdzewski G, Strangman G, Wagner J, Kwong K, Poldrack R, Boas D. Differences in the hemodynamic response to event-related motor and visual paradigms as measured by near-infrared spectroscopy. Neuroimage. 2003;20:479–88.
11. Jordan G, Angermeier K. Preoperative evaluation of erectile function with dynamic infusion cavernosometry/cavernosography in patients undergoing surgery for Peyronie's disease: correlation with postoperative results. J Urol. 1993;150:1138–42.
12. Glina S, Virag R, Luis Rhoden E, Sharlip ID. Intracavernous Injection of Papaverine for Erectile Failure R. Virag. J Sex Med. 2010;7:1331–5.
13. Virag R, Frydman D, Legman M, Virag H. Intracavernous injection of papaverine as a diagnostic and therapeutic method in erectile failure. Angiology. 1984;35:79–87.
14. Swindle RW, Cameron AE, Lockhart DC, Rosen RC. The psychological and interpersonal relationship scales: assessing psychological and relationship outcomes associated with erectile dysfunction and its treatment. Arch Sex Behav. 2004;33:19–30.
15. Gallagher A, Lassonde M, Bastien D, Vannasing P, Lesage F, Grova C, et al. Non-invasive pre-surgical investigation of a 10 year-old epileptic boy using simultaneous EEG-NIRS. Seizure. 2008;17:576–82.
16. Hock C, Villringer K, Muller-Spahn F, Wenzel R, Heekeren H, Schuh-Hofer S, et al. Decrease in parietal cerebral hemoglobin oxygenation during performance of a verbal fluency task in patients with Alzheimer's disease monitored by means of near-infrared spectroscopy (NIRS)–correlation with simultaneous rCBF-PET measurements. Brain Res. 1997;755:293–303.
17. Stothers L, Shadgan B, Macnab A. Urological applications of near infrared spectroscopy. Can J Urol. 2008;15:4399–409.

18. Irani F, Platek SM, Bunce S, Ruocco AC, Chute D. Functional Near Infrared Spectroscopy (fNIRS): An Emerging Neuroimaging Technology with Important Applications for the Study of Brain Disorders. Clin Neuropsychol. 2007;21:9–37.

19. Farag FF, Martens FM, D'Hauwers KW, Feitz WF, Heesakkers JP. Near-infrared spectroscopy: a novel, noninvasive, diagnostic method for detrusor over-activity in patients with overactive bladder symptoms—a preliminary and experimental study. Eur Urol. 2011;59:757–62.

20. Burnett AL, Allen RP, Davis, Wright DC, Trueheart IN, Chance B. Near infrared spectrophotometry for the diagnosis of vasculogenic erectile dysfunction. Int J Impot Res. 2000;12:247–54.

21. Colier WN, Froeling FM, de Vries JD, Oeseburg B. Measurement of the blood supply to the abdominal testis by means of near infrared spectroscopy. Eur Urol. 1995;27:160–6.

22. Kim JG, Liu H. Variation of haemoglobin extinction coefficients can cause errors in the determination of haemoglobin concentration measured by near-infrared spectroscopy. Phys Med Biol. 2007;52:6295–322.

6

Scrotal extratesticular schwannoma

Giovanni Palleschi[1,2], Antonio Carbone[1,2], Jessica Cacciotti[3], Giorgia Manfredonia[4], Natale Porta[3], Andrea Fuschi[1], Cosimo de Nunzio[5], Vincenzo Petrozza[3] and Antonio Luigi Pastore[1,2]*

Abstract

Background: Schwannomas are tumours arising from Schwann cells, which sheath the peripheral nerves. Here, we report a rare case of left intrascrotal, extratesticular schwannoma. Although rare, scrotal localisation of schwannomas has been reported in male children, adult men, and elderly men. They are usually asymptomatic and are characterised by slow growth. Patients generally present with an intrascrotal mass that is not associated with pain or other clinical signs, and such cases are self-reported by most patients. Imaging modalities (such as ultrasonography, computed tomography, and magnetic resonance imaging) can be used to determine tumour size, exact localisation, and extension. However, the imaging findings of schwannoma are non-specific. Therefore, only complete surgical excision can result in diagnosis, based on histological and immunohistochemical analyses. If the tumour is not entirely removed, recurrences may develop, and, although malignant change is rare, this may occur, especially in patients with a long history of an untreated lesion. Thus, follow up examinations with clinical and imaging studies are recommended for scrotal schwannomas.

Case presentation: A 52-year-old man presented with a 3-year history of asymptomatic scrotal swelling. Physical examination revealed a palpable, painless, soft mass in the left hemiscrotum. After surgical removal of the mass, its histological features indicated schwannoma.

Conclusions: Schwannoma should be considered in cases of masses that are intrascrotal but extratesticular. Ultrasonography provides the best method of confirming the paratesticular localisation of the tumour, before surgical removal allows histopathological investigation and definitive diagnosis. Surgery is the standard therapeutic approach. To prevent recurrence, particular care should be taken to ensure complete excision. This case report includes a review of the literature on scrotal schwannomas.

Keywords: Scrotal schwannoma, Diagnosis, Histopathology

Background

Schwannomas are tumours arising from Schwann cells, which sheath the peripheral nerves. Schwannomas can develop in any region of the human body, either sporadically or in association with neurofibromatosis [1]. Most clinical findings associated with schwannoma are not specific to the disease, because schwannomas grow slowly and do not result in symptoms until they enlarge and compress the surrounding structures [2]. The exact incidence of schwannoma is not known [3]. Scrotal localisation of schwannoma is rare, but has been the occasional subject of reports in the literature [4,5]. We recently treated a case of intrascrotal, extratesticular schwannoma, which was found in an adult man who had a 3-year history of an asymptomatic lesion in the left hemiscrotum. Here, we describe the case with a complete report, including intraoperative findings. We also provide a review of the literature, which was performed to collect and summarise the present state of knowledge on this type of tumour.

* Correspondence: antopast@hotmail.com
[1]Sapienza University of Rome, Department of Medical and Surgical Biotechnologies, Unit of Urology, ICOT, Via Franco Faggiana 1668, 04100 Latina, Italy
[2]Uroresearch Association, non profit association, Via Franco Faggiana 1668, 04100 Latina, Italy
Full list of author information is available at the end of the article

Case presentation

Clinical history

A 52-year-old man presented with a 3-year history of asymptomatic scrotal swelling. He had a body mass index of 28 kg/m2 at the time of presentation. The patient reported that his scrotum had significantly enlarged during the last 6 months. Physical examination revealed a palpable, painless, soft mass in the left hemiscrotum, approximately the size of an egg. Further, an adhesion had formed between the mass and the left testicle. The lesion appeared not to be attached to the skin of the scrotum or the underlying tissues. The abdominal examination findings were unremarkable, and rectal exploration showed enlargement of the prostate gland without any palpatory pathological findings. The patient did not report any systemic symptoms. Accordingly, the initial diagnostic hypothesis was suspicion of a left testicular tumour. Written informed consent was obtained from the patient for publication of this case report and any accompanying images.

Imaging

The patient underwent scrotal ultrasonography (US), which revealed a hypoechoic solid mass. The mass was 4 × 7 cm in size and had a nodular appearance. It was found in the mid-left hemiscrotum, behind the left testicle, which appeared reduced in size (Figure 1). Left varicocele was observed, whereas hydrocele was absent bilaterally. Colour Doppler evaluation showed poor perilesional and intralesional hypervascularisation. Quantitative elastography revealed that the lesion had a low elastic modulus relative to the left testicular parenchyma

and low intralesional vascularity (Figure 2). The patient's right testicle was normal. To better examine the patient, contrast-enhanced computed tomography (CT) of the abdomen, scrotum, and chest was performed. The scan identified a 7.1 × 3.9 cm mass, which was localised medially in the left testicle, without extension into the tunica vaginalis. Lymphadenopathy was not present.

Laboratory findings

Blood tests showed normal levels of alpha-fetoprotein, beta-human chorionic gonadotropin, and carcinoembryonic antigen. Prostate specific antigen levels were also normal.

Therapeutic approach

Based on this evidence, we decided to surgically remove the mass, and the patient agreed. A left inguinal 4-cm incision was made, the spermatic cord was clamped, and the testicle was tractioned from the left inguinal ring. The mass presented with some adhesions to the left testicle, but did not infiltrate the testicle (Figure 3). Surgical removal appeared to be simple and was performed using monopolar scissors in a few minutes. The spermatic cord was then released, and the left testicle was pushed back into the scrotum. The patient was discharged 48 hours after surgery, without complications. After 12 months of follow-up, physical examination and scrotal ultrasound were negative.

Macroscopic findings

The surgical specimen was immediately measured and found to be 7.1 × 3.8 cm. It comprised a white mass,

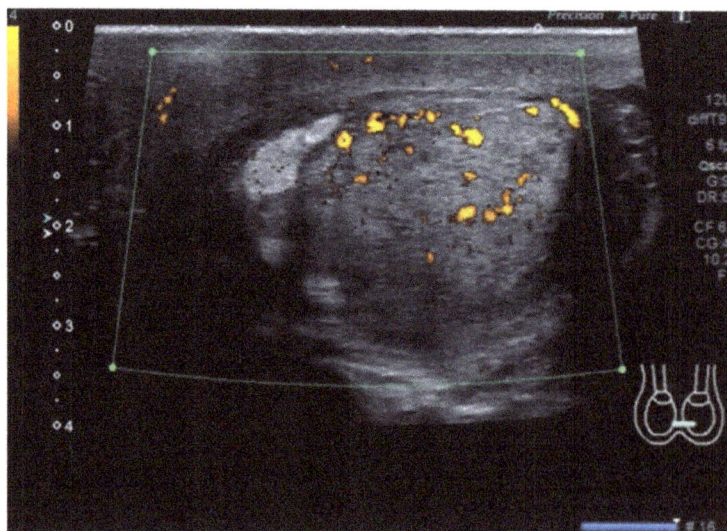

Figure 1 Ultrasonography and colour Doppler examination of the schwannoma. The lesion appeared inhomogeneous, was partially hypoechogenic, and had poor hypervascularisation.

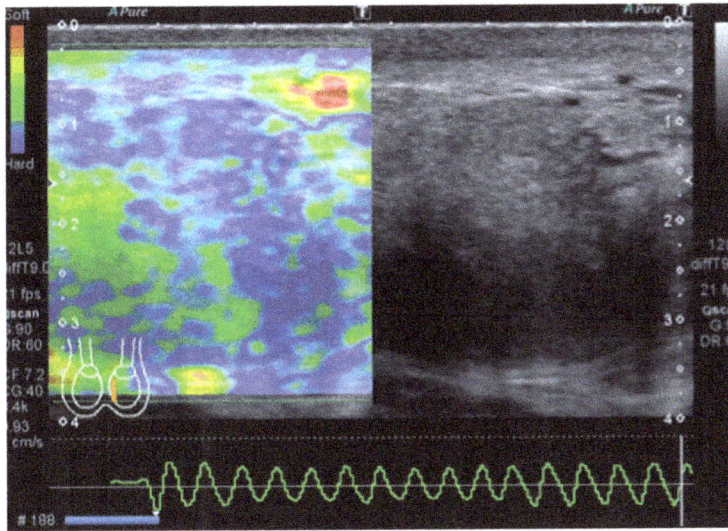

Figure 2 Elastographic investigation of the lesion. Quantitative elastography showed that the lesion had a low elastic modulus, as represented by the green area. After compression induced by the operator, there was no modification in the elastographic waves.

which was soft and had a regular and translucent external surface (Figure 4A). The specimen was sectioned at the midline along the longest diameter. The inner tissue presented a multinodular appearance with haemorrhagic areas (Figure 4B).

Microscopic findings

Considerable cellular proliferation was observed, comprising spindle elements with elongated hyperchromatic nuclei and poorly eosinophilic cytoplasm, separated by abundant oedematous fluid. A myxoid appearance was noted focally (the so-called 'Antoni B pattern'). These elements were occasionally arranged concentrically around vessels with thin walls. Areas of necrosis and mitoses were not observed (Figure 5A). Immunohistochemically, the tumour cells showed intense immunoreactivity for S-100 protein and vimentin. Further, tumour cells were negative for smooth-muscle actin, desmin, and CD-34, supporting

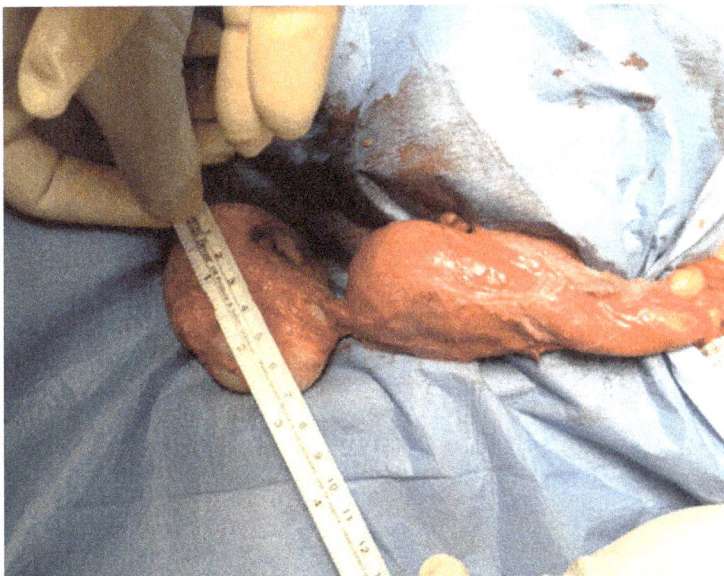

Figure 3 Intraoperative appearance of the lesion. The mass presented with some adhesions to the left testicle, but did not infiltrate the testicle.

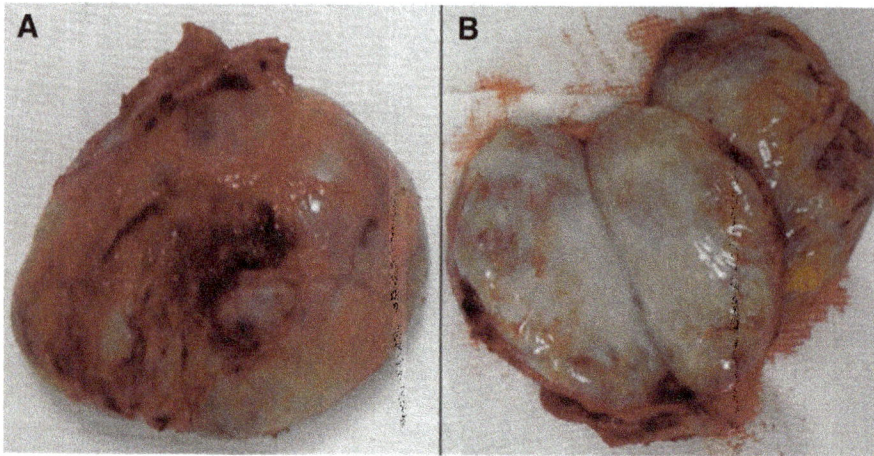

Figure 4 Macroscopic examination and sectioning of the lesion. (A) Macroscopic examination after surgical removal showed a white mass that was soft and had a regular, translucent external surface. **(B)** After sectioning, the specimen was multinodular in appearance, with haemorrhagic areas.

the neural differentiation of the tissue (Figure 5B and C). These histological features were suggestive of schwannoma.

Literature review and comparison with previous cases (Table 1)

Scrotal masses require a precise diagnosis to prevent therapeutic errors. Among various types of intrascrotal extratesticular lesions, schwannomas have been described previously and have always represented a diagnostic challenge for clinicians. During differential diagnosis of these tumours, clinicians must also consider benign and malignant neoplasms of supporting structures of the scrotum: leiomyoma, leiomyosarcoma, and adenosarcoma [3].

The clinical history of the disease was similar in each of the previous reports that we examined [3-6]. Each of the subjects presented with painless scrotal swelling, which had been present for between a few months [3] and 3 years, as in our case. The ages of patients varied considerably across the reports, although older ages (>60 years) were most common. Physical examination usually revealed a soft mass without adhesion to the scrotal skin or the surrounding tissues. Yet, examining the patient does not entirely clarify whether the lesion originated from the testicle or another location. In previously reported cases, therefore, US, magnetic resonance imaging (MRI), and CT have variously been used to arrive at more

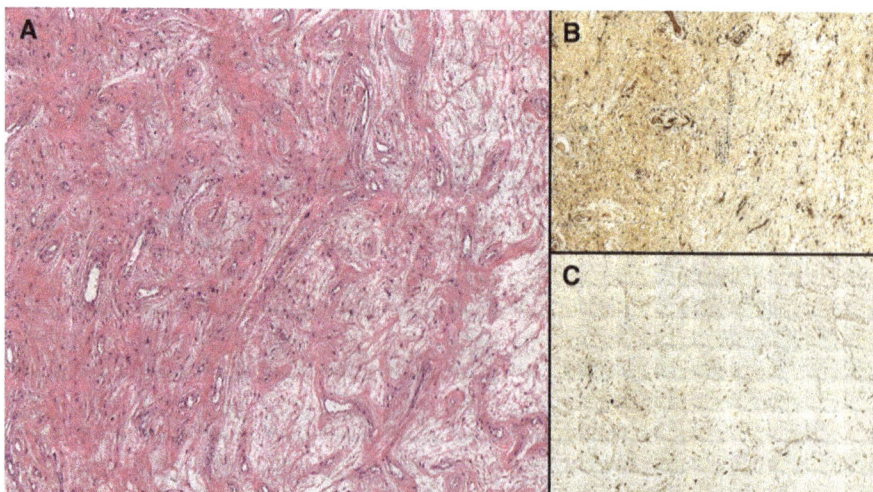

Figure 5 Microscopic findings. (A) Proliferation was characterised by spindle elements with elongated hyperchromatic nuclei and poorly eosinophilic cytoplasm, separated by abundant oedematous fluid. These elements were occasionally arranged concentrically around vessels with thin walls (magnification × 4). **(B)** The cells show intense immunoreactivity for vimentin (magnification × 20) and **(C)** S-100 protein (magnification × 20).

Table 1 Literature review with onset symptoms, management, and final diagnosis

Authors	Onset symptoms	Management	Diagnosis
Sighinolfi MC et al. [2]	Presence of a small and painless swelling with elastic consistency	Orchifunicolectomy	Intratesticular neurilemoma
Chan PT et al. [3]	Asymptomatic scrotal swelling	Surgical excision	Extratesticular schwannoma
Arciola AJ et al. [4]	Supratesticular intrascrotal mass clinically mimicking a spermatocele	Surgical excision	Intrascrotal schwannoma
Fernandez MJ et al. [5]	Intrascrotal giant painless mass	Surgical excision	Giant neurilemoma of the scrotum
Kim YJ et al. [6]	Episode of multiple slowly growing masses in the scrotum	Surgical excision	Schwannomas of the scrotum
Matsui F et al. [9]	Painless, solid and elastic-hard scrotal mass	Tumor resection	Giant scrotal schwannoma
Safak M et al. [10]	Painless, solid scrotal mass	Surgical excision	Intrascrotal extratesticular malignant schwannoma
Muzac A and Mendoza E [11]	Inguinal scrotal painless solid mass	Surgical excision	Malignant schwannoma

exact diagnoses [2,3,6]. However, none of these options have allowed schwannoma to be identified, because there is no pathognomonic finding for this disease [6]. On US, schwannoma generally appears as a well-circumscribed mass with a hypoechoic pattern [2], and on colour Doppler imaging, poor hypervascularisation is noted. In our case, we also performed quantitative elastography, which showed that the mass had a lower elastic modulus than the testicle, as the result of a higher tissue density, which is typical of tumours. However, despite some evidence that it contributes to a diagnostic algorithm for scrotal masses, the value of elastography is still under investigation and should only be used if combined with standard methods [7,8]. Nevertheless, because of the lack of specific findings that can identify schwannomas, many clinicians have used MRI and CT to confirm the extratesticular localisation of the lesion. For this purpose, MRI appears to be more capable of identifying the tumour and distinguishing it from testicle parenchyma [3], showing a peripheral rim-enhancement of the pathologic tissue in T2 weighted sequences [1]. In addition, laboratory examinations are not helpful for diagnosing scrotal schwannoma, and none of the previous reports found alterations to testicular tumour markers. Surgical excision remains the mainstay of treatment for scrotal schwannomas, as the authors of all previous reports have noted. In a previous case, the schwannoma was localised intratesticularly and required orchiectomy [2]. In another case, scrotectomy was required due to an extension of the tumour superficial to the tunica vaginalis, testis, and corpus spongiosum [3]. In all cases, definitive diagnosis was achieved only by histopathological examination, combined with positive immunostaining for S-100 protein and negative staining for CD-34 [2,3]. Immunohistochemical evidence is needed for the diagnosis of schwannoma. However, fine-needle aspiration biopsy cannot be considered helpful, even though it has been performed in some previously reported cases; information on the tissue's architecture is required for diagnosis, but cannot be obtained from the cytology specimen [3]. Macroscopically, the largest scrotal schwannoma reported in the literature was described by Matsui et al., who surgically removed a $13 \times 7.5 \times 3.0$ cm intrascrotal tumour, which weighed 285 g [9]. Cases of multiple scrotal schwannomas have also been reported. Kim et al. reported multiple schwannomas of the scrotum (with the largest lesion measuring 3.5 cm) in a 67-year-old man. In this case, some lesions had invaded the penile root without reducing erectile function or causing penile deviation. The author reported no recurrence for at least 6 months after surgery. For patients with the systemic disease of schwannomatosis, the development of a single or multiple scrotal masses should lead the clinician to suspect peripheral localisation of schwannoma. In another case, reported by Ikary et al., a scrotal schwannoma developed in a 66-year-old man who had previously undergone surgical excision of a brain tumour, which itself originated from the glossopharyngeal nerve [1]. The patient's histological diagnosis was schwannoma. Therefore, regular surveillance is needed for patients with schwannomatosis, because they are at a high risk of developing multiple schwannomas. However, follow-up is also required for patients who have undergone surgical removal of a scrotal schwannoma. Indeed, as has generally been reported for schwannomas located in other regions of the body, incomplete removal can be followed by local recurrence, even many years later. Safak et al. reported a case of late recurrence in the scrotum in 1998. The authors reported late local recurrence after treatment of an intrascrotal extratesticular malignant schwannoma with rhabdomyoblastic features in an adult man [10]. Muzac and Mendoza reported a case of malignant schwannoma in 1992 [11]. Malignant degeneration of schwannomas is extremely rare, and when present, such cases have a sarcomatoid-like behaviour. The diagnosis of malignant peripheral nerve sheath tumour lacks standardised criteria and is usually based on evaluations of mitosis, pleomorphism, and blood vessel infiltration. Therefore, it is very important to remove the tumour completely, which allows the most precise histopathological investigation. From a histopathological perspective, the microscopic appearance of schwannoma is distinctive, with 2 recognisable patterns, which are not always present together: Antoni A areas and Antoni B areas. Antoni A areas are composed of compacted spindle cells that are arranged in palisades or in an organoid arrangement (Verocay bodies). Antoni B areas consist of tumour cells suspended in a myxomatous matrix that may appear microcystic. Several histological variants have been described previously: cellular, glandular, epithelioid, and ancient, which involves bizarre hyperchromatic nuclei without mitosis [3]. However, each of these variants is benign, and the ancient type is rare, especially in the scrotum (most cases occur in the head and neck region).

Conclusion

Our experience with the reported case and our review of the literature strongly suggest that schwannoma should be considered in cases involving masses that are intrascrotal and extratesticular. US (followed by MRI) is the best modality with which to confirm the paratesticular localisation of the tumour, before surgical removal allows histopathological investigation and definitive diagnosis. Surgery is the standard therapeutic approach, which allows the testicle to be spared in most cases. To prevent recurrence, particular care should be taken to ensure complete excision, especially in cases that involve large or multiple masses. Eventhough it is hard to establish a specific follow-up plan considering the limited number of cases reported in literature, basing on all the experiences reported in literature, in case of benign lesions completely removed it might be suggested a clinical post-operative evaluation at 6 and 12 months. Differently, in case of histopathological suspicious or clear evidence of malignancy, a MRI after 6 months from surgery should be proposed.

Early diagnosis can help limit the extent of surgical excision that is required. Further, early diagnosis can prevent the onset of malignant degeneration, which is rare, but has been reported in the literature.

Consent

Patient has given his consent for the case report to be published. A copy of the written consent is available, at anytime, for review by the Editor of this journal.

Abbreviations
CT: Computed tomography; MRI: Magnetic resonance imaging; US: Ultrasound.

Competing interests
No financial support has been received for this study, and none of the authors have any conflicts of interest pertinent to the content of the manuscript.

Authors' contributions
AC and VP ideated the study. GP, NP, JC, GM, ALP acquired the data. GP and NP drafted the manuscript. AC, GP, ALP, VP critically revised the manuscript. All authors read and approved the final manuscript.

Acknowledgements
None source of funding supported the study.

Author details
[1]Sapienza University of Rome, Department of Medical and Surgical Biotechnologies, Unit of Urology, ICOT, Via Franco Faggiana 1668, 04100 Latina, Italy. [2]Uroresearch Association, non profit association, Via Franco Faggiana 1668, 04100 Latina, Italy. [3]Department of Medical and Surgical Biotechnologies, Histopathology Unit, ICOT Latina, via Faggiana 1668, Latina, Italy. [4]ICOT Hospital, CADI Centre, via Faggiana 1668, Latina, Italy. [5]Sapienza University of Rome, Department of Urology, Sant'Andrea Hospital, Rome, Italy.

References
1. Ikari R, Keisei Okamoto K, Tetsuya Yoshida T, Johnin K, Okabe H, Okada Y: A rare case of multiple Schwannomas presenting with scrotal mass: a probable case of Schwannomatosis. *Int J Urol* 2010, 17:734–736.
2. Sighinolfi MC, Mofferdin A, De Stefani S, Celia A, Micali S, Saredi G, Rossi G, Bianchi G: Benign intratesticular schwannoma: a rare finding. *Asian J Androl* 2006, 8(1):101–103.
3. Chan PT, Tripathi S, Low SE, Robinson LQ: Case report – ancient schwannoma of the scrotum. *BMC Urol* 2007, 7(I):1–4.
4. Arciola AJ, Golden S, Zapinsky J, Fracchia JA: Primary intrascrotal nontesticular schwannoma. *Urology* 1985, 26:304–306.
5. Fernandez MJ, Martino A, Khan H, Considine TJ, Burden J: Giant neurilemoma: unusual scrotal mass. *Urology* 1987, 30:74–76.
6. Kim YJ, Kim SD, Huh JS: Intrascrotal and extratesticular multiple schwannoma. *World J Mens Health* 2013, 31(2):179–181.
7. Cantisani V, Olive M, Di Segni M, Di Leo N, Grazdhani H, D'Ettorre G, Ceccarelli G, Fioravanti C, Ricci P: Contrast-enhanced ultrasonographic (CEUS) and elastosonographic features of a case of testicular Leydig tumor. *Ultraschall Med* 2012, 33(5):407–409.
8. Aigner F, De Zordo T, Pallwein-Prettner L, Junker D, Schäfer G, Pichler R, Leonhartsberger N, Pinggera G, Dogra VS, Frauscher F: Real-time sonoelastography for the evaluation of testicular lesions. *Radiology* 2012, 263(2):584–589.
9. Matsui F, Kobori Y, Takashima H, Amano T, Takemae K: A case of intrascrotal schwannoma. *Hinyokika Kiyo* 2002, 48(12):749–751.
10. Safak M, Baltaci S, Ozer G, Turkolmez K, Uluoglu O: Long-term outcome of a patient with intrascrotal extratesticular malignant schwannoma. *Urol Int* 1998, 60(3):202–204.
11. Muzac A, Mendoza E: Malignant schwannoma presenting as an inguinoscrotal mass. *Eur Urol* 1992, 21(4):340–342.

7

Penile metastasis of sigmoid colon carcinoma

Zhengbang Dong[1†], Chao Qin[2†], Qijie Zhang[2†], Lei Zhang[2], Haijing Yang[1], Jingdong Zhang[1] and Fei Wang[1*]

Abstract

Background: Metastasis to penis usually arises from genitourinary organs, but in rare cases, metastasis comes from the sigmoid colon. Furthermore, very few cases of penile metastasis of primary sigmoid colon carcinoma have been reported.

Case presentation: We described a case of a 53-year-old man with penile metastasis of sigmoid colon carcinoma along with a review of the literature. Physical examination revealed two subcutaneous nodules on the glans penis. Biopsy of the nodules showed that penile metastasis of sigmoid colon carcinoma.

Conclusion: Metastasis of sigmoid colon carcinoma to the penis is extremely rare, which presents an advanced form of sigmoid colon carcinoma, therefore survival is extremely shortened. Although treatment of penile metastasis is almost always palliative, it is important to recognize this unusual manifestation so that timely appropriate treatment can be initiated. Early recognition may enhance survival rate of these patients.

Keywords: Carcinoma, Penile metastasis, Sigmoid colon

Background

Colorectal cancer commonly metastasizes to regional lymph nodes, the liver, the lung, and the peritoneum, but rarely to the penis. The vast majority of secondary penile tumors originate from genitourinary organs, among which the prostate and the bladder are the most common sites of primary cancer. Less than 400 cases of penile metastases have been reported since 1870 when Eberth discovered the first case [1]. Penile metastasis from sigmoid colon carcinoma rarely occurs. Here is a case of secondary penile metastasis from sigmoid adenocarcinoma, followed by discussion of its possible metastatic mechanisms and clinical implications.

Case presentation

A 53-year-old Chinese man complaining of two painless lesions on the glans penis presented in December 2010. Five years ago, he had undergone a sigmoidectomy with a moderately well-differentiated adenocarcinoma. Postoperative histopathological examination revealed metastases in six regional lymph nodes (6 out of 13 nodes). After surgery he received adjuvant chemo-radiotherapy and regular follow-ups. In March 2008, serum car左髋臼cinoembryonic antigen level (CEA) markedly elevated (210.7 ng/ml). Computed tomographic (CT) [Figure 1] scan showed metastases to the lung and the pelvic cavity. Clinical examination revealed two painless nodules on his glans penis with angiotelectasis of its surface. The nodules were pink, hard, and immobile, with a diameter of approximately 2 cm [Figure 2].

Senile malignancy was suspected, and a biopsy of the glans penis was performed. The biopsy of the left nodule led to a diagnosis of adenocarcinoma [Figure 3]. The cells exhibited pleomorphic, hyperchromatic nuclei with prominent nucleoli. Slides of the primary tumor were similar to those of the penile lesion, which was supported by immunohistochemistry in the metastatic deposit. The immunohistochemistry of tumor cells showed remarkable positive for cytokeratin 20 [Figure 4] and negative for cytokeratin 7. The cells were also positive for caudal-related homeobox transcription factor 2(CDX2) [Figure 5] and villin, while negative for cytokeratin 5/6 and cytokeratin 14. Therefore, it was concluded that the patient had penile metastasis from sigmoid colon carcinoma. Without further specific treatment, the patient just under symptomatic care survived for 2 months after being diagnosed with penile metastasis.

* Correspondence: ffwangfei@163.com
†Equal contributors
[1]Department of Dermatology, Zhongda Hospital, Southeast University, Nanjing, Jiangsu 210009, China
Full list of author information is available at the end of the article

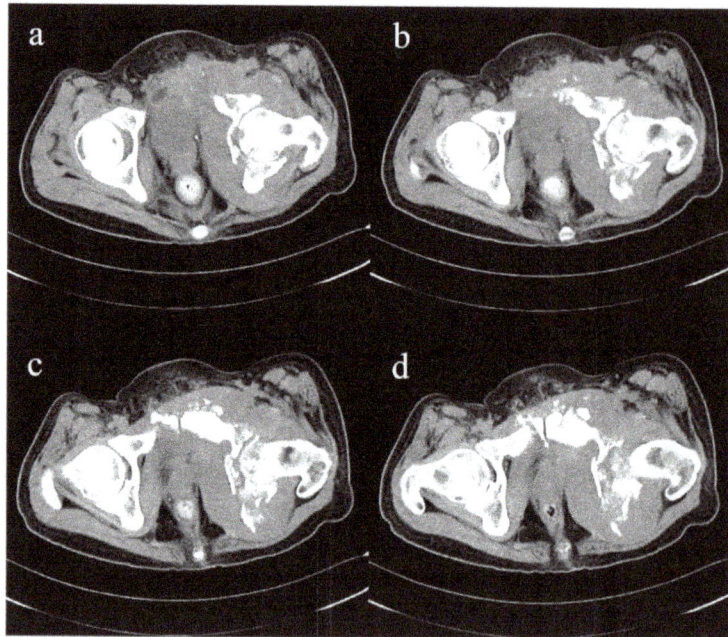

Figure 1 CT indicates that the sigmoid colon carcinoma metastasizes to the bone and soft tissues. **a**. The surrounding soft tissues of the left hip joint swell significantly and the spatium intermusculare disappears. **b**. The surrounding soft tissues of the left hip joint swell significantly and the spatium intermusculare disappears. **c**. Left acetabulum and pubic symphysis appear multiple bone destructions. **d**. Left acetabulum and pubic symphysis appear multiple bone destructions.

Discussion

In spite of sufficient blood supply and close proximity to pelvic malignancies, penile metastasis rarely occurs, and the spread route is still in controversy. Cherian *et al.* explained as follows: (1) retrograde venous route, (2) retrograde lymphatic route, (3) direct extension, (4) implantation and secondary to instrumentation, (5) arterial spread [2]. More than one spread routes may occur in a single case, and it is very difficult to elucidate their exact mode of spread.

Metastasis of gastric carcinoma to the skin may manifest as cutaneous nodules, cellulitis, carcinoma en cuirasse, infiltrated skin plaques, carcinoma erysipelatoides,

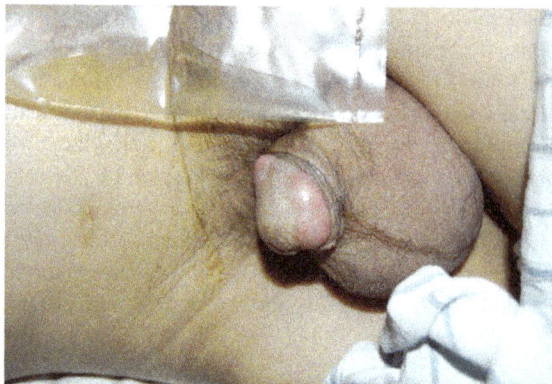

Figure 2 Subcutaneous nodules on the glans penis.

nodules, or large cauliflower-like papillomatous mass [3]. There is no characteristic symptom complex for secondary tumors of penis. The most common chief complaint was penile mass, followed by priapism. In up to 60% of the cases, the metastatic lesion presents as multiple infiltrative mass that is rigid, smooth, immobile, and painless. The penile shaft is the most affected anatomical site [1]. Priapism is a prominent feature in nearly 27% of patients. It could be caused either by tumor infiltration of cavernosal spaces, or by occlusion of draining veins due to infiltrating tumor cells. Irritation of neural pathways responsible for erection may be another mechanism [4]. Pain is not a prominent symptom in most of the patients. Other manifestations of penile metastasis include ulceration, obstructive or irritating voiding symptoms, hematuria, enlargement of inguinal lymph nodes, and penile or perineal pain [5,6].

The main differential diagnosis focuses on primary benign tumors, syphilitic chancre, venereal or other infectious ulcerations, idiopathic priapism, Peyronie's plaque, candidiasis, cavernositis, tuberculosis of penis, sclerosing lipogranuloma [7]. Compared with ultrasound or computed tomographic scans alone, MRI (magnetic resonance imaging) is a favorable imaging modality to delineate the degree of involvement in the penis [8]. MRI is being increasingly used to state the disease; but accurate diagnosis of metastasis to penis must rely on penile lesion biopsy. In particular, immunohistochemistry is helpful in determining

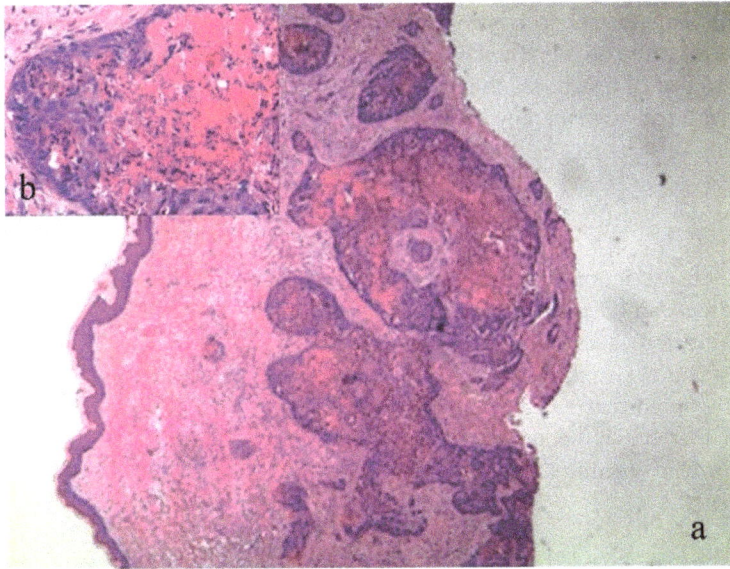

Figure 3 Biopsy from a nodule of glans penis showing metastatic adenocarcinoma. (H&E; **a** × 40, **b** × 400).

the primary site. Persistent painful penile nodule could raise suspicion of the existence of metastatic lesion. To achieve a diagnostic approach to these penile nodules, fine-needle aspiration (FNA) rather than complicated and invasive procedures can be performed, which can also be complemented by immunocytochemical phenotypical characterization to distinguish the primary site of origin [9].

About 90% of the reported penile metastases are part of widespread diseases. In the previously reported cases, the patients' average survival is 9 months approximately, with a maximum of 18 months. The longest survival reported is 9 years [6]. Longer survival occurs in patients without other apparent metastatic sites. Clinical evidence of penile metastasis in a patient with a known malignancy is an ominous sign that should alert the clinicians of the dismal prognosis. The patient studied in

this paper died of metastatic disease 2 months after penile metastases.

Given the poor prognosis, a stopgap measure to improve the patients' life is usually taken into consideration. Treatment options include surgical excision, radiotherapy, and chemotherapy. The choice depends mainly on patients' general clinical situation: type and extent of the primary tumor, presence of widespread metastatic disease, and type of symptoms [10]. Local surgical excision or radiotherapy is usually the most preferred. Penile ulcer has to be taken out by local excision. Radiotherapy is used to reduce the size of lesion as well as to control pain. Second-line chemotherapy with docetaxel, paclitaxel, vinorelbine, gemcitabine, irinotecan, and gefitinib has anindefinite curative effect [5]. Some patients only receive

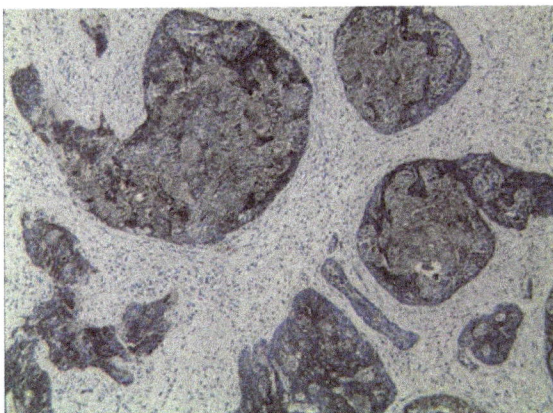

Figure 4 Immunohistochemically the malignant cells were positive for cytokeratin 20. (×100).

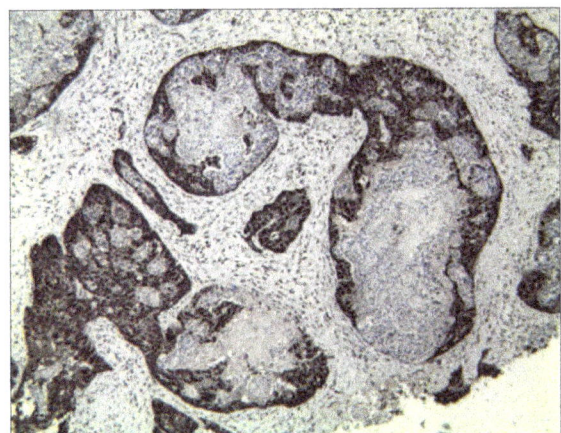

Figure 5 Immunohistochemically the malignant cells were positive for CDX2. (×100).

symptomatic treatment. A penile dorsal nerve block using local anesthesia may be of some benefit to control pain. Anxiety and pain can be dealt with parenteral opioids and anxiolytics. In the case with dismal prognosis, the patient has to be treated mainly with palliative therapy to relieve the intolerable symptoms.

Conclusion

Metastasis of sigmoid colon carcinoma to the penis is extremely rare, which presents an advanced form of sigmoid colon carcinoma, therefore survival is extremely shortened. Although treatment of penile metastasis is almost always palliative, it is important to recognize this unusual manifestation so that timely appropriate treatment can be initiated. Early recognition may enhance survival rate of these patients.

Consent statement

The patient has signed his written informed consent to participate in the study. The data do not contain any information that could identify the patient.

Competing interests
The authors declare that they have no competing interests.

Authors' contributions
ZBD, CQ and QJZ drafted the manuscript and revised it. HJY, LZ and JDZ participated in data collection. FW collected cases and do the check. All authors read and approved the final manuscript.

Acknowledgments
This work was supported by the National Natural Science Foundation of China [grant number 81201571], by the natural science foundation of Jiangsu Province (BK2012748), and Nanjing City Science And Technology Development Plan item (201104028).

Author details
[1]Department of Dermatology, Zhongda Hospital, Southeast University, Nanjing, Jiangsu 210009, China. [2]Department of Urology, First Affiliated Hospital of Nanjing Medical University, Nanjing, Jiangsu 210029, China.

References
1. Chaux A, Amin M, Cubilla AL, Young RH. Metastatic tumors to the penis: A report of 17 cases and review of the literature. Int J Surg Pathol. 2011;19:597–606.
2. Cherian J, Rajan S, Thwaini A, Elmasry Y, Shah T, Puri R. Secondary penile tumours revisited. Int Semin Surg Oncol. 2006;3:33.
3. Hussein MR. Skin metastasis: a pathologist's perspective. J Cutan Pathol. 2010;37:e1–20.
4. Chan PT, Bégin LR, Arnold D, Jacobson SA, Corcos J, Brock GB. Priapism secondary to penile metastasis: A report of two cases and a review of the literature. J Surg Oncol. 1998;68:51–9.
5. Karanikas C, Ptohis N, Mainta E, Baltas CS, Athanasiadis D, Lechareas S, et al. Pulmonary adenocarcinoma presenting with penile metastasis: A case report. J Med Case Rep. 2012;6:252.
6. Lin YH, Kim JJ, Stein NB, Khera M. Malignant priapism secondary to metastatic prostate cancer: A case report and review of literature. Rev Urol. 2011;13:90–4.
7. Zheng FF, Zhang ZY, Dai YP, Liang YY, Deng CH, Tao Y. Metastasis to the penis in a patient with adenocarcinoma of lung, case report and literature review. Med Oncol. 2009;26:228–32.
8. Andresen R, Wegner HE, Dieberg S. Penile metastasis of sigmoid carcinoma: Comparative analysis of different imaging modalities. Br J Urol. 1997;79:477–8.
9. Tsanou E, Sintou-Mantela E, Pappa L, Grammeniatis E, Malamou-Mitsi V. Fine-needle aspiration of secondary malignancies of the penis: A report of three cases. Diagn Cytopathol. 2003;29:229–32.
10. Pierro A, Cilla S, Digesù C, Morganti AG. Penile Metastases of Recurrent Prostatic Adenocarcinoma without PSA Level Increase: A case report. J Clin Imaging Sci. 2012;2:44.

8

Comparison of the complications of traditional 12 cores transrectal prostate biopsy with image fusion guided transperineal prostate biopsy

Haifeng Huang[1], Wei Wang[1], Tingsheng Lin[1], Qing Zhang[1], Xiaozhi Zhao[1], Huibo Lian[1] and Hongqian Guo[1,2*]

Abstract

Background: To compare the complications of traditional transrectal (TR) prostate biopsy and image fusion guided transperineal (TP) prostate biopsy in our center.

Methods: Two hundred and fourty-two patients who underwent prostate biopsy from August 2014 to January 2015were reviewed. Among them, 144 patients underwent systematic 12-core transrectal ultrasonography (TRUS) guided prostate biopsy (TR approach) while 98 patients underwent free-hand transperineal targeted biopsy with TRUS and multi-parameter magnetic resonance imaging (mpMRI) fusion images (TP approach). The complications of the two groups were presented and a simple statistical analysis was performed to compare the two groups.

Results: The cohort of our study include242 patients, including 144 patients underwent TR biopsies while 98 patients underwentTP biopsies. There was no significant difference of major complications, including sepsis, bleeding and other complication requiring admissionbetween the two groups ($P > 0.05$). The incidence rate of infection and rectal bleeding in TR was much higher than TP ($p < 0.05$), but the incidence rate of perineal swelling in TP was much higher than TR ($p < 0.05$). There were no significant differences of minor complications including hematuria, lower urinary tract symptoms (LUTS), dysuria, and acuteurinary retention between the two groups ($p > 0.05$).

Conclusion: The present study supports the safety of both techniques. Free-handTP targeted prostate biopsy with real-time fusion imaging of mpMRI and TR ultrasound is a good approach for prostate biopsy.

Keywords: Prostate biopsy, Prostate cancer, Fusion image, Magnetic resonance imaging, Complications

Background

Biopsies of the prostate have been used to diagnose prostate cancer since the beginning of the last century [1]. The field of prostate diagnostics, especially biopsy techniques develops rapidly [2]. Transrectal ultrasonography (TRUS) guided prostate biopsy, which isperformed with a core biopsy needle passing through the rectum, was first applied for the biopsy of prostate in 1968 [3]. Since the introduction of the systematic 12-core transrectal prostate biopsy guided by TRUS, it has become awidely accepted, routinely performed technique for prostate cancer detection [4]. The transperineal prostate biopsy, which is performed with the core biopsy needle passing through the skin of the perineum, is far less common compared with transrectal biopsy [5].

Several studies have demonstrated that the transrectal technique is a faster and convenient approach for prostate biopsy. Though the minor complications rate of hematuria, rectal bleeding, hematospermia, vasovagal episodes, infection was reported to be similar in these two techniques [6], transrectal prostate biopsy had more major complicationse.g. sepsis, bleeding or other complications requiring admission compared with the transperineal biopsy [7, 8]. More importantly, an increasing risk of septic shock was reported in the transrectal biopsy, which might be life-threatening [9, 10].

* Correspondence: dr.guohongqian@gmail.com
[1]Department of Urology, Affiliated Drum Tower Hospital, Medical School of Nanjing University, Nanjing 210008, China
[2]Institute of Urology, Nanjing University, Nanjing 210008, China

Recently, transperineal prostate biopsy has been becoming an increasingly popular approach for accurate diagnosis and risk stratification of prostate cancer [11]. MRI/US-fusion-guided biopsyis a potential approach to offer improved diagnostic information over systematic 12-core transrectal prostate biopsy guided by TURS alone [12, 13]. We have previously described free-hand transperineal targeted biopsy guided by TRUS and mpMRI fusion images [14]. The targeted biopsy is a precise, faster and more accessible technique for prostate biopsy compared to systematic biopsy. In the present study, we reported the complications of transperineal targeted biopsy guided by TRUS-mpMRI fusion images and traditional 12 cores systematic transrectal biopsy guided by TURS in our center.

Methods

The study protocol was approved by the local institutional review board at Nanjing University (NJU201500987), and informed written consent was received from patients, including acquiring essential medical images for publication. Research was carried out in compliance with the Helsinki Declaration.

Patients

Procedures

The present study was performed by reviewing a total of 262 patients who underwent prostate biopsy from August 2014 to January 2015. At the time of analysis, the database contained 262 patients of whom 20 were excluded because of <10 cores taken in systematic biopsies. Thus, 242 patients were available for analysis. These patients with PSA level greater than 4.0 ng/mL underwent mpMRI prospectively. All these patients were assessed with prostate mpMRI in the radiology department of our hospital, and 98 patients had at least one suspicious areas in mpMRI images who underwent free-hand transperineal targeted biopsy with TRUS and multi-parameter magnetic resonance imaging (mpMRI) fusion images (TP approach). The

other 144 patients underwent systematic 12-core Transrectal Ultrasonography (TRUS) guided prostate biopsy (TR approach). No patients had any previous history of prostate biopsy. All patients had given informed consent. Patient demographics including age, digital rectal examination (DRE) findings (recorded as benign, suspicious, malignant or unknown), Body Mass Index (BMI, kg/m2), prostate volume, serum total prostate specific antigen (PSA), biopsy technique (transperineal or transrectal), total number of cores taken, number of cores positive for prostate adenocarcinoma from histology, Gleason grade and score, positive biopsies, complications (The major complications included sepsis and severe hematuria, the minor complications included minor hematuria, LUTS (lower urinary tract symptoms), dysuria, acute urinary retention, infection, rectal bleeding, perineal swelling) and treatments of the study cohort are shown in Table 1. In our study, rectal bleeding was defined as the passage of bright red blood rectally > 12 h after biopsy, or any bleed requiring active management irrespective of the time of occurrence. Major hameaturia was defined as obvious gross hematuria with or without blood clot, minor hameaturia was defined as no obvious gross hematuria and was confirmed microscopic hematuria.

All prostate biopsies were performed by an experienced urologist. (W. W). We used the cefuroxime sodium (1.5g, intravenous drip) for anti-infective prophylactic therapy. Systematic 12-core prostate biopsy were performed under transrectal ultrasound guidance, a standard of twelve cores was taken using TR approach. TR approach were performed with the patient in the left decubitus position, using an 18-G automatic biopsy gun with a specimen size of 22 mm (Bard Magnum; Bard Medical, Covington, GA, USA), 20 ml of Lidocaine gel was introduced intra-rectally 15 min before the procedure, the sextant biopsies were taken laterally in the prostate from the base, midline and apex, 3 cores were taken from each side from the far lateral areas of the prostate at the base, midline and near the apex. TP approach was performed according

Table 1 Characteristics of patients

Parameter	TR	TP	P
Patients (n)	144	98	–
Age, yr (range)	65.61 ± 11.21 (51~86)	63.40 ± 9.81 (50~77)	0.107
BMI, kg/m^2 (range)	27.81 ± 4.86 (23.5~34.7)	28.60 ± 5.17 (22.4~35.1)	0.221
PSA, ng/ml (range)	11.23 ± 6.82 (6.3~46.7)	9.61 ± 7.94 (4.6~36.6)	0.104
Prostate volume, ml (range)	32.62 ± 9.11 (20.5~67.8)	34.21 ± 6.42 (23.5~59.8)	0.110
Suspicious DRE findings (rate)	9 (6.3%)	6 (6.1%)	0.968
biopsy time, min (range)	11.55 ± 6.71 (10~26)	16.61 ± 7.82 (12~39)	<0.001
biopsy number (range)	12	15.16 (13~17)	<0.001
Gleason score (range)	6.89 ± 0.75 (6~9)	7.10±0.89 (6~9)	0.057
Follow up, months (range)	7.51 ± 4.26 (1~12)	8.12±5.15 (1.5~13)	0.337

to our previous study. Multi-parametric MRI examination and TRUS-mpMRI image fusion were shown in Additional file 1. Biopsy protocol: The biopsy started with target biopsy to the center of cancer-suspicious lesions without the guide of template using the free-hand transperineal technique, and then, standard 12-core stand biopsy (blinded to the MRI target lesions) was carried out in all patients. Lesions suspicious of cancer identified on MRI were semi automatically displayed on the real-time TRUS image [13]. All target lesions were sampled once in both axial and sagittal planes, with at least two core biopsies per target. An 18-G automatic biopsy gun with a specimen size of 22 mm (Bard Magnum; Bard Medical, Covington, GA, USA) was used to take biopsy cores. All patients underwent general anesthesia using a larynx mask during the biopsy procedure.

Statistical analysis

Data are presented as the Mean ± SD. Statistical analysis involved use of SPSS 17.0 (SPSS Inc, Chicago, IL). Between-group comparisons involved t test and chi-square test. $P<0.05$ was considered statistically significant.

Results

Patients demographics are shown in Table 1. The patients were divided into two groups based on the different prostate biopsy techniques. A total of 242 patients were included in the study. Among them, 144 men underwent transrectal biopsies while 98 men underwent transperineal biopsies. The mean age of the TR biopsies and TP biopsies was 65.61 ± 11.2 years (range 51–86 years) and 63.40 ± 9.81 years (range 50–77 years)respectively. The mean BMI of TR and TP was 27.81 ± 4.86 kg/m^2 (range $23.5 \sim 34.7$ kg/m^2) and 28.60 ± 5.17 kg/m^2 (range $22.4 \sim 35.1$ kg/m^2) respectively. The mean preoperative PSA value of TR and TP was 11.23 ± 6.82 ng/mL (range $6.3 \sim 46.7$ ng/mL) and 9.61 ± 7.94 ng/mL (range $4.6 \sim 36.6$ ng/mL) respectively. The mean preoperative prostate volume of TR and TP, calculated using the ellipsoid formula, was 32.62 ± 9.11 mL (range $20.5 \sim 67.8$ mL) and 34.21 ± 6.42 mL (range $23.5 \sim 59.8$ mL), respectively. Nine patients in TR (6.3%) had a recognized palpable nodule in the prostate based on digital rectal examination (DRE), and six patients in TP (6.1%) had suspicious DRE findings. The mean biopsy time of TR was 11.55 ± 6.71 min (range 10–26 min). The mean

biopsy time of TP, including the MRI-TRUS fusion time and needle puncture time without anesthesia, was 16.61 ± 7.82 min (range 12–39 min). The biopsy time of TR was shorter than TP ($p < 0.001$). The mean Gleason score of TR was 6.89 ± 0.75 (range $6 \sim 9$) whilethe mean Gleason score of TP was 7.10 ± 0.89 (range $6 \sim 9$). The mean follow-up of TR was 7.51 ± 4.26 months (range $1 \sim 12$ months) while the mean follow-up of TP was 8.12 ± 5.15 months (range $1.5 \sim 13$ months). There were no significant differences between TR and TP in age, BMI, PSA, prostate volume, suspicious DRE findings, Gleason score, during the follow-up period ($p > 0.05$).

The comparative pathological results of prostate biopsies in TR and TP are shown in Table 2. The TR and TP detected prostate cancer (PCa) in 57 (39.6%) and 51 (52.0%) patients, respectively. The TR detected High-grade PIN, Low-grade prostatic intraepithelial neoplasia (PIN) in 10 (6.9%) and 7 (4.9%) patients, respectively. The TP detected High-grade PIN, Low-grade PIN in 5 (5.1%) and 6 (6.1%) patients, respectively. The TR and TP detected benign prostate hyperplasia (BPH) in 59 (40.9%) and 32 (32.7%) patients, respectively. The TR and TP detected chronic prostatit is in 11 (7.6%) and 4 (4.1%) patients, respectively.

Comparison of the positive (detected PCa) and negative (undetected PCa) results of TR and TP according to PSA classification is shown in Table 3. In patients who's PSA level lower than 10ng/ml, The TR and TP detected PCain 8 and 4patients, respectively. ($p = 0.401$). In patients who'sPSA between 10 to 20ng/ml, The TR and TP detected PCain13 patients, respectively ($p = 0.895$). In patients who'sPSA higher than 20ng/ml, The TR and TP detected PCain36 and 40 patients, respectively ($p = 0.029$). The PCa detection rate of TP was much higher than TR in patients who'sPSA higher than 20ng/ml ($p < 0.05$).

Complications rates of the two groups were recorded and the results are presented in Table 4. The major complications included sepsis and severe hematuria. The minor complications included minor hematuria, lower urinary tract symptoms (LUTS), dysuria, acute urinary retention, infection, rectal bleeding, perineal swelling. In the TR group, one patient (0.7%) had sepsis and treated with admitted intravenous (IV) antibiotics. Two patients (1.38%) had severe hematuria. In the TP group, no patient had major complications. However, there was no significant difference between two groups of major

Table 2 Comparison of the pathological results TR biopsy and TP biopsy

Group	PCa n (%)	High-grade PIN n (%)	Low-grade PIN n (%)	BPH n (%)	Chronic prostatitis n (%)	Total n (%)
TR	57 (39.6)	10 (6.9)	7 (4.9)	59 (40.9)	11 (7.6)	144
TP	51 (52.0)	5 (5.1)	6 (6.1)	32 (32.7)	4 (4.1)	98
P value	0.055	0.559	0.669	0.189	0.259	/

PIN prostate intraepithelial neoplasm

Table 3 Comparison of the positive and negative results of TR and TP

PSA	Positive, n		Negative, n		P value
	TR	TP	TR	TP	
<10	8	4	37	32	0.401
10~20	13	7	26	11	0.895
>20	36	40	20	8	0.029

complications ($P > 0.05$). There were significant differences between the two groups of minor complications in infection, rectal bleeding, and perineal swelling. As shown in Table 4,there were 16 patients in TR (11.11%) and 3 patients in TP (3.06%) with infection.2 patients in TR (1.4%) and no patients in TP (0%) had rectal bleeding. 3 patients in TR (2.08%) and 10 patients in TP (10.2%) had perineal swelling. The rate of infection and rectal bleeding in TR were much higher than TP ($p < 0.05$) However, the rate of perineal swelling in TP was much higher than TR ($p < 0.05$). There were no significant differences of minor complications including minor hematuria, LUTS dysuria, acute urinary retention between thetwo groups ($p > 0.05$), in spite of more biopsy cores in TP biopsy.

Total complications in each patient of TR and TP were shown in Table 5. There were 18 patients (12.5%) without any complication after biopsy in TR and 29 patients (29.59%) without any complication after biopsy in TP. There were more patients without any complications in TP group than that in TR ($p < 0.001$). 43 patients (29.86%) with one complication were detected in TR and 41 patients (41.83%) in TP. 45 patients (31.25%) with two complications after biopsy were found in TR group and 21 patients (21.42%) in TP.34 patients (23.61%) were found with more than three complications after biopsy in TR and 7 patients (7.14%) in TP. The rate of multiple complications after biopsy in TR were much higher than TP ($p < 0.001$).

Table 4 Comparison of the incidence of complications of TR and TP biopsy

Group	TR (n, %)	TP (n, %)	P value
Major			
sepsis	1 (0.70)	0 (0.00)	0.408
Severe haematuria	2 (1.38)	0 (0.00)	0.241
Minor			
Minor hematuria	45 (31.25)	35 (35.71)	0.468
LUTS	24 (16.67)	25 (25.51)	0.091
Dysuria	9 (6.25)	11 (11.22)	0.168
Acute urinary retention	13 (9.03)	10 (10.20)	0.759
Infection	16 (11.11)	3 (3.06)	0.022
Rectal bleeding	2 (1.4)	0 (0)	<0.001
Perineal swelling	3 (2.08)	10 (10.20)	0.006

Table 5 Total complications in each patient of TR and TP

Total complications	TR (n, %)	TP (n, %)	P value
0	18 (12.5)	29 (29.59)	<0.001
1	43 (29.86)	41 (41.83)	0.055
2	45 (31.25)	21 (21.42)	0.092
≥3	34 (23.61)	7 (7.14)	<0.001

Discussion

The present results showed that cancer detection rate of TP group were higher than TR group (Table 2). This might be due tothat the TP group had at least one suspicious area in mp MRI images and included at least one targeted biopsy, but the TP group had notargeted biopsy.

Complication rate of prostate biopsies varies widely in medical literature. Several studies reveal major complications (sepsis, bleeding or other complication requiring admission) rates of around 1–2% in transrectal prostate biopsy, with the following rates of minor complications: hematuria 10–84%; rectal bleeding 1.3–45%; hematospermia 1.1–93%; vasovagal episodes 0–5%; infective complications 0–6.3% [7, 15]. Studies also reveal similar wide-ranging rates of minor complications in transperineal biopsies. Recently, a systematic review showed that the rate of sepsis after TRUS biopsy is as high as 5%, and appears to be rising with increasing rates of multiresistant bacteria found in rectal flora. However, the rate of sepsis from published series of TP biopsy approached zero [10], andour results was consistent with the conclusions from the literature.

In our study, the major complications rate following TR was 2%, whereas no patient had a major complication following TP (Table 4). However, there was no significant difference between the rate of major complications in the two groups ($P > 0.05$). Of note, there was one case of sepsis in the TR approach, and cured by admitted intravenous drip antibiotics. Visible hematuria following prostate biopsy is common, with reported rates of 10–84% [15]. Bleeding post procedure is usually self-limiting and rarely life threatening. Two patients had severe hematuria and cured by continuous bladder irrigation. Mortality after prostate biopsy is extremely rare, and most reported deaths are the result of septic shock. In fact, there was no patient died after prostate biopsy in the present study.

Minor complication rates in both techniques were comparable. Infection is a well-established risk of prostate biopsy. Various strategies to reduce infectious complications have been explored, as were recently reviewed [9]. Recently, several studies have shifted from the transrectal to the transperineal technique with anecdotal reports of very low rates of sepsis, even without the use of prophylactic antibiotics [10, 16]. In this study, we also found that the rate of infection in TR was significantly higher than TP ($p < 0.05$). The rate of infection and rectal bleeding in TR were much higher than TP ($p < 0.05$), while the rate of perineal swelling in TP was much higher than TR ($p < 0.05$). This might be due to the different approaches since more biopsy cores were taken in TP procedure. Bleeding is the most frequently reported complication after biopsy, but it is usually minor and resolves spontaneously. The present study was unable to prove any significant difference of minor complications including minor hematuria, LUTS, dysuria, acute urinary retention between the two groups ($p > 0.05$).

The TR approach is a much easier procedure and can prevent patients' discomfort by using only local anesthesia. This changed after several reports of fatalities following septic complications of transrectal biopsy [17]. Image fusion guided TP biopsy is increasingly popular as a mean for accurate diagnosis and risk stratification [11, 18]. An increasing number of studies have showed that MRI/US image-fusion guided TP is an effective and accurate method for prostate cancer diagnosis. Our study also showed a higher prevalence of MRI/US image-fusion guided TP proven cancers in suspicious areas, which can result in better prostate cancer characterization via precise localization, prediction of Gleason grade, and more accurate cancer core length. Moreover, the incidence rate of infection and rectal bleeding after biopsy in TP was much less than TR.

There were some limitations in the present study. The first is the retrospective study design was absence of randomization. Second, there was inadequate sample size in this study. Third, the procedure of TR with local anesthesia was simplicity, but the procedure of TP with general anesthesia was complexity. It is unknown whether this difference has clinical significance, and how it affects the complication rates. Further prospective multi-center randomized controlled trials will be conducted.

Conclusion

The present study supports the safety of both transrectal prostate biopsy and free-hand transperineal targeted prostate biopsy with real-time fusion imaging of mpMRI/US in the diagnosis of prostate cancer. Transperineal prostate biopsy is safe with no cases of sepsis recorded, and the rate of infection and rectal bleeding in TP is much lower than TR, in spite of more biopsy cores in TP biopsy. This suggests that free-hand transperineal targeted prostate biopsy with real-time fusion imaging of mpMRI/US can be a good approach for prostate biopsy.

Abbreviations

DRE: Digital rectal examination; mpMRI: Multi-parameter magnetic resonance imaging; TP: Transperineal; TR: Transrectal; TRUS: Transrectal Ultrasonography

Acknowledgements
The authors would like to thank all our participants for their gracious participation in this study.

Funding
This study was supported by a grant from the National Natural Science Foundation of China (81302542, 81371207, and 81171047), China Postdoctoral Science Foundation (2014M551562), and Fundamental Research Funds for theCentral Universities (20620140532).

Authors' contributions
All authors made substantial contributions to the conception, design, analysis and interpretation of the data; HH drafted the first draft of the manuscript and WW provided critical revision; all authors give final approval for the manuscript and agree to be accountable for all aspects of the work herein.

Competing interests
The authors declare that they have no competing interests

References
1. Denmeade SR, Isaacs JT. A history of prostate cancer treatment. Nat Rev Cancer. 2002;2:389–96.
2. Yacoub JH, Verma S, Moulton JS, Eggener S, Oto A. Imaging-guided prostate biopsy: conventional and emerging techniques. Radiographics. 2012;32:819⁻37.
3. Lee F, Torp-Pedersen S, Siders D, Littrup P, McLeary R. Transrectal ultrasound in the diagnosis and staging of prostatic carcinoma. Radiology. 1989;170:609–15.
4. Hara R, et al. Optimal approach for prostate cancer detection as initial biopsy: prospective randomized study comparing transperineal versus transrectal systematic 12-core biopsy. Urology. 2008;71:191–5.
5. Moran BJ, Braccioforte MH. Stereotactic transperineal prostate biopsy. Urology. 2009;73:386–8.
6. Bittner N, Merrick GS, Butler WM, Bennett A, Galbreath RW. Incidence and pathological features of prostate cancer detected on transperineal template guided mapping biopsy after negative transrectal ultrasound guided biopsy. J Urol. 2013;190:509–14.
7. Loeb S, et al. Systematic review of complications of prostate biopsy. Eur Urol. 2013;64:876⁻92.
8. Selvanayagam A, Perera M, Roberts MJ, Pretorius CF. Perforated Rectal Diverticulum following Prostate Biopsy Resulting in Peri-Rectal Abscess and Sepsis. Surg Infect Case Rep. 2016;1:2⁻3.
9. Williamson, D.A., et al. Infectious complications following transrectal ultrasound⁻guided prostate biopsy: new challenges in the era of multidrug-resistant Escherichia coli. Clinical infectious diseases, cit193 (2013).
10. Grummet JP, et al. Sepsis and 'superbugs': should we favour the transperineal over the transrectal approach for prostate biopsy? BJU Int. 2014;114:384–8.
11. Scott S, Samaratunga H, Chabert C, Breckenridge M, Gianduzzo T. Is transperineal prostate biopsy more accurate than transrectal biopsy in determining final Gleason score and clinical risk category? A comparative analysis. BJU international. 2015;116:26–30.
12. Siddiqui MM, et al. Magnetic resonance imaging/ultrasound–fusion biopsy significantly upgrades prostate cancer versus systematic 12-core transrectal ultrasound biopsy. Eur Urol. 2013;64:713–9.

13. Rastinehad AR, Durand M. A comparison of magnetic resonance imaging and ultrasonography (MRI/US)-fusion guided prostate biopsy devices: too many uncontrolled variables. BJU Int. 2016;117:548–9.

14. Zhang Q, et al. Free-hand transperineal targeted prostate biopsy with real-time fusion imaging of multiparametric magnetic resonance imaging and transrectal ultrasound: single-center experience in China. Int Urol Nephrol. 2015;47:727–33.

15. Patel U, et al. Infection after transrectal ultrasonography-guided prostate biopsy: increased relative risks after recent international travel or antibiotic use. BJU Int. 2012;109:1781–5.

16. Zhou, Y., Yan, W. & Li, H. Re: Eduard Baco, Erik Rud, Lars Magne Eri, et al. A Randomized Controlled Trial to Assess and Compare the Outcomes of Two-core Prostate Biopsy Guided by Fused Magnetic Resonance and Transrectal Ultrasound Images and Traditional 12-core Systematic Biopsy. Eur Urol 2016; 69: 149–56. European urology (2016).

17. Ogino, H., et al. Transperineal Approach Versus Transrectal Approach for Fiducial Marker Placement in Proton Beam Therapy of Prostate Cancer: A Prospective Comparison. International Journal of Radiation Oncology Biology Physics 90, S405 (2014).

18. Dowrick, A.S., Wootten, A.C., Howard, N., Peters, J.S. & Murphy, D.G. A prospective study of the short-term quality of life outcomes of patients undergoing transperineal prostate biopsy. BJU international (2016).

9

Computer-aided transrectal ultrasound: does prostate HistoScanning™ improve detection performance of prostate cancer in repeat biopsies?

Moritz Franz Hamann[*], C. Hamann, A. Trettel, K P Jünemann and C M Naumann

Abstract

Background: An imaging tool providing reliable prostate cancer (PCa) detection and localization is necessary to improve common diagnostic pathway with ultrasound targeted biopsies. To determine the performance of transrectal ultrasound (TRUS) augmented by prostate HistoScanning™ analysis (PHS) we investigated the detection of prostate cancer (PCa) foci in repeat prostate biopsies (Bx).

Methods: 97 men with a mean age of 66.2 (44 – 82) years underwent PHS augmented TRUS analysis prior to a repeat Bx. Three PHS positive foci were defined in accordance with 6 bilateral prostatic sectors. Targeted Bx (tBx) limited to PHS positive foci and a systematic 14-core backup Bx (sBx) were taken. Results were correlated to biopsy outcome. Sensitivity, specificity, predictive accuracy, negative predictive value (NPV) and positive predictive value (PPV) were calculated.

Results: PCa was found in 31 of 97 (32 %) patients. Detection rate in tBx was significantly higher (p < .001). Detection rate in tBx and sBx did not differ on patient level(p ≥ 0.7). PHS sensitivity, specificity, predictive accuracy, PPV and NPV were 45 %, 83 %, 80 %, 19 % and 95 %, respectively.

Conclusions: PHS augmented TRUS identifies abnormal prostatic tissue. Although sensitivity and PPV for PCa are low, PHS information facilitates Bx targeting to vulnerable foci and results in a higher cancer detection rate. PHS targeted Bx should be considered in patients at persistent risk of PCa.

Keywords: Prostate, Prostate cancer, Transrectal ultrasonography, HistoScanning, Prostate biopsy

Background

Transrectal ultrasound (TRUS) imaging and systematic TRUS-guided biopsies (Bx) are gold standard procedures for prostate diagnostics and detection of prostate cancer (PCa) [1, 2]. However, the power to identify - and in particular to exclude - cancer reliably is limited due to low PCa specificity of grey scale ultrasound patterns [3]. Up to one-third of men with an initial negative systematic Bx are found to have prostate cancer in subsequent Bx [3, 4]. The question whether to pursue further repeat TRUS guided Bx in patients with a rising prostate-specific antigen (PSA) level subsequent to an initially negative Bx is a common clinical dilemma and remains a diagnostic challenge in urology. On the other hand, multiparametric magnetic resonance imaging (mp MRI) of the prostate is rapidly gaining significance due to its capability to detect PCa. Targeted biopsies of suspicious lesions, using MRI fused with real-time ultrasound, show encouraging rates of detection of clinically significant PCa [5]. In contrast to widely-used ultrasound, MRI hardware is expensive and time-consuming diagnostic protocols limit its availability. Further developments in ultrasound techniques, like contrast enhancement, elastography or prostate HistoScanning™ (PHS), improve TRUS capability to detect pathology confined to the prostatic gland and increase the validity of TRUS-guided Bx [6]. Initial data on PHS computer-aided ultrasonography have

* Correspondence: moritz.hamann@uksh.de
Department of Urology and Pediatric Urology, University Hospital Schleswig Holstein, Campus Kiel, Arnold Heller Str. 3, 24105 Kiel, Germany

shown favorable results [7]. But evidence from existing Bx studies is scarce and controversial [8–11].

To generate a greater diagnostic yield than systematic needle Bx, we integrated the results of HS into our repeat prostate biopsy program. We report the cancer detection rate and characteristics of this approach in a prospective series of 97 consecutive patients with previous negative prostate Bx.

Methods

At one center, data was collected from 97 consecutive men with a mean age of 66.2 (44 – 82) years [Table 1]. All of them were at a persistent risk of prostate cancer and had at least one previous set of TRUS-guided prostate Bx, yielding a non-cancerous diagnosis. All of them had suspicious findings at the digital rectal examination (DRE), or serum prostate-specific antigen (PSA) level >10 ng/mL, or both. Elevated serum PSA levels >4 ng/mL a PSA-velocity of >0.75 ng/mL p.a. and free-to-total PSA ratio < 15 % were seen as the indication for prostate biopsies. Rescanning of the prostate was scheduled at least three months after the previous manipulation of the gland in order to minimize impairment of data quality through earlier diagnostic procedures. All patients were informed of the mode of the extended prostate Bx scheme and its potential complications. All patients provided written informed consent for the procedures. Patients were advised that information collected from their Bx would be used for internal analysis and medical research as approved by the local Ethics Committee of the medical faculty of the University of Schleswig-Holstein, and was subsequently analyzed retrospectively.

HistoScanning technique and prostate biopsy technique
After indication diagnostics and before starting the Bx procedure, all patients underwent an automatic standardized 3-dimensional (3D) transrectal ultrasound (TRUS) using a BK ProFocus UV ultrasound system with 8818 tri-plane probe (Analogic Corp, Peabody MA, USA). To facilitate appropriate data acquisition and a standardized scanning process, an external motor sweeps the ultrasound probe's sagittal array. Beside the signals from macroscopic tissue boundaries, which are used to create anatomical images, ultrasound produces a continuous stream of echoes emanating from the tissue's underlying microscopic features, known as

Table 1 Patient characteristics

Mean (range) patient age	66.24 (44–82)
Mean (range) PSA level ng/mL	10.42 (1.02–35.00)
DRE pos / neg (%)	86/11 (89/11)
Prostate volume ml Mean (range)	51.43 (17.00/105.00)
Previous Biopsy sessions Mean (range)	1.46 (1–5)

ultrasound backscatter. PHS analyses these backscatter signals by using numerical descriptors of multiparametric measures from the individual 3D raw data scan, which vary in its properties due to suspicious (malignant) or normal prostatic tissue characteristics. A statistical classifier categorizes corresponding prostatic regions as normal or suspicious. Displaying these informations as a colored (red) overlay in the ultrasound images complements the conventional ultrasound greyscale diagnostics.

Computer-aided analysis of the data was performed on a PHS workstation with software version 2.3 (Advanced Medical Diagnostics, Waterloo BE). Based on the PHS image, the physician defined the most prominent (largest) target regions, up to a maximum of three. In turn, a structured scaffold was created from PHS projection reports of the prostate, which was used at a later point for guidance of targeted Bx procedures (Fig. 1). The location of the suspicious/target regions was defined according to 12 peripheral sectors and two central sectors: a bilateral transition zone, apex, center, and base (each of the latter three medially and laterally).

The biopsy procedures were performed consecutively during a single visit with the patient in a dorsal lithotomy position under general anesthesia. Three targeted cores were taken transperineally from each suspicious region based on PHS analysis (maximum of 3). A brachytherapy template grid fixed to a cradle was placed next to the perineum and used as a guide. Using the information from the PHS projection reports, the biopsy needle was directed through the brachytherapy template to obtain the Bx under direct TRUS guidance using a BK 8848 ultrasound probe (Analogic Corp, Peabody MA, USA). Sampling a target lesion, neither the needle position (grid perforation) nor the depth of the biopsies was changed (Fig. 1). Thereafter, three targeted cores were taken by a transrectal approach from each suspicious region using the tri-plane 8818 probe. Using the information from PHS analysis, Bx was directed cognitively to the PHS positive volumes. Finally, a standardized 14-core transrectal-guided Bx was performed by sampling the corresponding seven sectors bilaterally, as mentioned above. Biopsies were performed randomly by four senior surgeons with at least five years of biopsy experience.

The local pathologists of the University Hospital Schleswig Holstein, Campus Kiel, performed histopathology analysis of Bx cores.

Statistical analysis
All data were registered in a Microsoft Access database (2010) and tabulated subsequently in Microsoft Excel (2010), with statistical analysis performed using PC SAS (Version 9.3 or higher) and R (version 3.0.1). For

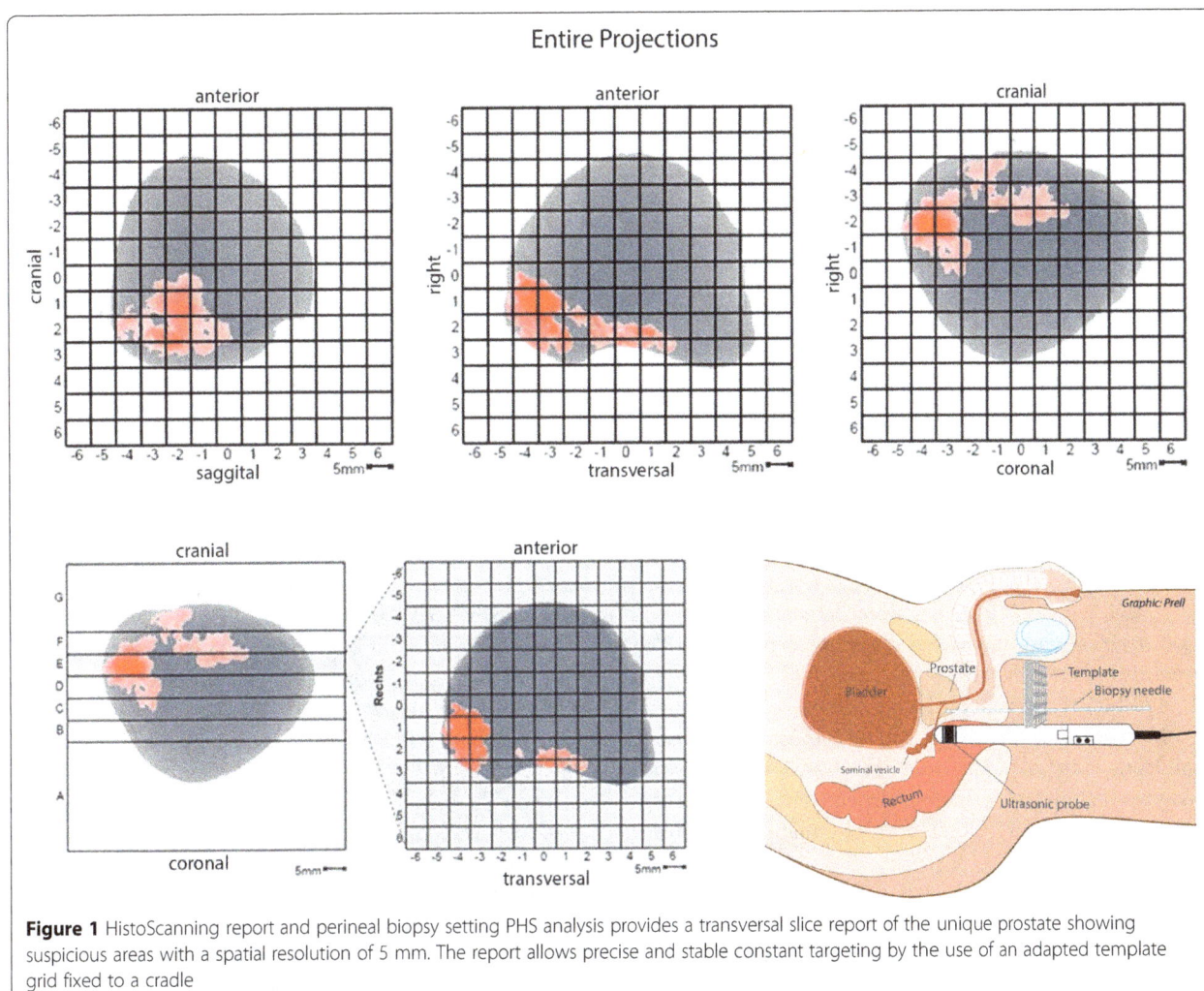

Figure 1 HistoScanning report and perineal biopsy setting PHS analysis provides a transversal slice report of the unique prostate showing suspicious areas with a spatial resolution of 5 mm. The report allows precise and stable constant targeting by the use of an adapted template grid fixed to a cradle

calculation on paired data the McNemar test was used. A two-sample Chi-squared test of proportions was used for binomial data. Differences in total PHS suspicious volume were compared using the Wilcoxon signed rank test. A p-value of 0.05 was considered to indicate statistical significance.

The cancer detection rate and procedure characteristics for all cases were evaluated. Table 1 summarizes the patient characteristics.

Results

PHS analysis detected abnormalities in all prostate scans of the 97 patients included. 224 sectors contained PHS positive ultrasound patterns. In 31 of 97 (32 %) patients prostate adenocarcinoma was diagnosed, and 40 of 248 (16 %) sectors harbored cancer with respect to biopsy results. Additionally, histopathological examination detected atypical small acinar proliferation in seven patients (7 %), high-grade prostatic intraepithelial neoplasia in 20 (21 %) and chronic active inflammation in 72 (74 %) respectively. Based on the combined outcome,

diagnostic performance of PHS to detect cancer at sector level shows sensitivity, specificity, predictive accuracy, a positive predictive value (PPV) and a negative predictive value (NPV) of 45 %, 83 %, 80 %, 19 % and 95 %, respectively. Table 2 summarizes the histological findings for all patients. The median PHS sum of the suspicious volume of 3 regions was 1.32 ml (range 0.20-9.32). Eighty seven patients (90 %) had a PHS sum ≥0.50 ml. Bx outcome and Gleason sum in relation to PHS suspicious volume is presented in Table 3. With respect to biopsy results, PHS volumes of benign prostate sectors and prostate sectors harboring cancer did not differ significantly. In 32 out of 77 (42 %) positive biopsies, the cancerous tissue was found in the anterior zone. 34 (44 %) respectively 21 (27 %) cancerous cores were harvested from the medial and basal parts of the gland. The occurrence of PHS positive ultrasound patterns did not differ significantly at sector level. Although the targeted biopsies originated from a maximum of three prostatic sectors, the detection rate per patient was not significantly different from systematic Bx. The detection

Table 2 Histopathological results in prostate biopsies

		Systematic	HS-template targeted transperineal	HS- targeted transrectal	All biopsies
Bx+		23	20	21	31
GS sum in Bx+	Mean (range)	6.5 (5–9)	6.5 (5–9)	6.38 (5–9)	6.35 (5–9)
GS sum ≥7 in Bx+	N (%)	5 (5)	10(10)	8(8)	11 (11)
GS I = 2/3 in Bx+	N (%)	19(19)	14(14)	16(16)	24 (25)
GS I = 4/5 in Bx+	N (%)	4(4)	6(6)	5(5)	7 (7)
ASAP	N (%)	3(3)	2(2)	2(2)	7 (7)
HG-PIN positive	N (%)	12(12)	9(9)	12(12)	20 (21)
Prostatitis	N (%)	68(70)	59(61)	59(61)	72 (74)

Bx+, prostate cancer positive biopsy; GS, Gleason Score; ASAP, atypical small acinar proliferations; HG PIN, high-grade intra epithelial proliferations

rate for each PHS positive region was significantly higher in both targeted transperineal and targeted transrectal Bx compared to systematic Bx(p < .001). Table 4 shows an analysis of the detection rates of different procedures. Twenty two cancers were detected by systematic biopsies, while 20 and 21 cancers were detected in PHS targeted perineal and transrectal biopsies, respectively. The detection rate of significant cancer (GS ≥ 7) in PHS-targeted biopsies was superior in comparison to systematic biopsies. Perineal PHS targeted biopsies missed 1 significant cancer, PHS targeted transrectal biopsies missed 3 significant cancers, respectively. Most of the cancers (18/23, 78 %) detected by systematic biopsy were insignificant.

Discussion

Cancer specific accuracy in standard prostate Bx tends to be determined by PSA, prostate texture recorded by digital rectal examination as well as the number of biopsy cores in relation to prostate size, rather than by transrectal grey scale ultrasound displaying malignant foci [12]. Thus, a substantial number of patients undergo repeat biopsy, indicated by weak prognostic factors, still facing the same limited cancer-specific imaging characteristics of TRUS. With respect to initial data, PHS seems to overcome these limitations by analyzing radiofrequency backscattered raw data of prostatic ultrasound [13]. Our data is unable to confirm a comparable high prognostic validity for prostate cancer. In the present study, PHS revealed at least 2 to 3

aberrations in 94 % and 59 % of the ultrasound scans, but histopathological analysis confirms malignant tissue in only 32 % of the patients. Although, these detection results are within the range of previous studies on repeat biopsies [4], calculations of PHS predictive characteristics show weak results with respect to PPV (17 %) and sensitivity (44 %). These findings are in line with recent studies which also failed to show significant accuracy for PHS to predict positive biopsy results: According to sextant analysis, PHS had a sensitivity, specificity, PPV and NPV of 32.0-100 %, 5.9-32.7 %, 19.6-22.7 % and 86.4-84 %, respectively [9, 10]. Further analysis found no correlation between pathology and the whole gland tumor volumes estimated by PHS, nor between the PHS volumes and prostate cancer GS [10, 14]. Table 3 shows comparable results. It has to be taken into account, that PHS algorithms allow exclusively two opposed classifications (suspicious vs. non-suspicious) for ultrasound properties in virtual subvolumes. Based on a repeated but uniform calculation, the number of decisions as displayed by the PHS volume does not display varying characteristics or allow risk stratification concerning Gleason grading. Additionally, it must be assumed that acoustic similarity in the ultrasound backscatter properties of malignant and nonmalignant structures might account for further limitations in the analysis. With respect to specificity and NPV of 83 % and 95 %, respectively, PHS results need careful interpretation before the results can make a contribution to decision-making like biopsy indication or planning.

Table 3 Relation between Prostate HistoScanning™ suspicious volume and Bx outcome

		Bx +	Bx-	p-value
Total PHS suspicious volume in ml	N	31	66	
	median(range)	1.58 (0.20-9.32)	1.26 (0.22-6.59)	n.s.
		Gleason sum <7	Gleason sum > =7	
Total PHS suspicious volume in ml	N	20	11	
	median (range)	1.55 (0.20-9.32)	1.86 (0.22-4.35)	n.s.

PHS, prostate HistoScanning; Bx, prostate biopsy; Bx+, prostate cancer positive biopsy; Bx-, prostate cancer negative biopsy; p-values Bx + vs Bx- (Wilcoxon rang sum test)

Table 4 Analysis of detection rate per prostate region of different procedures

N = 97	Systematic Bx	PHS-template targeted transperineal Bx		PHS- targeted transrectal Bx	
patients with Bx+	23	20	n.s.	21	n.s.
regions biopsied	1358	248		248	
regions with Bx+	73	32		28	
detection rate per region	5 %	13 %	<0.001	11 %	<0.001

Biopsy Bx, prostate cancer positive biopsy Bx+, Pca negative biopsy Bx-, p-values compared with systematic biopsy (Chi-squared test)

On the other hand, the detection rate in our cohort improved significantly by PHS-targeted biopsies. On patient level, the PHS template-targeted biopsies account for a 27 % increase in the detection rate, transrectal-targeted biopsies for 23 %, and the combined targeted biopsies for an increase by 41 % compared to systematic biopsy alone. PHS perineal targeted biopsies detect twice as much significant cancer foci than systematic ultrasound-guided biopsies. De Coninck et al. reported comparable findings in 41 men who underwent prostate biopsies supplemented with cognitive-targeted biopsies in suspicious regions based on prostate PHS. Targeted biopsies were 4.5-fold more likely to be positive than the random biopsies [11]. In our series, the rate of non-significant cancers detected by PHS-targeted perineal vs. systematic Bx was lower (Table 2). This rebuts potential concerns of an increased detection of clinically insignificant cancers caused by more substantial sampling. PHS-targeted biopsies detected 6 significant prostate cancers that were overseen by systematic biopsy. Additionally, the absolute numbers of atypical histopathological findings like ASAP, HG PIN and prostatitis in PHS-positive sectors do not differ significantly from systematic Bx despite the limited sampling.

Our data might suggest a reduction of biopsies in non-PHS positive sectors and to focus on more vulnerable or suspect regions in the prostate. The corresponding PB scheme would theoretically achieve appropriate sampling by targeting certain locations rather than by increasing the core numbers. In an analysis of 164 autopsies, which had not previously undergone clinical biopsy, step-section analysis revealed that the common 12-core biopsy technique detects the majority of clinically significant cancers with a sensitivity of 80 % [15]. The authors conclude that the chance of detecting cancer was correlated more closely to the location of the sampling (peripheral, lateral and apical cores) than to the number of biopsy cores taken.

Prostate cancer detection rates from perineal targeted biopsies differed from the transrectal targeted biopsy regime. This difference occurred independently from previous tissue analysis, for the reason that both targeted approaches are aligned to the same scanning process. In comparison to the transrectal approach, the perineal biopsy technique might reduce variables that can influence the needle placement. Furthermore, longitudinal biopsy punches following the axis of the prostate seem to allow more accurate sampling of the anterior part. Theoretically, because previous studies reported inhomogeneous results comparing transrectal and transperineal prostate biopsies [8, 16].

There are several limitations in this study. Firstly, the analysis was performed on a regional basis. Dependencies between neighboring regions, as well as correlation of the different biopsy procedures with the HS results are difficult to account for and may incur misleading results. Secondly, there is no minimum threshold defining when a PHS signal is to be called positive; this may also affect the results. For example, the targeted regions could stretch across different sections meaning that even a small amount in one sector would lead to it being seen as a positive PHS sector, but it might still yield negative biopsies because the few cores would not necessarily pick up the cancer. Moreover, the knowledge of "abnormal" regions might influence the surgeon's decisions during the subsequent systematic biopsy as a result of the non-blinded, single-surgeon biopsy procedure. Nevertheless, we did not find any significant interoperator variability with respect to the detection rate or the biopsy approach.

Generally, it is difficult to compare the diagnostic accuracy of Bx techniques in different patient series. Ethical concerns will always prevent verification of negative Bx results by radical prostatectomy, and positive biopsies are not always and necessarily followed by prostatectomy. Therefore, the clinical setting will always account for a potential verification bias, not knowing what the exact location of the cancer is and how many cancers were missed by biopsy.

Finally, recent results from multi-parametric MRI procedures pull into question all ultrasound-based techniques including color Doppler imaging, real-time elastography, C-TRUS / ANNA and Prostate HS. The application of integrated interpretation strategies for mp MRI variables, such as the PIRADS score, improves the risk stratification for prostate cancer and allows for effective fusion guidance of targeted prostate biopsy [17, 18]. Likewise, all ultrasound modalities have been devised to increase the diagnostic yield of prostate biopsy, using ultrasound data to visualize and locate tissues suspected of harboring prostate cancer [19–21]. Despite their promising characteristics, none of them are established in clinical practice because of missing evidence, lack of standardization and significant user-dependent performance. Similarity in the prostate tissue features such as the degree of elasticity/firmness, irregular patterns of blood vessels and ultrasound backscatter properties of malignant and other non-malignant microstructures might account for these limitations. So far, each technique in itselfis limited in its predictive impact on prostate cancer diagnostics, but might be combined into an effective diagnostic tool. Accordingly, a multiparametric approach similar to MRI algorithms might improve future performance and increase the diagnostic yield by specifically visualizing and locating prostate cancer tissue.

Conclusions

HS-augmented ultrasound analysis improves the interpretation of transrectal prostate imaging by identification of abnormal prostatic tissue. Although prostate cancer specificity remains low, the additional information facilitates improved biopsy targeting and results in a higher cancer detection rate in selective prostate sectors. The high NPV might help to reduce biopsies in PHS-negative prostate sectors and to focus on more vulnerable regions in the prostate. With the help of this strategy, increased but unsought detection of clinically insignificant cancers through too substantial sampling can be avoided. The PHS technique should be considered at leastwith respect to patients who had previously negative prostate biopsy results despite elevated PSA levels. Further multicenter analysis has to confirm the advantages of PHS in primary Bx-settings.

™; PCa: Prostate

Abbreviations
TRUS: Transrectal ultrasound; PHS: Prostate HistoScanning cancer; Bx: Prostate biopsies; tBx: Targeted prostate biopsies; sBx: Systematic prostate biopsies; NPV: Negative predictive value; PPV: Positive predictive value; PSA: Prostate specific antigen; mp MRI: Multiparametric magnet resonance imaging.

Competing interests
The authors declare that they have no competing interests.

Authors' contributions
All of the authors have made substantial contributions to the study. MH has developed the concept and design of the study, performed the statistical analysis and interpretation of data and drafted the manuscript. CH has made substantial contributions to concept of the study, data acquisition and was involved in drafting the manuscript. AT was involved in acquisition, analysis and interpretation of data. KJ has made substantial contributions to concept

of the study and was involved in revising the manuscript critically and adding important content. MN has participated in the design of the study, the interpretation of data and was involved in drafting the manuscript and revising it critically and substantially. All authors have read and approved the final manuscript.

Acknowledgements
We thank Almut Kalz who has provided medical writing services and linguistic amendments. Further, we thank Felix Prell who set up the figures. They both belong to our institutional study center, a part of the department of Urology and pediatric Urology, University Hospital Schleswig Holstein, Campus Kiel.

References
1. Heidenreich A, Bastian PJ, Bellmunt J, Bolla M, Joniau S, van der Kwast T, et al. EAU guidelines on prostate cancer. part 1: screening, diagnosis, and local treatment with curative intent-update 2013. Eur Urol. 2014;65(1):124–37.
2. Carter HB, Albertsen PC, Barry MJ, Etzioni R, Freedland SJ, Greene KL, et al. Early detection of prostate cancer: AUA Guideline. J Urol. 2013;190(2):419–26.
3. Ukimura O, Coleman JA, de la Taille A, Emberton M, Epstein JI, Freedland SJ, et al. Contemporary role of systematic prostate biopsies: indications, techniques, and implications for patient care. Eur Urol. 2013;63(2):214–30.
4. Roehl KA, Antenor JA, Catalona WJ. Serial biopsy results in prostate cancer screening study. J Urol. 2002;167:2435–9.
5. Kasivisvanathan V, Dufour R, Moore CM, Ahmed HU, Abd-Alazeez M, Charman SC, et al. Transperineal magnetic resonance image targeted prostate Biopsy versus transperineal template prostate Biopsy in the detection of clinically significant prostate cancer. J Urol. 2013;189:860–6.
6. Aigner F, Pallwein L, Schocke M, Lebovici A, Junker D, Schäfer G, et al. Comparison of Real-time Sonoelastography With T2-weighted endorectal magnetic resonance imaging for prostate cancer detection. JUM. 2011;30:643–9.
7. Simmons LA, Autier P, Zát'ura F, Braeckman J, Peltier A, Romic I, et al. Detection, localisation and characterisation of prostate cancer by Prostate HistoScanningTM. BJU Int. 2011;110:28–35.
8. Hamann MF, Hamann C, Schenk E, Al-Najar A, Naumann CM, Jünemann KP. Computer-aided (HistoScanningTM) Biopsies versus conventional transrectal ultrasound-guided prostate biopsies: Do targeted biopsy schemes improve the cancer detection rate? Urology. 2013;81:370–5.
9. Schiffmann J, Tennstedt P, Fischer J, Tian Z, Beyer B, Boehm K, et al. Does HistoScanning™ predict positive results in prostate biopsy? A retrospective analysis of 1,188 sextants of the prostate. World J Urol. 2014;32(4):925–30.
10. Javed S, Chadwick E, Edwards AA, Beveridge S, Laing R, Bott S, et al. Does HistoScanningTM play a role in detecting prostate cancer in routine clinical practice? Results from three independent studies. BJU Int. 2014;114(4):541–8.
11. De Coninck V, Braeckman J, Michielsen D. Prostate HistoScanning: a screening tool for prostate cancer? Int J Urol. 2013;20:1184–90.
12. Chun FK, Epstein JI, Ficarra V, Freedland SJ, Montironi R, Montorsi F, et al. Optimizing performance and interpretation of prostate biopsy: a critical analysis of the literature. Eur Urol. 2010;58:851–64.
13. Braeckman J, Autier P, Soviany C, Nir R, Nir D, Michielsen D, et al. The accuracy of transrectal ultrasonography supplemented with computer-aided ultrasonography for detecting small prostate cancers. BJU Int. 2008;102:1560–5.
14. Schiffmann J, Fischer J, Tennstedt P, Beyer B, Böhm K, Michl U, et al. Comparison of prostate cancer volume measured by HistoScanning and final histopathological results. World J Urol. 2014;32(4):939–44.
15. Haas GP, Delongchamps NB, Jones RF, Chandan V, Serio AM, Vickers AJ, et al. Needle biopsies on autopsy prostates: sensitivity of cancer detection based on true prevalence. J Natl Cancer Inst. 2007;99:1484–9.
16. Abdollah F, Novara G, Briganti A, Scattoni V, Raber M, Roscigno M, et al. Trans-rectal versus trans-perineal saturation rebiopsy of the prostate: is there a difference in cancer detection rate? Urology. 2011;77:921–5.

17. Somford DM, Hoeks CM, de Kaa CA H-v, Hambrock T, Fütterer JJ, Witjes JA, et al. Evaluation of diffusion-weighted MR imaging at inclusion in an active surveillance protocol for low-risk prostate cancer. Invest Radiol. 2013;48:152–7.

18. Barentsz JO, Richenberg J, Clements R, Choyke P, Verma S, Villeirs G, et al. ESUR prostate MR guidelines 2012. Eur Radiol. 2012;22:746–57.

19. Moore CM, Robertson NL, Arsanious N, Middleton T, Villers A, Klotz L, et al. Image-guided prostate biopsy using magnetic resonance imaging-derived targets: a systematic review. Eur Urol. 2013;63(1):125–40.

20. Salomon G, Drews N, Autier P, Beckmann A, Heinzer H, Hansen J, et al. Incremental detection rate of prostate cancer by real-time elastography targeted biopsies in combination with a conventional 10-core biopsy in 1024 consecutive patients. BJU Int. 2014;113(4):548–53.

21. Grabski B, Baeurle L, Loch A, Wefer B, Paul U, Loch T. Computerized transrectal ultrasound of the prostate in a multicenter setup (C-TRUS-MS): detection of cancer after multiple negative systematic random and in primary biopsies. World J Urol. 2011;29(5):573–9.

10

46,XX testicular disorder of sexual development with *SRY*-negative caused by some unidentified mechanisms

Tian-Fu Li[1†], Qiu-Yue Wu[1†], Cui Zhang[1], Wei-Wei Li[1], Qing Zhou[1], Wei-Jun Jiang[1], Ying-Xia Cui[1], Xin-Yi Xia[1*] and Yi-Chao Shi[2*]

Abstract

Background: 46,XX testicular disorder of sex development is a rare genetic syndrome, characterized by a complete or partial mismatch between genetic sex and phenotypic sex, which results in infertility because of the absence of the azoospermia factor region in the long arm of Y chromosome.

Case presentation: We report a case of a 14-year-old male with microorchidism and mild bilateral gynecomastia who referred to our hospital because of abnormal gender characteristics. The patient was treated for congenital scrotal type hypospadias at the age of 4 years. Semen analysis indicated azoospermia by centrifugation of ejaculate. Levels of follicle-stimulating hormone and luteinizing hormone were elevated, while that of testosterone was low and those of estradiol and prolactin were normal. The results of gonadal biopsy showed hyalinization of the seminiferous tubules, but there was no evidence of spermatogenic cells. Karyotype analysis of the patient confirmed 46,XX karyotype and fluorescent *in situ* hybridization analysis of the sex-determining region Y (*SRY*) gene was negative. Molecular analysis revealed that the *SRY* gene and the AZFa, AZFb and AZFc regions were absent. No mutation was detected in the coding region and exon/intron boundaries of the *RSPO1*, *DAX1*, *SOX9*, *SOX3*, *SOX10*, *ROCK1*, and *DMRT* genes, and no copy number variation in the whole genome sequence was found.

Conclusion: This study adds a new case of *SRY*-negative 46,XX testicular disorder of sex development and further verifies the view that the absence of major regions from the Y chromosome leads to an incomplete masculine phenotype, abnormal hormone levels and infertility. To date, the mechanisms for induction of testicular tissue in 46, XX *SRY*-negative patients remain unknown, although other genetic or environmental factors play a significant role in the regulation of sex determination and differentiation.

Keywords: 46,XX testicular disorder of sex development, Ambiguous genitalia, *SRY*-negative

* Correspondence: xinyixia78@gmail.com; yichaoshi71@gmail.com
†Equal contributors
[1]Department of Reproduction and Genetics, Institute of Laboratory Medicine, Jinling Hospital, Nanjing University School of Medicine, Nanjing 210002, PR China
[2]Center for Reproduction and Genetics, Suzhou Municipal Hospital, Nanjing Medical University Affiliated Suzhou Hospital, 26 Daoqian Street, Suzhou 215002, PR China

Background

46,XX testicular disorder of sex development (DSD) is a rare genetic syndrome, which is characterized by a complete or partial mismatch between genetic sex and phenotypic sex [1]. In addition, 46,XX testicular DSD always presents as one of three phenotypes: (1) classic XX males, infertility with normal male internal and external genitalia; (2) XX males with ambiguous genitalia, which is usually apparent at birth by external genital ambiguities, such as hypospadias, micropenis, or hyperclitoridy, and (3) XX true hermaphrodites with internal or external genital ambiguities detected at birth [2-4]. The sex-determining region Y (SRY) gene plays a major role in encoding a testis determining factor (TDF), which is located on the Y chromosome [5,6]. Approximately 80% of patients with 46,XX testicular DSD are SRY-positive and usually have a normal male phenotype at birth. Other SRY-negative 46,XX males exhibit different degrees of masculinization [7]. However, even though 46,XX males carry different phenotypes, these patients are often infertile because of the absence of the AZFa, AZFb and AZFc regions [8].

Here, we analyzed the clinical characteristics, chromosomal karyotype, and related genes in a male with 46,XX testicular DSD, who referred to our hospital because of abnormal gender characteristics. The aim of the present study was to investigate the different clinical characteristics in different categories of sex reversed 46,XX individuals and the relationships with variable clinical phenotypes and expression levels of the SRY, RSPO1, DAX1, SOX9, SOX3, SOX10, ROCK1, and DMRT genes. We also reviewed the literature to identify proposed mechanisms to explain the etiology of SRY-negative 46,XX sex reversal (Table 1).

Case presentation

Participant and clinical data

A 14-year-old male with microorchidism and mild bilateral gynecomastia was referred to our outpatient clinic because of abnormal gender characteristics. A physical examination included measurement of height, assessment of potential gynecomastia, and inspection of the external sex organs. Bilateral volume was calculated as the sum of the volume of both testes. Semen analysis was assessed according to the guidelines of the World Health Organization. Serum levels of follicle-stimulating hormone (FSH), luteinizing hormone (LH), estradiol (E2), prolactin (PRL), and testosterone (T) were also assessed.

Methods

Histopathological examination of gonadal tissue

A gonadal biopsy was performed and specimens were obtained, sliced into 4 μm-thick histological sections, and stained with hematoxylin-eosin (HE) for microscopic analysis [9].

Immunohistochemical staining of gonadal tissue for inhibin and vimentin

Gonadal tissue from the patient was fixed in 10% buffered formalin solution, embedded in paraffin, and sliced into 3-μm sections for immunostaining with monoclonal antibodies against inhibin and vimentin (HZ817454; dilution, 1:400; Enzyme Chain Biotechnology Co., Ltd., Shanghai, China). The tissue sections were dewaxed and subjected to antigen retrieval (pressure cooking for 1 min, 15 psi, in 0.001 M EDTA, pH 8.0). Immunohistochemical staining of inhibin and vimentin was performed using the EnVision™ + System (K5007; Dako Denmark A/S, Glostrup, Denmark) [9].

Table 1 Milestones of 46,XX testicular DSD

Year	Viewpoints		References
1964	46,XX testicular DSD was first described.		Delachapelle et al. [1]
1992	SRY-positive	The SRY gene plays a major role in encoding TDF and indicated that SRY-positive 46,XX males were infertile.	McElreavey et al. [4]
2001; 2004	SRY-negative	Hidden mosaicism was reported to cause TH in some 46,XX SRY-negative patients, but the results were differed.	Nieto et al. [14] Domenice et al. [15]
2008; 2011		Up/down regulation of the testis/ovarian signaling pathways was found.	Smith et al. [17] Tomaselli et al. [18]
2010–2013	Described the function of the genes located downstream of the SRY gene.	DAX1, SOX9, SOX3, SOX10, ROCK1, DMRT	Mizuno et al. [13] Sukumaran et al. [23] Moalem et al. [24] Sutton et al. [25] Laronda et al. [26] Polanco et al. [27]

Karyotype analysis of G-banding in lymphocytes and fluorescence in situ hybridization (FISH)

Karyotyping of 100 metaphase lymphocytes from peripheral blood was performed by conventional techniques. The X chromosome, Y chromosome, and SRY gene were located using FISH with probes specific for the centromeres of the X and Y chromosomes (item no.: 32-111051CEP X with Spectrum Green and CEP Y with Spectrum Orange; Vysis, Inc., Downers Grove, IL, USA) and SRY gene (item no.: 30–190079, SRY with Orange; Vysis, Inc.) [10].

Molecular analysis

Genomic DNA from peripheral blood was extracted using the QIAamp DNA Blood Kit (Qiagen GmbH, Hilden, Germany). Three discrete regions (AZFa, AZFb, and AZFc) located on the long arm of Y chromosome were amplified by multiplex polymerase chain reaction (PCR) using primers specific for the diagnosis of microdeletion of the AZFa, AZFb, and AZFc regions, which included sY84, sY86, sY127, sY134, sY254, sY255, SRY, and ZFX/ZFY. Then, the RSPO1, DAX1, SOX9, SOX3, SOX10, ROCK1, and DMRT genes were amplified and sequenced [10]. We also analyzed the presence of SRY sequence in fresh gonadal tissues from this 46,XX male case.

Single nucleotide polymorphism array

Genomic DNA of the patient was extracted and analyzed using the Cytogenetics Whole-Genome 2.7 M Array (Affymetrix, Inc., Santa Clara, CA, USA), especially for the SOX9 gene, located between 64000 kb and 72000 kb on chromosome 17q24.2–25.1, according to the manufacturer's protocols. Briefly, genomic DNA was denatured, neutralized, and then amplified by PCR. The PCR products were then purified, fragmented, and end-labeled with biotin. The fragmented, labeled PCR products were then hybridized overnight to the arrays. The variation in copy number was analyzed using Chromosome Analysis Suite software (v1.2.2; Affymetrix, Inc.) [11].

Ethics statement

The research adhered to the tenets of the Declaration of Helsinki. The Ethics Committee of Jinling Hospital approved the protocols used in this study. Written informed consent was obtained from the parent of the patient for publication of this case report and any accompanying images. A copy of the written consent is available for review by the Editor of this journal.

Results

The patient was treated for congenital scrotal type hypospadias at the age of 4 years. On physical evaluation, the patient's weight was 51 kg (age-appropriate mean weight, 53.37 ± 9.29 kg) and height was 155 cm (age-appropriate mean height, 165.90 ± 7.21 cm). The grade of

gynecomastia was IA [12]. Pubic hair was normal, the length of stretched penile was 3 cm and bilateral testicular volume was 2 mL. The results of laboratory analysis were as follows: T = 5.8 nmol/L (normal range, 9.4–37 nmol/L), E2 = 0.142 nmol/L (normal range, 0.129–0.239 nmol/L), FSH = 24.4 IU/L (normal range, 1.5–11.5 IU/L), LH = 15.7 IU/L (normal range, 1.1–8.2 IU/L), and PRL = 174.2 mIU/L (normal range, 89.04–826.8 mIU/L). Semen analysis by centrifugation of the ejaculate indicated azoospermia and no spermatogenic cells were observed. The levels of seminal plasma fructose, α-glucosidase, and acid phosphatase were 2.08 g/L (normal range, 0.87–3.95 g/L), 51.93 U/mL (normal range, 35.1–87.7 U/mL), and 12.37 U (normal range, 48.8–208.6 U), respectively.

The gonadal biopsy results showed hyalinization of the seminiferous tubules, but without evidence of spermatogenic cells (Figure 1). Consistent with gonadal biopsy, immunohistochemical analysis also confirmed that the gonadal tissue was immunoreactivity positive to inhibin and vimentin, respectively (Figure 2), which indicated the presence of Leydig cells. Karyotype analysis of the patient confirmed a 46,XX karyotype and FISH analysis was negative for the SRY gene (Figure 3). Molecular analysis revealed locus deletions at SY84, SY86, SY127, SY134, SY254, and SY255 within the AZF sequence on chromosome Y, with the absence of the SRY gene (Figure 4). Sequencing of the coding regions and exon/intron boundaries of the RSPO1, DAX1, SOX9, SOX3, SOX10, ROCK1, and DMRT genes detected no mutations. No copy number variation in the whole genome sequence was found. In particular, there was no variation in copy number between positions 64000 kb and 72000 kb of chromosome 17q24.2-25.1. Duplication of this region, which codes for SOX9, can trigger sex reversal (Figure 5).

Discussion

46,XX testicular DSD is a rare form of sex reversal in infertile men, which was first described by la Chapelle et al. in 1964 with a frequency of 1:20,000 of newborn males [1]. Most males have normal phenotypes at birth and are usually diagnosed in adolescence because of delayed puberty, gynecomastia, or infertility. Moreover, some XX males have hypospadias, cryptorchidism, or more severe genital ambiguity. However, all 46,XX males are infertile because of the absence of the azoospermia factor region in the long arm of the Y chromosome. 46,XX males can be classified into two subgroups, SRY-positive and SRY-negative, according to the presence or absence of the SRY gene, which is located in the Y chromosome and regulates testicular differentiation [10]. Patients with SRY-positive, which always translocates to the X chromosome or to an autosome, are usually more likely to have a normal male phenotype at birth and are

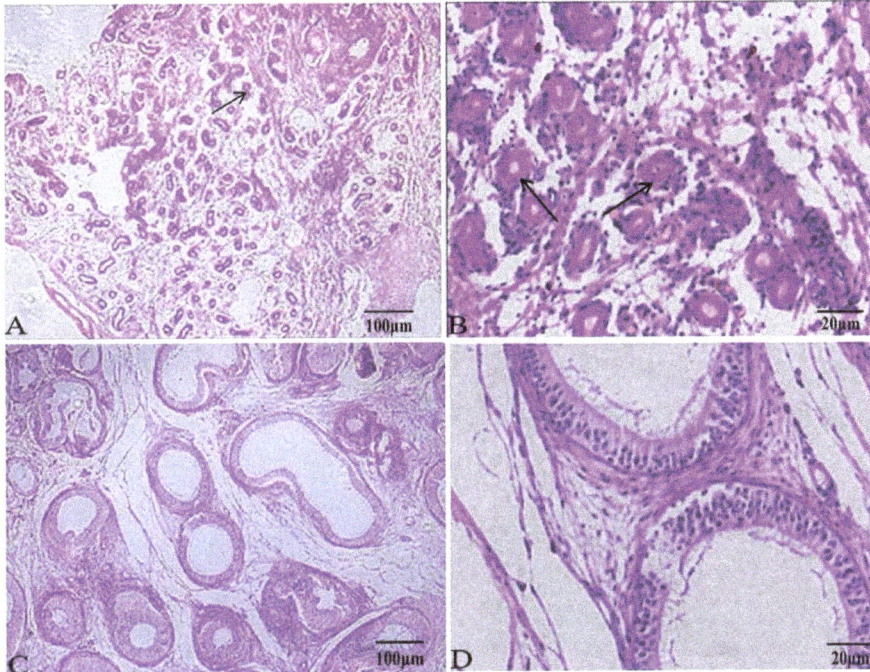

Figure 1 Histological examination of gonadal tissue by HE staining under light microscopy. The results of gonadal biopsy showed the appearance of hyalinization of the seminiferous tubules, but without evidence of spermatogenic cells. **(A)** and **(B)** are testis tissue; **(C)** and **(D)** are epididymis tissue. The black arrows show hyalinization of seminiferous tubules in **(A)** and **(B)**.

referred for infertility treatment after puberty. *SRY*-negative patients include those with ovotesticular-DSD, which is characterized by the presence of testicular and ovarian tissue in the same individual. Testicular-DSD is characterized by full development of both gonads as testes without evidence of ovarian tissue [13].

The mechanisms of testicular tissue induction in *SRY*-negative patients remain unknown, although several hypotheses have been proposed, as follows: (1) hidden gonadal mosaicism for *SRY*; (2) mutations in some auto-somal or X-linked genes that repress the male pathway can result in de-repression of the male pathway in XX

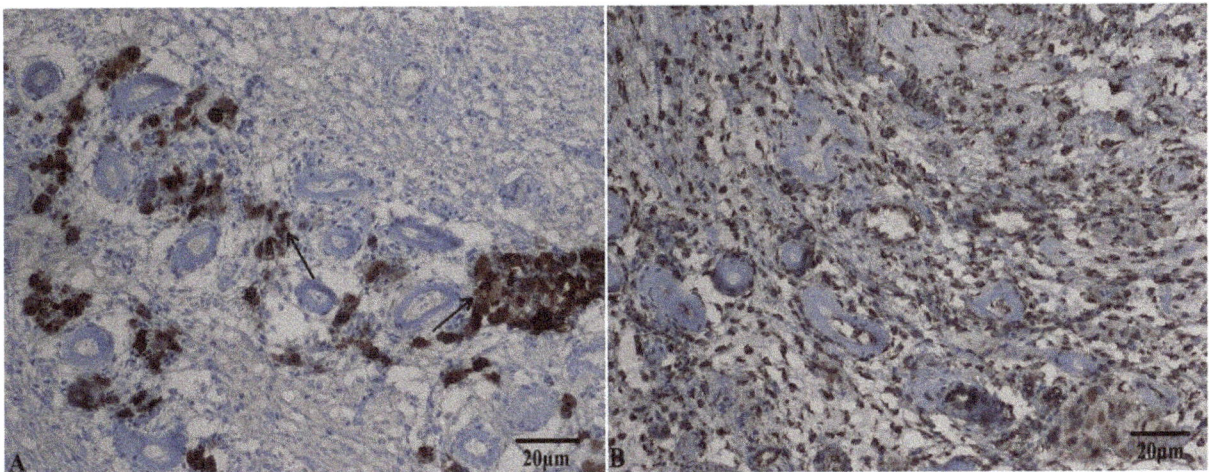

Figure 2 Immunohistochemical staining of inhibin and vimentin was observed by light microscopy. Immunohistochemical analysis also confirmed the gonadal tissue had positive immunoreactivity to inhibin **(A)** and vimentin **(B)**, which indicated the presence of Leydig cells. The black arrows in **(A)** indicated that the tissue was positive for inhibin by immunohistochemical staining.

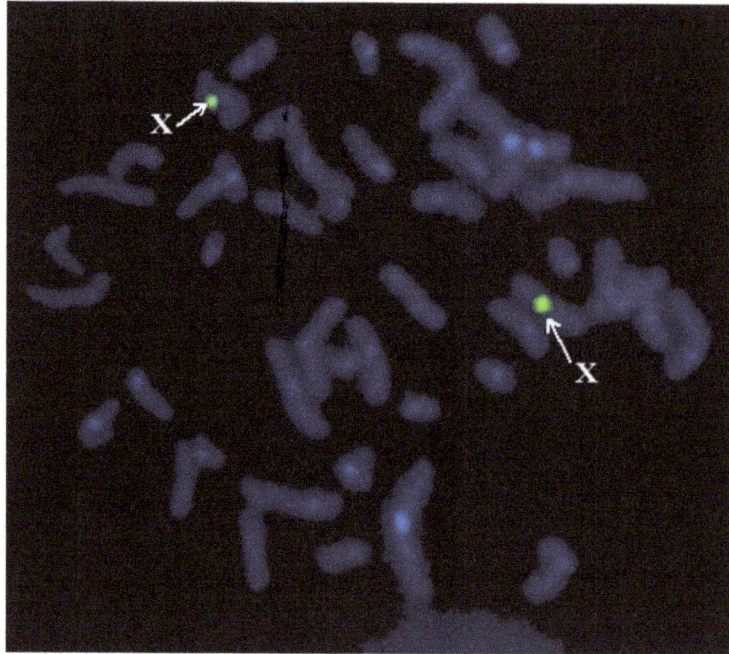

Figure 3 FISH was used to analysis of metaphase chromosomes of a second case using the LSI *SRY* (orange) / CEP X (green) probes. FISH showed the absence of the SRY gene in our patient, while there were two green signals of the X chromosome (white arrows).

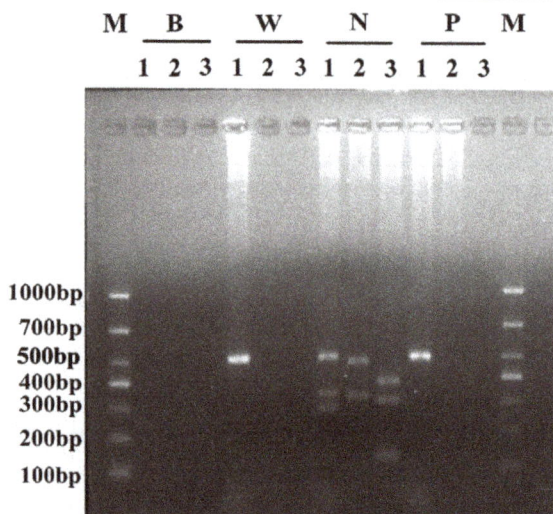

Figure 4 Result of multiplex polymerase chain reaction (PCR). Multiplex 1: ZFX/ZFY (690 bp), sY84 (320 bp), and sY127 (274 bp); Multiplex 2: SRY (472 bp) and sY86 (326 bp); Multiplex 3: sY254 (400 bp), sY134 (301 bp), and sY255 (126 bp). M: DL1000 DNA Marker; W: a DNA sample from a woman as a negative control; N: a DNA sample from a normal fertile man as a positive control; P: a DNA sample from the patient; B: a blank (water) control.

gonads; and (3) altered expression of other sex determining genes downstream of the *SRY*.

True hermaphroditism (TH), also known as ovotesticular-DSD, is a rare form of intersexuality characterized by the presence of testicular and ovarian tissue in the same individual. Genetic heterogeneity has been proposed as a cause of dual gonadal development in some cases and recently, hidden mosaicism was reported to cause TH in some *SRY*-negative 46,XX patients [14]. However, Domenice *et al.* [15] reported the absence of the SRY sequence in DNA from blood samples of all true hermaphrodites and in testicular and ovarian tissues of a 46,XX true hermaphrodite case and a 46,XX male with ambiguous genitalia, which indicated that cryptic SRY mosaicism in gonadal tissues is not the usual mechanism responsible for testicular development in patients with 46,XX true hermaphroditism.

R-Spondin1 (*RSPO1*) is a novel regulator of ovary development through the up-regulation of the Wnt/β-catenin signaling pathway to oppose testis formation [16,17]. Loss-of-function mutations in human *RSPO1* lead to reduced β-catenin protein and WNT4 mRNA levels, consistent with downregulation of ovarian pathways, which cause testicular differentiation in 46,XX females [18].

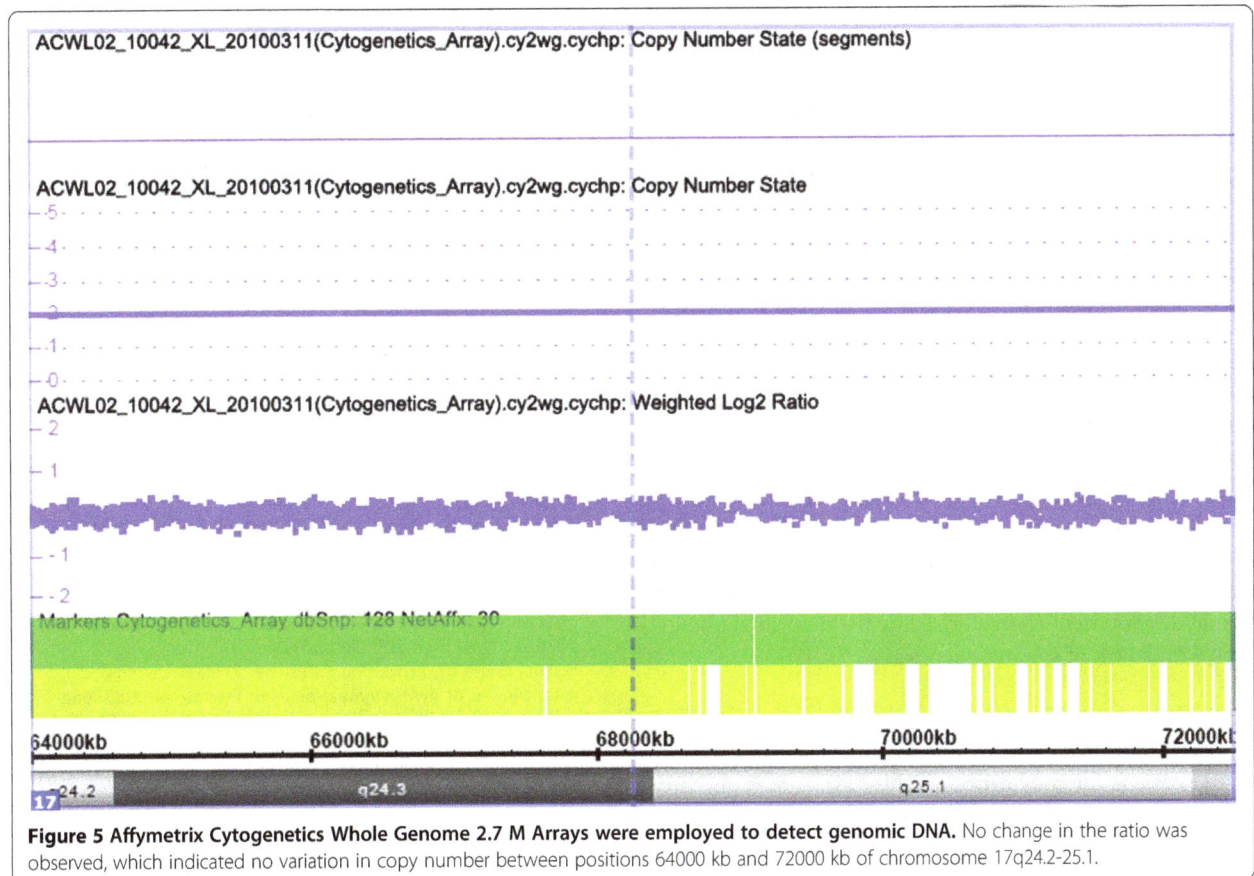

Figure 5 Affymetrix Cytogenetics Whole Genome 2.7 M Arrays were employed to detect genomic DNA. No change in the ratio was observed, which indicated no variation in copy number between positions 64000 kb and 72000 kb of chromosome 17q24.2-25.1.

Previous reports have identified gene dysregulation in 46,XX *SRY*-negative DSD. The *SRY*-box 9 (*SOX9*) gene is a widely expressed transcription factor that plays several relevant functions during development and essential for testes differentiation, which is considered to be the direct target gene of the *SRY* [19]. The essential role of *SOX9* in male gonadal development was initially described in mice and subsequent reports stated that *SOX9* duplications were a relevant cause of *SRY*-negative XX sex reversal in dogs [20]. *SOX9* duplication was reported for the first time in Korea in a case involving a 4.2-year-old SRY-negative 46,XX boy with complete sex reversal, which indicated that *SOX9* duplication was a rare cause of 46,XX testicular DSD in humans [21]. The genomic domain regulating SOX9 expression spans more than 1 Mb upstream of SOX9 [11]. Benko *et al*. [22] revealed that a non-coding regulatory region located far upstream of the *SOX9* promoter was critical for gonadal *SOX9* expression and subsequent normal sexual development and copy number variations were the genetic basis of isolated 46,XX testicular DSD of variable severity. Moreover, the minimum critical region associated with gonadal development, about a 67-kb region located 584–517 kb upstream of *SOX9*, was confirmed to induce *SOX9* overexpression in female-to-male sex reversal [11].

Regulatory elements in the duplication region might enhance SOX9 expression through complex mechanisms. It has been suggested that changes in SOX9 expression resulting from disruptions in some regions upstream of SOX9 could be important in 46,XX testicular disorder of sexual development. However, other groups have suggested that duplication in the region of 17q that contains *SOX9* is not a common cause of testis development in subjects with *SRY*-negative 46,XX testicular or ovotesticular DSD [23].

Consistent with *SOX9*, the *DAX1* gene might also function downstream of the *SRY* gene in the sex-determination pathway. Overexpression of the *DAX1* gene could cause female-to-male sex reversal [24]. *ROCK1* (Rho-associated, coiled-coil protein kinase 1) phosphorylates and activates *SOX9* in Sertoli cells to initiate testes formation [13]. *SOX3* was recently shown to upregulate *SOX9* expression via a similar mechanism to *SRY* and modulate XX male sex reversal in humans through gain-of-function mutations mediated by genomic rearrangements around *SOX3*, possibly leading to its altered regulation [25-27]. Overexpression of the *SOX10* gene at 22q13 might be the cause of sex reversal [28].

However, the above mechanisms were not applicable in this case, as any hidden gonadal mosaicism for *SRY* or mutations to autosomal or sex-linked genes that repress the male pathway and alter expression of other sex determining genes downstream of *SRY* were found in our case. These findings suggest that other unidentified genetic or environmental factors play significant roles in the regulation of sex determination and differentiation.

Conclusions

46,XX *SRY*-negative individuals with complete masculinization are rare and usually exhibit phenotypic differences. Our patient had incomplete masculinization, which was characterized by microorchidism and mild bilateral gynecomastia, and was diagnosed with abnormal gender characteristics. His T level was low and levels of FSH and LH were elevated. Furthermore, we detected locus deletions at SY84, SY86, SY127, SY134, SY254, and SY255 within the AZF sequence on chromosome Y, with the absence of the *SRY* gene. Further studies are needed to explain the mechanisms of 46,XX testicular disorder of sexual development characterized by the described phenotype with a lack of spermatogenesis.

Consent

Written informed consent was obtained from the parent of the patient for publication of this case report and any accompanying images. A copy of the written consent is available for review by the Editor of this journal.

Abbreviations
DSD: Disorder of sex development; *SRY*: Sex-determining region Y; TDF: Testis determining factor; FSH: Follicle-stimulating Hormone; LH: Luteinizing Hormone; E2: Estradiol; PRL: Prolactin; T: Testosterone; PCR: Polymerase Chain Reaction; FISH: Fluorescent in situ hybridization; TH: True hermaphroditism; Rspo1: R-Spondin1; *SOX9*: *SRY*-box 9; *ROCK1*: Rho-associated, coiled-coil protein kinase 1.

Competing interests
The authors declare that they have no competing interests.

Authors' contributions
TFL, QYW, XYX and YCS conceived and designed the experiments. WWL, CZ, QZ, WJJ and YXC performed the experiments. YCS and QYW analyzed the data. TFL and XYX wrote the paper. All authors read and approved the final manuscript.

Acknowledgments
This work was supported by Natural Science Foundation of Jiangsu Province (BK2011660 and BK2012601), Key Foundation of Jiangsu Science and Technology Bureau (BM2013058) and Nature Science Foundation of China (81170611).

References
1. Delachapelle A, Hortling H, Niemi M, Wennström J: XX sex chromosomes in a human male. First case. *Acta Med Scand* 1964, 175(Suppl 412):25–28.
2. Abbas NE, Toublanc JE, Boucekkine C, Toublanc M, Affara NA, Job J-C, Fellous M: A possible common origin of "Y-negative" human XX males and XX true hermaphrodites. *Hum Genet* 1990, 84(4):356–360.
3. Boucekkine C, Toublanc J, Abbas N, Chaabouni S, Ouahid S, Semrouni M, Jaubert F, Toublanc M, McElreavey K, Vilain E: Clinical and anatomical spectrum in XX sex reversed patients. Relationship to the presence of Y specific DNA-sequences. *Clin Endocrinol* 1994, 40(6):733–742.
4. McElreavey K, Rappaport R, Vilain E, Abbas N, Richaud F, Lortat-Jacob S, Berger R, LeConiat M, Boucekkine C, Kucheria K: A minority of 46, XX true hermaphrodites are positive for the Y-DNA sequence including SRY. *Hum Genet* 1992, 90(1–2):121–125.
5. Anık A, Çatlı G, Abacı A, Böber E: 46, XX male disorder of sexual development: a case report. *J Clin Res Pediatr Endocrinol* 2013, 5(4):258–260.
6. Jain M, V V, Chaudhary I, Halder A: The Sertoli Cell Only Syndrome and Glaucoma in a Sex-Determining Region Y (SRY) Positive XX Infertile Male. *J Clin Diagn Res* 2013, 7(7):1457–1459.
7. Vorona E, Zitzmann M, Gromoll J, Schuring AN, Nieschlag E: Clinical, endocrinological, and epigenetic features of the 46, XX male syndrome, compared with 47, XXY Klinefelter patients. *J Clin Endocrinol Metab* 2007, 92(9):3458–3465.
8. Rizvi AA: 46, XX man with SRY gene translocation: cytogenetic characteristics, clinical features and management. *Am J Med Sci* 2008, 335(4):307–309.
9. Eghbali M, Sadeghi MR, Lakpour N, Edalatkhah H, Zeraati H, Soltanghoraee H, Akhondi MM, Hashemi SB, Modarressi MH: Molecular analysis of testis biopsy and semen pellet as complementary methods with histopathological analysis of testis in non-obstructive azoospermia. *J Assist Reprod Genet* 2014, 31(6):707–715.
10. Wu QY, Li N, Li WW, Li TF, Zhang C, Cui YX, Xia XY, Zhai JS: Clinical, molecular and cytogenetic analysis of 46, XX testicular disorder of sex development with SRY-positive. *BMC Urol* 2014, 14(1):70.
11. Xiao B, Ji X, Xing Y, Chen YW, Tao J: A rare case of 46, XX SRY-negative male with approximately 74-kb duplication in a region upstream of SOX9. *Eur J Med Genet* 2013, 56(12):695–698.
12. Rohrich RJ, Ha RY, Kenkel JM, Adams WP Jr: Classification and management of gynecomastia: defining the role of ultrasound-assisted liposuction. *Plast Reconstr Surg* 2003, 111(2):909–923.
13. Mizuno K, Kojima Y, Kamisawa H, Moritoki Y, Nishio H, Kohri K, Hayashi Y: Gene expression profile during testicular development in patients with SRY-negative 46,XX testicular disorder of sex development. *Urology* 2013, 82(6):1453. e1-e7.
14. Nieto K, Peña R, Palma I, Dorantes LM, Eraña L, Alvarez R, García-Cavazos R, Kofman-Alfaro S, Queipo G: 45, X/47, XXX/47, XX, del (Y)(p?)/46, XX mosaicism causing true hermaphroditism. *Am J Med Genet A* 2004, 130A(3):311–314.
15. Domenice S, Nishi MY, Billerbeck AE, Carvalho FM, Frade EM, Latronico AC, Arnhold IJ, Mendonca BB: Molecular analysis of SRY gene in Brazilian 46, XX sex reversed patients: absence of SRY sequence in gonadal tissue. *Med Sci Monit* 2001, 7(2):238–241.
16. De Lau WB, Snel B, Clevers HC: The R-spondin protein family. *Genome Biol* 2012, 13(3):242.
17. Smith CA, Shoemaker CM, Roeszler KN, Queen J, Crews D, Sinclair AH: Cloning and expression of R-Spondin1 in different vertebrates suggests a conserved role in ovarian development. *BMC Dev Biol* 2008, 8(1):72.
18. Tomaselli S, Megiorni F, Lin L, Mazzilli MC, Gerrelli D, Majore S, Grammatico P, Achermann JC: Human RSPO1/R-spondin1 is expressed during early ovary development and augments β-catenin signaling. *PLoS One* 2011, 6(1):e16366.
19. Vetro A, Ciccone R, Giorda R, Patricelli MG, Della Mina E, Forlino A, Zuffardi O: XX males SRY negative: a confirmed cause of infertility. *J Med Genet* 2011, 48(10):710–712.
20. Rossi E, Radi O, De Lorenzi L, Vetro A, Groppetti D, Bigliardi E, Luvoni GC, Rota A, Camerino G, Zuffardi O: Sox9 duplications are a relevant cause of Sry-negative XX sex reversal dogs. *PLoS One* 2014, 9(7):e101244.
21. Lee GM, Ko JM, Shin CH, Yang SW: A Korean boy with 46, XX testicular disorder of sex development caused by SOX9 duplication. *Ann Pediatr Endocrinol Metab* 2014, 19(2):108–112.
22. Benko S, Gordon CT, Mallet D, Sreenivasan R, Thauvin-Robinet C, Brendehaug A, Thomas S, Bruland O, David M, Nicolino M, Labalme A, Sanlaville D, Callier P, Malan V, Huet F, Molven A, Dijoud F, Munnich A, Faivre L, Amiel J, Harley V, Houge G, Morel Y, Lyonnet S: Disruption of a long distance regulatory region upstream of SOX9 in isolated disorders of sex development. *J Med Genet* 2011, 48(12):825–830.
23. Temel SG, Cangul H: Duplication of SOX9 is not a common cause of 46, XX testicular or 46, XX ovotesticular DSD. *J Pediatr Endocrinol Metab* 2013, 26(1–2):191.

24. Sukumaran A, Desmangles JC, Gartner LA, Buchlis J: **Duplication of dosage sensitive sex reversal area in a 46, XY patient with normal sex determining region of Y causing complete sex reversal.** *J Pediatr Endocrinol Metab* 2013, **26**(7–8):775–779.

25. Moalem S, Babul-Hirji R, Stavropolous DJ, Wherrett D, Bägli DJ, Thomas P, Chitayat D: **XX male sex reversal with genital abnormalities associated with a de novo SOX3 gene duplication.** *Am J Med Genet A* 2012, **158A**(7):1759–1764.

26. Sutton E, Hughes J, White S, Sekido R, Tan J, Arboleda V, Rogers N, Knower K, Rowley L, Eyre H, Rizzoti K, McAninch D, Goncalves J, Slee J, Turbitt E, Bruno D, Bengtsson H, Harley V, Vilain E, Sinclair A, Lovell-Badge R, Thomas P: **Identification of SOX3 as an XX male sex reversal gene in mice and humans.** *J Clin Invest* 2011, **121**(1):328–341.

27. Laronda MM, Jameson JL: **Sox3 functions in a cell-autonomous manner to regulate spermatogonial differentiation in mice.** *Endocrinology* 2011, **152**(4):1606–1615.

28. Polanco JC, Wilhelm D, Davidson TL, Knight D, Koopman P: **Sox10 gain-of-function causes XX sex reversal in mice: implications for human 22q-linked disorders of sex development.** *Hum Mol Genet* 2010, **19**(3):506–516.

11

Targeting *HOX* transcription factors in prostate cancer

Richard Morgan[1*], Angie Boxall[1], Kevin J Harrington[2], Guy R Simpson[1], Agnieszka Michael[1] and Hardev S Pandha[1]

Abstract

Background: The *HOX* genes are a family of transcription factors that help to determine cell and tissue identity during early development, and which are also over-expressed in a number of malignancies where they have been shown to promote cell proliferation and survival. The purpose of this study was to evaluate the expression of *HOX* genes in prostate cancer and to establish whether prostate cancer cells are sensitive to killing by HXR9, an inhibitor of *HOX* function.

Methods: *HOX* function was inhibited using the HXR9 peptide. *HOX* gene expression was assessed by RNA extraction from cells or tissues followed by quantitative PCR, and siRNA was used to block the expression of the *HOX* target gene, *cFos*. *In vivo* modelling involved a mouse flank tumour induced by inoculation with LNCaP cells.

Results: In this study we show that the expression of *HOX* genes in prostate tumours is greatly increased with respect to normal prostate tissue. Targeting the interaction between HOX proteins and their PBX cofactor induces apoptosis in the prostate cancer derived cell lines PC3, DU145 and LNCaP, through a mechanism that involves a rapid increase in the expression of *cFos*, an oncogenic transcription factor. Furthermore, disrupting HOX/PBX binding using the HXR9 antagonist blocks the growth of LNCaP tumours in a xenograft model over an extended period.

Conclusion: Many *HOX* genes are highly over-expressed in prostate cancer, and prostate cancer cells are sensitive to killing by HXR9 both *in vitro* and *in vivo*. The *HOX* genes are therefore a potential therapeutic target in prostate cancer.

Keywords: Prostate cancer, HXR9, *HOX*, PBX

Background

Prostate cancer is the most prevalent male malignancy with just under one million new cases worldwide each year [1]. Treatment pathways for this disease are relatively well defined and include surgery, radiotherapy and/or hormonal therapy. While the majority of patients with early stage disease are cured, 10-15% patient still develop locally recurrent or metastatic disease and have a significantly reduced survival rate [2]. Despite the general adoption of docetaxel chemotherapy agents and novel agents such as abiraterone [3], there is still an urgent need to develop effective new treatments, and therefore it is necessary to explore new target proteins and intracellular signalling pathways.

Recently, considerable interest has been shown in genes that play key roles in defining the identity of cells and tissues in early development and which therefore also have important regulatory roles in cell proliferation and survival. One group of genes that fit into this category are the *HOX* family of transcription factors [4]. HOX proteins are characterised in part by a highly conserved homeodomain that mediates DNA binding, together with a defined set of co-factors that modify their function including members of PBX family [5-7]. The pro-proliferative and anti-apoptotic roles of some *HOX* genes in development make them potential oncogenes, and indeed there are numerous reports of *HOX* overexpression in a range of malignancies, including prostate cancer [4,8-11]. Although definitive oncogenic roles for some *HOX* genes have been described, in general studies on the function of individual *HOX* genes in cancer have

* Correspondence: r.morgan@surrey.ac.uk
[1]Faculty of Health and Medical Sciences, University of Surrey, Guildford, UK
Full list of author information is available at the end of the article

been complicated by the high levels of sequence identity and functional redundancy exhibited by most members [12,13]. This functional redundancy in particular has made the results of conventional knock-down studies (using for example siRNA) hard to interpret. As an alternative approach we developed a peptide, HXR9 that acts as a competitive antagonist of the interaction between HOX proteins and their PBX co-factor. This interaction is mediated by a conserved hexapeptide sequence shared by the majority of HOX proteins, and HXR9 can globally repress HOX function through mimicking this peptide [14-22]. In this study we show that prostate tumours have a highly dysregulated pattern of *HOX* expression and that HXR9 induces apoptosis in prostate cancer derived cell lines through a mechanism that involves a rapid increase in expression of the *cFos* gene. Furthermore, HXR9 can block prostate tumour growth *in vivo* for an extended period, suggesting that HXR9 or its derivatives might represent a possible therapeutic option for locally recurrent prostate cancer.

Methods
Cell lines and culture
The cell lines used in this study were DU145 (derived from a prostate carcinoma brain metastasis) [23], PC3 (derived from a prostate adenocarcinoma bone metastasis) [24], LNCaP (derived from a prostate carcinoma lymph node metastasis)[25], and WPMY-1 (derived from normal prostate stroma and immortalised with SV40 Large T antigen) [26]. They were obtained from the ATCC through LGC Standards Ltd (UK), and were cultured according to the instructions on the LGC Standards website.

Synthesis of HXR9 and CXR9 peptides
HXR9 is an 18 amino acid peptide consisting of the previously identified hexapeptide sequence that can bind to PBX and nine C-terminal arginine residues (R9) that facilitate cell entry. The N-terminal and C-terminal amino bonds are in the D-isomer conformation, which has previously been shown to extend the half-life of the peptide to 12 hours in human serum [19]. CXR9 is a control peptide that includes the R9 sequence but lacks a functional hexapeptide sequence due to a single alanine substitution. All peptides were synthesized using conventional column based chemistry and purified to at least 80% (Biosynthesis Inc, USA). The sequences of the peptides are as follows:

HXR9: WYPWMKKHHRRRRRRRRR (2700.06 Da)
CXR9: WYPAMKKHHRRRRRRRRR (2604.14 Da)

Primary prostate tumour RNA
Total RNA from prostate tumours and normal prostate tissue was obtained from OriGene Technologies Ltd, Rockville, USA. Six normal prostate tissue samples (median age of donor 56 years, range 52–71 years), and 17 prostate tumour samples (median age of donor 60 years, range 48–73 years) were included in the analysis. Of the prostate tumour samples, 5 were Gleason grade 6, 8 were Gleason grade 7, 1 was Gleason grade 8, and 3 were Gleason grade 9. Reverse transcription and QPCR were performed as described below.

RNA purification and reverse transcription
Total RNA was isolated from cells using the RNeasy Plus Mini Kit (Qiagen) by following the manufacturer's protocol. The RNA was denatured by heating to 65°C for 5 minutes. cDNA was synthesized from RNA using the Cloned AMV First Strand Synthesis Kit (Invitrogen) according to the manufacturer's instructions.

Quantitative PCR
Quantitative PCR was done using the Stratagene MX3005P real-time PCR machine and the Brilliant SYBR Green QPCR Master Mix (Stratagene). Oligonucleotide primers were designed to facilitate the unique amplification of β-actin, c-Fos, and each *HOX* gene. The expression of each gene was calculated using the $^{\Delta\Delta}Ct$ method.

Mice and *in vivo* trial
All animal experiments were conducted in accordance with the United Kingdom Co-ordinating Committee on Cancer Research (UKCCCR) guidelines for the Welfare of Animals in Experimental Neoplasia [27]. The experimental protocol was approved by the University of Surrey Animal Welfare Ethical Review Board, and by the UK Home Office (licence number 70/7347).

Athymic nude mice were kept in positive pressure isolators in 12 hour light/dark cycles and food and water were available *ad libitum*. Mice were inoculated subcutaneously with a suspension of 2.5×10^6 LNCaP cells in culture media (100 µl). Once tumours reached volumes of approximately 100 mm^3, mice received an initial, single intratumoural dose of 100 mg/Kg CXR9 or HXR9 dissolved in 0.1 ml PBS, with subsequent dosing when or if the tumour reoccurred. The HXR9 and CXR9 treatment groups contained 9 and 8 mice, respectively. The mice were monitored carefully for signs of distress, including behavioural changes and weight loss.

Results
Multiple *HOX* genes are dysregulated in prostate tumours and cell lines
Previous studies have revealed that *HOX* genes are generally dysregulated in malignant tissue compared to normal adult cells, and we investigated whether this is also the case in prostate cancer. In order to do this we

obtained RNA from three cell lines derived from prostate cancer; DU145 [23], PC3 [24] and LNCaP [25], and a cell line derived from non-malignant prostate stromal cells, WPMY-1 [26]. QPCR analysis of expression levels of all 39 *HOX* genes shows that the tumour derived cell lines have significantly different patterns of *HOX* expression compared to WMPY-1. In particular, the cancer-derived lines all show higher expression of the *HOXC* genes and of *HOXB5* and *HOXB7*, whilst WMPY-1 expresses *HOX* genes closer to the 5′ (posterior) end of each *HOX* cluster (Figure 1).

The HOX/PBX antagonist HXR9 is cytotoxic to prostate cancer derived cell lines

Given the elevated expression of *HOX* genes in both primary prostate tumours and cell lines, we assessed whether the prostate cancer-derived cell lines LNCaP, DU145 and PC3 were sensitive to killing by the HOX/PBX antagonist HXR9. HXR9 is an 18 amino acid peptide that can enter cells via endocytosis mediated by a polyarginine sequence. A fluorescently labelled version of this peptide was taken up by all of the cell lines tested (Figure 2a), and could be detected in both the cytoplasm and the nucleus. As a negative control, we used a second peptide, CXR9, which is identical to HXR9 with the exception of a single alanine substitution in the hexapeptide sequence. PC3 cells treated with 60 μM CXR9 for two hours do not exhibit any apparent cytotoxicity compared to untreated cells (Figure 2b, c), whilst the same

concentration of HXR9 results in extensive cell death (Figure 2d).

The cytotoxicity of HXR9 and CXR9 was determined for all three cancer-derived lines and the non-malignant line WPMY-1 using an MTS assay. This revealed that all three of the lines were sensitive to killing by HXR9, whilst WPMY-1 cells were significantly less sensitive (Figure 2e, f).

HXR9 induces apoptosis in prostate cancer derived cell lines

To further understand the mechanism of HXR9-induced cell death, we studied the activity of caspase 3 in HXR9-treated cells. Caspase 3 is a key component of both the intrinsic and extrinsic apoptotic pathway, and can cleave a group of proteins involved in cell survival and proliferation. All of the prostate cancer derived cell lines showed a significant increase in caspase 3 activity when treated with 60 μM HXR9 for two hours (3.7 fold for PC3 cells and 4.8 fold for both DU145 and LNCaP cells), whilst WPMY-1 cells do not (1.4 fold increase, p = 0.0972). Treatment with CXR9 did not change caspase 3 activity in any of the cell lines (Figure 3a).

To further explore whether HXR9 induces cell death primarily through apoptosis, we also used a FACS based analysis for changes in the cell membrane that are characteristic of process and which can be detected by fluorescently labelled Anexxin. The assay also utilises a fluorescent DNA label (7AAD) to measure the membrane

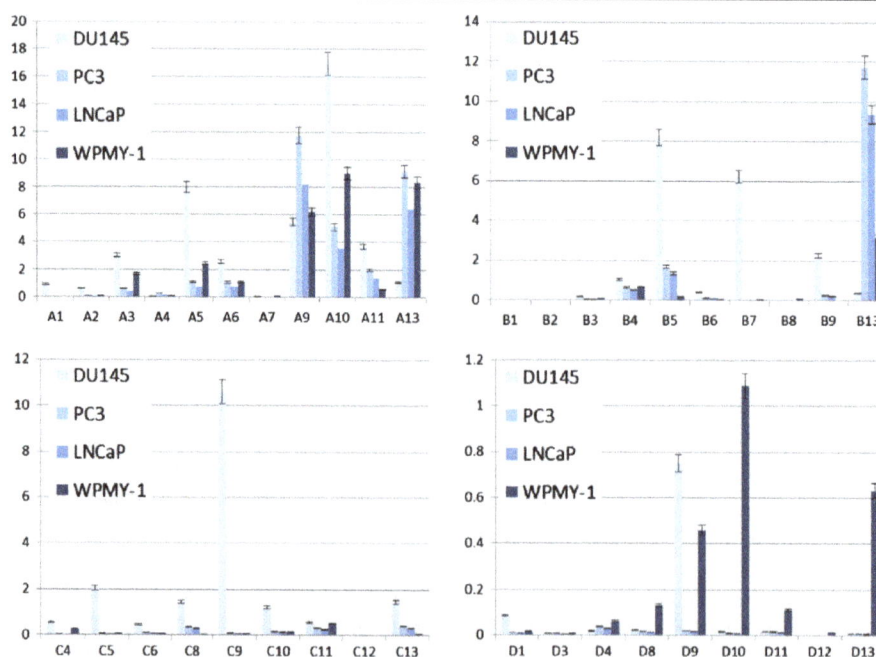

Figure 1 *HOX* gene expression in prostate cancer derived cell lines and in WPMY-1, which is derived from normal prostate cells. The expression of each gene was determined by semi-quantitative PCR and is shown relative to the house keeping gene *GAPDH* (x10000). The values shown are the mean of three independent experiments and the error bars represent the standard error of the mean (SEM).

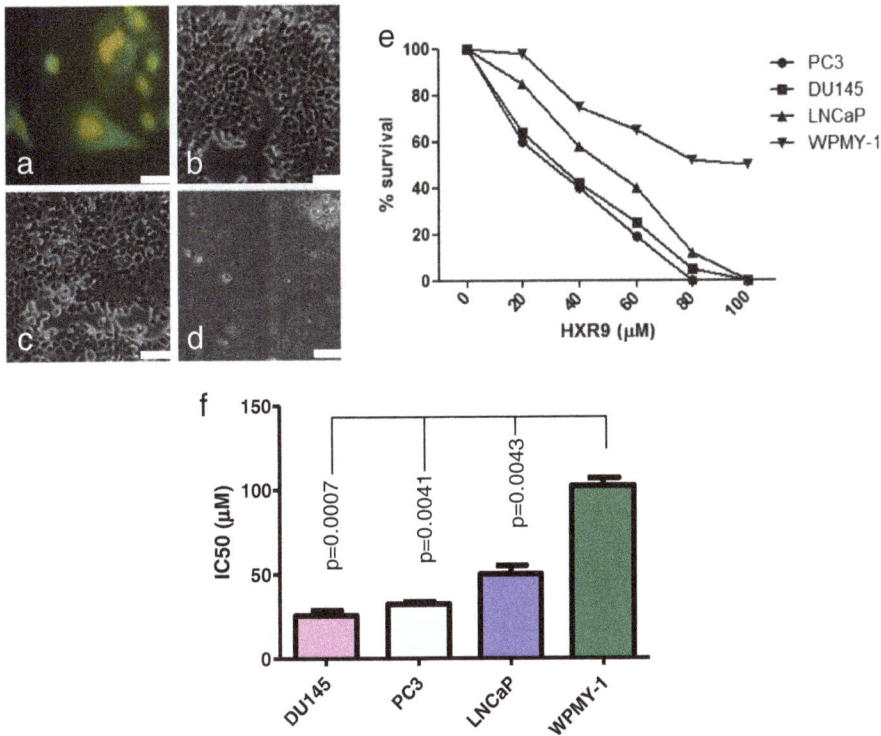

Figure 2 Prostate cancer-derived cell lines are sensitive to killing by the *HOX*/PBX antagonist HXR9. (a) HXR9 enters the cytoplasm and nuclei of PC3 cells *in vitro*. PC3 cells were incubated with 5 µM FITC labelled HXR9 (green) for two hours and then stained with Hoechst S769121 (a fluorescent dye staining nuclei yellow). Scale bar: 20 µm **(b-d)** Light micrographs of PC3 cells either untreated **(b)** or incubated with 60 µM CXR9 **(c)** or HXR9 **(d)** for two hours. Scale bar: 100 µm **(e)** Survival curves for PC3, DU145, LNCaP and WPMY-1 cells treated with HXR9. **(f)** IC50 values for HXR9 treatment. The negative control peptide CXR9 was not toxic at any of the concentrations tested for any of the cell lines (i.e. the IC50 > 100 µM). Error bars represent the SEM (n = 3), the p values are with respect to WPMY-1.

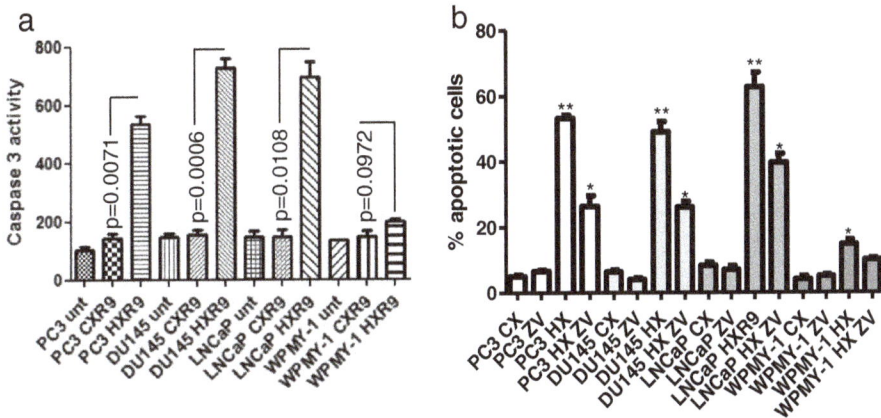

Figure 3 HXR9 induces apoptosis in prostate cancer cells. (a) Caspase 3 activity in PC3, DU145, LNCaP and WPMY-1 cells treated with 60 µM HXR9 or CXR9 for two hours. 'Unt' - untreated cells; Y axis units: relative fluorescence **(b)** PC3, DU145, LNCaP and WPMY-1 cells were treated with 60 µM HXR9 (HX) or CXR9 (CX) for two hours and cells were assessed for apoptosis through Annexin/7AAD staining. The % of cells in apoptosis is shown. Cells were also treated with the Caspase inhibitor ZVAD (ZV) alone or in combination with HXR9 (HX ZV). Error bars show the SEM. *p < 0.05, **p < 0.01 with respect to untreated cells.

integrity of cells, thus allowing cells to be divided into those undergoing early or late stage apoptosis depending on the relative binding of the two labels (Figure 3b). All of the cell lines tested had significantly increased levels of apoptosis after a two hour treatment with 60 µM HXR9, compared to CXR9 treated cells. Apoptosis was considerably higher in the prostate cancer derived cell lines PC3, DU145 and LNCaP (10.6, 8.2 and 7.9 fold, respectively) than in WPMY-1 (3.8 fold).

To provide further confirmation that cells were undergoing apoptosis, HXR9 and CXR9 treated cells were also treated with 50 µM Z-VAD, a caspase inhibitor that blocks the apoptotic cascade. This caused a significant reduction in the proportion of cells undergoing apoptosis (Figure 3b), with the exception of WPMY-1 cells.

HXR9 induced cell death is mediated by cFos

Previous studies have suggested that HXR9-induced apoptosis might be mediated by the elevated expression of the *cFos* gene [19,21]. To further explore this, and determine whether it is true for prostate cancer derived cells, we used QPCR to assess the expression level of *cFos* in HXR9 and CXR9 treated cells. A two hour treatment with 60 µM HXR9 caused a 6.2, 10.3 and 19.1 fold increase in *cFos* levels in DU145, PC3 and LNCaP cells, respectively (Figure 4a). In contrast, no significant increase was observed in WPMY-1 cells.

In order to establish whether increased *cFos* levels were directly responsible for inducing cell death, we used a siRNA knock down strategy to reduce *cFos* expression in HXR9 treated cells. DU145 cells were transfected with a random control siRNA (rnd siRNA), or one of two different siRNAs designed against the *cFos* sequence (siRNA1/2). Pre-treatment of DU145 cells with either of the *cFos* siRNAs was sufficient to block the increase in *cFos* expression upon subsequent treatment with HXR9, both at the mRNA and protein level (Figure 4b). This also resulted in a significant increase in

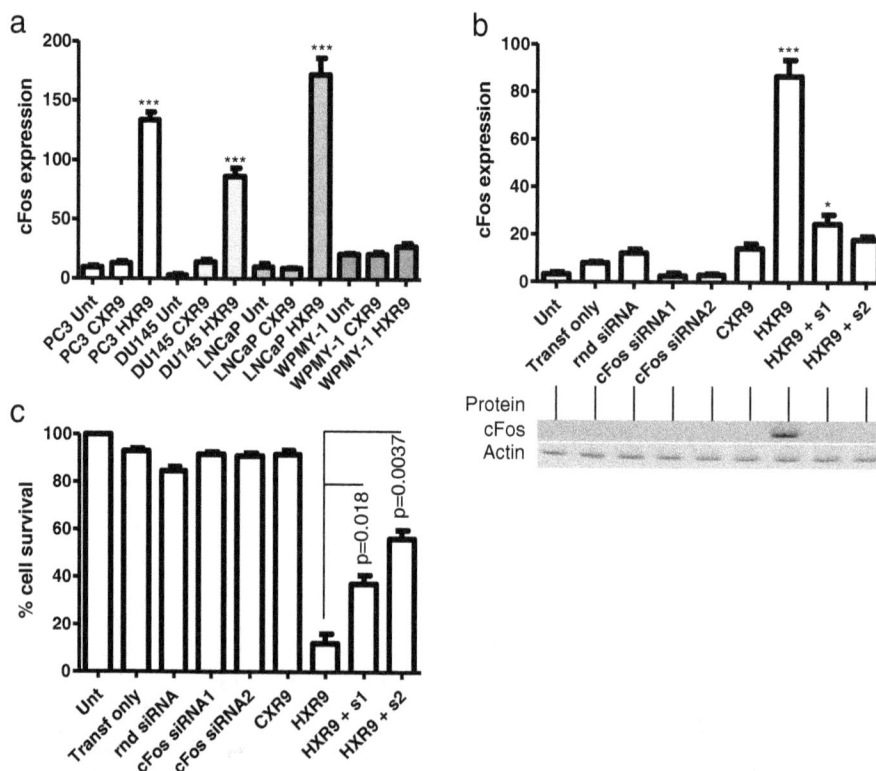

Figure 4 HXR9 induced apoptosis is mediated by *cFos*. (a) QPCR analysis of *cFos* expression in response to treatment of PC3, DU145, LNCaP and WPMY-1 cells with 60 µM HXR9 or CXR9 for two hours. 'Unt' – untreated cells; *cFos* expression is shown as a ratio with the β-actin gene (×10,000). **(b)** Knock down of *cFos* expression using siRNA. DU145 cells were incubated with transfection reagent alone ('Transf only'), or were transfected with a control siRNA with a random sequence ('rnd siRNA'), or with one of two siRNA targeting *cFos* ('cFos siRNA 1' and 'cFos siRNA 2'). Cells were also either treated with 60 µM HXR9 or CXR9, or with HXR9 in combination with one of the transfected *cFos* specific siRNAs ('HXR9 + s1' or 'HXR9 + s2'). The expression of *cFos* in treated cells was determined either at the RNA level using QPCR (upper section) or at the protein level using western blotting (lower section). **(c)** The % cell survival for each of the treatments described in **(b)**. Knock down of *cFos* in HXR9 treated cells results in a statistically significant decrease in cell death. Error bars show the SEM. *p < 0.05, ***p < 0.001 with respect to untreated cells.

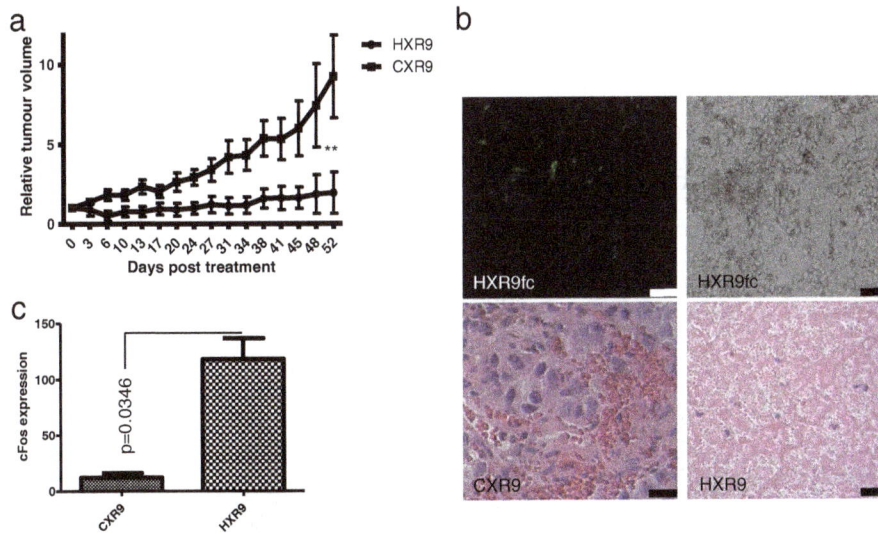

Figure 5 HXR9 retards LNCaP tumour growth *in vivo*. (a) Growth curve for LNCaP tumours treated intratumorally with a single dose of HXR9 (9 mice) or CXR9 (8 mice) when the tumour volume reached 100 mm³, followed by further doses if the tumour recurred. Error bars show the SEM. "Relative tumour volume" refers to the fold change in tumour size from the time of the first injection. **(b)** Top panels, sections through LNCaP tumours from mice treated with low dose (1 mg/Kg) FITC-HXR9. Top left, fluorescent view showing HXR9-FITC distribution (green). Top right, the same section under light microscopy. Scale bar: 100 μm. Bottom panels, sections through LNCaP tumours from mice treated with 100 mg/Kg HXR9 or CXR9. The CXR9 treated section shows highly undifferentiated tumour cells, whilst the HXR9 section shows the remains of dead tumour cells. Scale bar: 20 μm. **(c)** Expression of *cFos* in tumours treated with HXR9 or CXR9 2 hours prior to their excision, shown as a ratio between *cFos* and GAPDH transcripts detected by QPCR (x10,000).

cell survival (from 12% in cells treated with HXR9 only, to 37% and 56% in cells pre-treated with *cFos* siRNA1 and *cFos* siRNA2, respectively; Figure 4c).

HXR9 blocks the growth of LNCaP tumours *in vivo*
The sensitivity of prostate cancer derived lines to killing by HXR9 *in vitro* prompted us to test whether this sensitivity was also apparent *in vivo*. We initiated flank tumours in nude mice using a subcutaneous injection of LNCaP cells, which have been used in numerous studies as a murine model of prostate cancer. Tumours were injected directly with HXR9 or CXR9 once the mean tumour volume had reached 100 mm³. After 52 days the CXR9 injected tumours had, on average, increased in size 8 fold, whilst the average increase in HXR9 tumours was 1.5 fold (Figure 5a). Histological analysis of tumours revealed that whilst CXR9 treated tumours were composed principally of live, highly undifferentiated cells, those injected with HXR9 contained relatively few cells and were composed to a large extent of cellular debris (Figure 5b). Treating mice with a low dose of fluorescently labelled HXR9 revealed a widespread take up of the peptide by the tumour cells (Figure 5b). QPCR analysis of RNA extracted from tumours revealed that HXR9 induces an up regulation of *cFos* in a similar manner to that seen *in vitro*, suggesting that a similar mechanism of cell death may occur (Figure 5c).

HOX genes are globally overexpressed in primary prostate tumours
As previous studies on *HOX* gene expression in prostate cancer have focused only on single or small groups of genes, we undertook an analysis of all 39 *HOX* genes in prostate tumours and normal prostate tissue. This revealed a considerable over expression of many *HOX* family members, albeit in a heterogeneous manner with different *HOX* genes being overexpressed in different tumours. Only *HOXC4* and *HOXC6* showed consistently higher expression in the tumour compared to the normal prostate, with increases of 101 and 251 fold, respectively (Figure 6). Taking all of the *HOX* genes together also revealed a significantly higher global *HOX* expression in tumours (11.9 fold, Figure 6).

Discussion
In this study we have shown that *HOX* genes are highly deregulated in prostate tumours and in prostate cancer derived cell lines, which concurs with the findings of a number of previous studies [9-11]. It reveals that there is a very high level of deregulation with the majority of *HOX* genes being highly expressed in tumours but not in normal prostate tissue. This global increase in *HOX* expression makes it difficult to study those aspects of *HOX* function that are redundant throughout this highly conserved group. Here we have used HXR9, an inhibitor

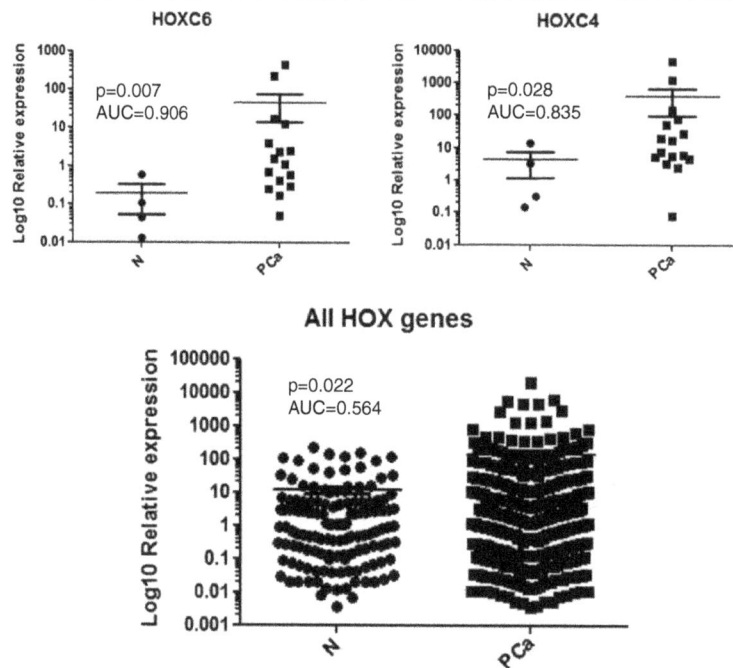

Figure 6 *HOX* gene expression in normal prostate tissue and prostate tumours. The expression of each gene was determined by semi-quantitative PCR and is shown relative to the house keeping gene *GAPDH* (x10000). The horizontal bar represents the mean and the error bars represent the SEM. AUC, area under the curve from a receiver-operator characteristics analysis.

of the interaction between HOX proteins and their common cofactor, PBX, to target a large subset of HOX proteins (i.e. members of paralogue groups 1-9) [19]. HXR9 causes apoptosis in all three of the prostate derived cells line studied, but only to a far lesser degree in a non-malignant cell line derived from prostate stroma (WPMY-1).

Disruption of HOX/PBX regulated transcription would be expected to cause changes in the expression of numerous target genes, and indeed previous studies have shown this to be the case. However only one of these targets – *cFos* – has been shown to be directly relevant to the induction of apoptosis by HXR9 [19]. It was previously shown that *cFos* up-regulation mediated the HXR9-induced apoptosis in melanoma B16F10 cells, and here we show that a similar mechanism exists in the prostate cancer-derived cell lines DU145, PC3 and LNCaP, as siRNA knock-down of *cFos* can partially rescue each of these cell lines from HXR9 –induced cell death. Although *cFos* is classically considered to be an oncogene, there are now a number of reports of it acting as a pro-apoptotic gene [19,28-31]. Our observation that HXR9 results in a rapid and very large increase in *cFos* expression indicates that the HOX/PBX dimer acts as a repressor of this gene. Whilst this could be a direct result of HOX/PBX binding to its regulatory sequences, a recent study showed that it could also be due to the increased

transcription of the oncogenic microRNAs miR221 and mir222, which in turn repress *cFos* expression [16].

The prevalence of *HOX* over expression in prostate cancer combined with the novel therapeutic mechanism exploited by HXR9 suggest that it could be a therapeutic approach where there is small volume, well defined disease. Local delivery of HXR9 into a range of tumours in mice has not resulted in a local inflammatory response [18,20,21]. Therefore delivery of HXR9 directly into the restricted confines of a primary or locally recurrent prostate cancer is feasible, and would not be limited due to the risk of prostatitis. Indeed a number of studies have evaluated intraprostatic gene therapy and oncolytic viral therapy and have reported no dose-limiting toxicity. These approaches utilised current imaging technology to achieve the precise delivery of reagents to small volume, well defined disease [32-34]. The application of HXR9 may be as a primary focal therapy, or where standard treatments approaches have failed, for example in cases of local recurrence following radical radiotherapy. The latter group of men currently receive ablative therapy which has low efficacy and is associated with significant toxicities [35]. In contrast to current treatments such as cryotherapy, the lack of inflammatory response associated with HXR9 treatment would potentially allow multiple, sequential intratumoral delivery.

Conclusions

The *HOX* genes are highly dysregulated, and generally over-expressed in prostate cancer. Targeting the interaction between HOX proteins and their PBX co-factor is a potential therapeutic strategy in this malignancy.

Competing interests

The authors declare that they have no competing interests.

Authors' contributions

RM designed the study and wrote the manuscript. AB performed the cell viability assays and gene expression analysis. KH critically reviewed the manuscript and helped with experimental design. GS performed the *in vivo* experiments. AM assisted in the primary tissue collection and the analysis of gene expression in these samples. HP helped to design the study and to write the manuscript. All authors read and approved the final manuscript.

Acknowledgment

The authors gratefully acknowledge the support of the Prostate Project charity (UK).

Author details

2Faculty of Health and Medical Sciences, University of Surrey, Guildford, UK. Targeted Therapy Team, Chester Beatty Laboratories, The Institute of Cancer Research, London, UK.

References

1. Ferlay J, Shin HR, Bray F, Forman D, Mathers C, Parkin DM: Estimates of worldwide burden of cancer in 2008: GLOBOCAN 2008. *Int J Cancer* 2010, 127:2893–2917.
2. DiBlasio CJ, Malcolm JB, Hammett J, Wan JY, Aleman MA, Patterson AL, Wake RW, Derweesh IH: Survival outcomes in men receiving androgen-deprivation therapy as primary or salvage treatment for localized or advanced prostate cancer: 20-year single-centre experience. *BJU Int* 2009, 104:1208–1214.
3. Mukherji D, Eichholz A, De Bono JS: Management of metastatic castration-resistant prostate cancer: recent advances. *Drugs* 2012, 72:1011–1028.
4. Shah N, Sukumar S: The *HOX* genes and their roles in oncogenesis. *Nat Rev Cancer* 2010, 10:361–371.
5. Chang CP, Brocchieri L, Shen WF, Largman C, Cleary ML: Pbx modulation of *HOX* homeodomain amino-terminal arms establishes different DNA-binding specificities across the *HOX* locus. *Mol Cell Biol* 1996, 16:1734–1745.
6. Knoepfler PS, Bergstrom DA, Uetsuki T, Dac-Korytko I, Sun YH, Wright WE, Tapscott SJ, Kamps MP: A conserved motif N-terminal to the DNA-binding domains of myogenic bHLH transcription factors mediates cooperative DNA binding with pbx-Meis1/Prep1. *Nucleic Acids Res* 1999, 27:3752–3761.
7. Morgan R, In der Rieden P, Hooiveld MH, Durston AJ: Identifying *HOX* paralog groups by the PBX-binding region. *Trends Genet* 2000, 16:66–67.
8. McGinnis W, Krumlauf R: Homeobox genes and axial patterning. *Cell* 1992, 68:283–302.
9. Miller GJ, Miller HL, van Bokhoven A, Lambert JR, Werahera PN, Schirripa O, Lucia MS, Nordeen SK: Aberrant *HOXC* expression accompanies the malignant phenotype in human prostate. *Cancer Res* 2003, 63:5879–5888.
10. Norris JD, Chang CY, Wittmann BM, Kunder RS, Cui H, Fan D, Joseph JD, McDonnell DP: The homeodomain protein *HOXB13* regulates the cellular response to androgens. *Mol Cell* 2009, 36:405–416.
11. Waltregny D, Alami Y, Clausse N, de Leval J, Castronovo V: Overexpression of the homeobox gene *HOXC8* in human prostate cancer correlates with loss of tumor differentiation. *Prostate* 2002, 50:162–169.
12. Eklund EA: The role of *HOX* genes in malignant myeloid disease. *Curr Opin Hematol* 2007, 14:85–89.
13. Huang L, Pu Y, Hepps D, Danielpour D, Prins GS: Posterior *HOX* gene expression and differential androgen regulation in the developing and adult rat prostate lobes. *Endocrinology* 2007, 148:1235–1245.
14. Ando H, Natsume A, Senga T, Watanabe R, Ito I, Ohno M, Iwami K, Ohka F, Motomura K, Kinjo S, Ito M, Saito K, et al: Peptide-based inhibition of the

HOXA9/PBX interaction retards the growth of human meningioma. *Cancer Chemother Pharmacol* 2014, 73:53–60.
15. Daniels TR, Neacato II, Rodriguez JA, Pandha HS, Morgan R, Penichet ML: Disruption of *HOX* activity leads to cell death that can be enhanced by the interference of iron uptake in malignant B cells. *Leukemia* 2010, 24:1555–1565.
16. Errico MC, Felicetti F, Bottero L, Mattia G, Boe A, Felli N, Petrini M, Bellenghi M, Pandha HS, Calvaruso M, Tripodo C, Colombo MP, et al: The abrogation of the *HOXB7/PBX2* complex induces apoptosis in melanoma through the miR-221&222-c-FOS pathway. *Int J Cancer* 2013, 133:879–892.
17. Li Z, Zhang Z, Li Y, Arnovitz S, Chen P, Huang H, Jiang X, Hong GM, Kunjamma RB, Ren H, He C, Wang CZ, et al: PBX3 is an important cofactor of *HOXA9* in leukemogenesis. *Blood* 2013, 121:1422–1431.
18. Morgan R, Boxall A, Harrington KJ, Simpson GR, Gillett C, Michael A, Pandha HS: Targeting the *HOX/PBX* dimer in breast cancer. *Breast Cancer Res Treat* 2012, 136:389–398.
19. Morgan R, Pirard PM, Shears L, Sohal J, Pettengell R, Pandha HS: Antagonism of *HOX/PBX* dimer formation blocks the *in vivo* proliferation of melanoma. *Cancer Res* 2007, 67:5806–5813.
20. Morgan R, Plowright L, Harrington KJ, Michael A, Pandha HS: Targeting *HOX* and PBX transcription factors in ovarian cancer. *BMC Cancer* 2010, 10:89.
21. Plowright L, Harrington KJ, Pandha HS, Morgan R: *HOX* transcription factors are potential therapeutic targets in non-small-cell lung cancer (targeting *HOX* genes in lung cancer). *Br J Cancer* 2009, 100:470–475.
22. Shears L, Plowright L, Harrington K, Pandha HS, Morgan R: Disrupting the interaction between *HOX* and PBX causes necrotic and apoptotic cell death in the renal cancer lines CaKi-2 and 769-P. *J Urol* 2008, 180:2196–2201.
23. Stone KR, Mickey DD, Wunderli H, Mickey GH, Paulson DF: Isolation of a human prostate carcinoma cell line (DU 145). *Int J Cancer* 1978, 21:274–281.
24. Kaighn ME, Narayan KS, Ohnuki Y, Lechner JF, Jones LW: Establishment and characterization of a human prostatic carcinoma cell line (PC-3). *Invest Urol* 1979, 17:16–23.
25. Horoszewicz JS, Leong SS, Kawinski E, Karr JP, Rosenthal H, Chu TM, Mirand EA, Murphy GP: LNCaP model of human prostatic carcinoma. *Cancer Res* 1983, 43:1809–1818.
26. Webber MM, Bello D, Quader S: Immortalized and tumorigenic adult human prostatic epithelial cell lines: characteristics and applications part 2. Tumorigenic cell lines. *Prostate* 1997, 30:58–64.
27. Workman P, Balmain A, Hickman JA, McNally NJ, Rohas AM, Mitchison NA, Pierrepoint CG, Raymond R, Rowlatt C, Stephens TC, et al: UKCCCR guidelines for the welfare of animals in experimental neoplasia. *Lab Anim* 1988, 22:195–201.
28. Sauvageau G, Lansdorp PM, Eaves CJ, Hogge DE, Dragowska WH, Reid DS, Largman C, Lawrence HJ, Humphries RK: Differential expression of homeobox genes in functionally distinct CD34+ subpopulations of human bone marrow cells. *Proc Natl Acad Sci U S A* 1994, 91:12223–12227.
29. Vider BZ, Zimber A, Hirsch D, Estlein D, Chastre E, Prevot S, Gespach C, Yaniv A, Gazit A: Human colorectal carcinogenesis is associated with deregulation of homeobox gene expression. *Biochem Biophys Res Commun* 1997, 232:742–748.
30. Kalra N, Kumar V: c-Fos is a mediator of the c-myc-induced apoptotic signaling in serum-deprived hepatoma cells via the p38 mitogen-activated protein kinase pathway. *J Biol Chem* 2004, 279:25313–25319.
31. Mikula M, Gotzmann J, Fischer AN, Wolschek MF, Thallinger C, Schulte-Hermann R, Beug H, Mikulits W: The proto-oncoprotein c-Fos negatively regulates hepatocellular tumorigenesis. *Oncogene* 2003, 22:6725–6738.
32. Patel P, Young JG, Mautner V, Ashdown D, Bonney S, Pineda RG, Collins SI, Searle PF, Hull D, Peers E, Chester J, Wallace DM, et al: A phase I/II clinical trial in localized prostate cancer of an adenovirus expressing nitroreductase with CB1954 [correction of CB1984]. *Mol Ther* 2009, 17:1292–1299.

33. Sonpavde G, Thompson TC, Jain RK, Ayala GE, Kurosaka S, Edamura K, Tabata K, Ren C, Goltsov AA, Mims MP, Hayes TG, Ittmann MM, *et al*: **GLIPR1 tumor suppressor gene expressed by adenoviral vector as neoadjuvant intraprostatic injection for localized intermediate or high-risk prostate cancer preceding radical prostatectomy.** *Clin Cancer Res* 2011, **17**:7174–7182.

34. Thirukkumaran CM, Nodwell MJ, Hirasawa K, Shi ZQ, Diaz R, Luider J, Johnston RN, Forsyth PA, Magliocco AM, Lee P, Nishikawa S, Donnelly B, *et al*: **Oncolytic viral therapy for prostate cancer: efficacy of reovirus as a biological therapeutic.** *Cancer Res* 2010, **70**:2435–2444.

35. Chou R, Dana T, Bougatsos C, Fu R, Blazina I, Gleitsmann K, Rugge JB: *Treatments for Localized Prostate Cancer: Systematic Review to Update the 2002 U.S. Preventive Services Task Force Recommendationed.* Rockville (MD): Agency For Healthcare Research and Quality; 2011.

12

Altered *PCA3* and *TMPRSS2-ERG* expression in histologically benign regions of cancerous prostates: a systematic, quantitative mRNA analysis in five prostates

Riina-Minna Väänänen[1*], Natalia Tong Ochoa[1], Peter J. Boström[2], Pekka Taimen[3] and Kim Pettersson[1]

Abstract

Background: *PCA3* and *TMPRSS2-ERG* are commonly overexpressed biomarkers in prostate cancer, but reports have emerged demonstrating altered expression also in areas outside the tumour foci in cancerous prostates. Our aim was to measure *PCA3* and *TMPRSS2-ERG* expression systematically in all regions of prostate cross-sections, matching the data to corresponding tissue morphology.

Methods: *TMPRSS2-ERG* and *PCA3* mRNA levels were measured with quantitative reverse-transcription PCR assays in 270 samples from cross-sections of five radical prostatectomy specimens. ERG expression was examined by immunohistochemistry.

Results: *TMPRSS2-ERG* mRNAs were detected in three patients and in 15 tissue samples in total. These included two carcinoma samples and 13 histologically benign samples, eight of which were located next to malignant tumours or PIN (prostatic intraepithelial neoplasia) lesions and five of which did not reside in the vicinity of any evident carcinoma foci. ERG protein expression was limited to areas of *TMPRSS2-ERG* mRNA expression, but did not identify all of them. *PCA3* expression was detected in all five cross-sections, with statistically significant, three-fold higher expression in carcinoma regions.

Conclusions: *TMPRSS2-ERG* expression was detected in carcinoma foci, regions next to them, and in samples not adjacent to carcinoma foci. Claimed as a cancer-associated phenomenon, this fusion gene measurement could, if validated with a larger cohort, be utilized as an addition to histological analysis to predict current or future cancer risk in men with negative biopsies. Molecular changes outside the carcinoma foci are also indicated for *PCA3*, as its expression was only moderately increased in the carcinoma regions.

Keywords: Prostate, Cancer, Biomarker, RNA, Reverse transcriptase polymerase chain reaction

Background

The proposed idea of field cancerization – phenomenon first described by Slaughter and colleagues in 1953 [1] – comprises the assumption that in cancers, originally a larger area of the tissue than merely the tumour focus can be changed due to inherent mutations or environmental factors. The hypothesis has been supported by several studies reporting molecular level alterations not only in the carcinoma tissue of an organ containing a malignant tumour, but also in the area outside the cancerous region [2, 3]. Both aberrant protein expression and mRNA transcript levels have been described [4]. Besides providing an interesting perspective to understanding carcinogenesis, detectable consequences of the field effect phenomenon could be used to supplement diagnostics.

Prostate cancer is a disease with a growing incidence and a heterogeneous nature, and the heterogeneity of the disease has made diagnostics and prognostics challenging. The currently used biomarker, PSA (prostate specific antigen) measured from blood, cannot reliably confirm the presence of cancer in the prostate since increased levels

* Correspondence: riinaminna.vaananen@gmail.com
[1]Department of Biotechnology, University of Turku, Turku, Finland
Full list of author information is available at the end of the article

are frequently found also in other prostatic diseases such as hyperplasia and prostatitis. Present routine to establish the prostate cancer diagnosis is based on the histological examination of core needle biopsies that are taken with trans-rectal ultrasound guidance. However, the biopsy cores represent a random sampling of the overall tumour load regarding the aiming of the biopsy needle to the estimated carcinoma location. A histologically benign biopsy result leads to a negative cancer diagnosis, but based on the previous reports on molecular level alterations in cancer-adjacent tissues, it may be premature in determining the status of the patient.

Alterations in the expression of prostate cancer marker candidate genes TMPRSS2-ERG (transmembrane protease, serine 2; ETV-related gene) and PCA3 (prostate cancer antigen 3) have previously been detected by us and others [5–9]. The changes were specifically seen in the histologically benign areas of cancerous prostates but not in similar areas of prostates that were free of clinical cancer. This study was designed to systematically locate the regions of differential expression of these genes in single cross-sections of five cancerous prostates and evaluate whether the location of the carcinoma was associated with TMPRSS2-ERG or PCA3 mRNA levels or ERG protein expression.

Methods

Sample collection

To measure the mRNA expression of the target genes by quantitative reverse-transcription PCR (qRT-PCR) in prostate tissue, prostate cross-sections covering the entire organ were obtained fresh from five prostates (hereafter referred to as prostates A, B, C, D, and E) from men undergoing robotic assisted laparoscopic radical prostatectomies due to prostate cancer at Turku University Hospital, Turku, Finland in June–September 2013. Five consecutive patients with previous diagnosis

of prostatic adenocarcinoma in transrectal biopsies were enrolled in the study. Patients with diagnosed adenocarcinoma in both lobes and patients with clinical suspicion of multifocal or large tumour were excluded from the study. The sample collection protocol is depicted in Fig. 1. Briefly, a horizontal tissue slice of 2 mm in thickness was removed from each prostate and further cut into 5x5x2 mm pieces systematically with sterile blades, avoiding cross-contamination between pieces. A Styrofoam plate with a 5x5 mm grid was used to record the two-dimensional location of each piece, resulting in a unique coordinate code for each piece of tissue. Depending on the size of the organ, this procedure yielded 48 individual samples for prostate A, 62 samples for prostate B, 44 samples for prostate C, 55 samples for prostate D, and 61 samples for prostate E. All pieces were stored separately in RNAlater RNA Stabilization Reagent (Qiagen, Hilden, Germany) at −20 °C.

Tissue immediately adjacent to the tissue cross-section used in mRNA measurements was fixed in formalin and embedded in macro paraffin blocks (FFPE) to enable examination of tissue morphology. Sections were cut directly from the superior and inferior side of the cross-section used in mRNA measurements, stained with hematoxylin and eosin (HE), and inspected for cancer foci and prostatic epithelial neoplasia (PIN) lesions by an experienced uro-pathologist. The locations of carcinoma areas and PIN lesions were marked and the slides were scanned into digital images. All five prostate cross-sections contained cancerous areas and cross-sections B and C contained also PIN lesions.

The study protocol was approved by the Ethics Committee of the Hospital District of Southwest Finland and it was in accordance with the Helsinki Declaration of 1975, as revised in 1996, with written informed consent obtained from each participant.

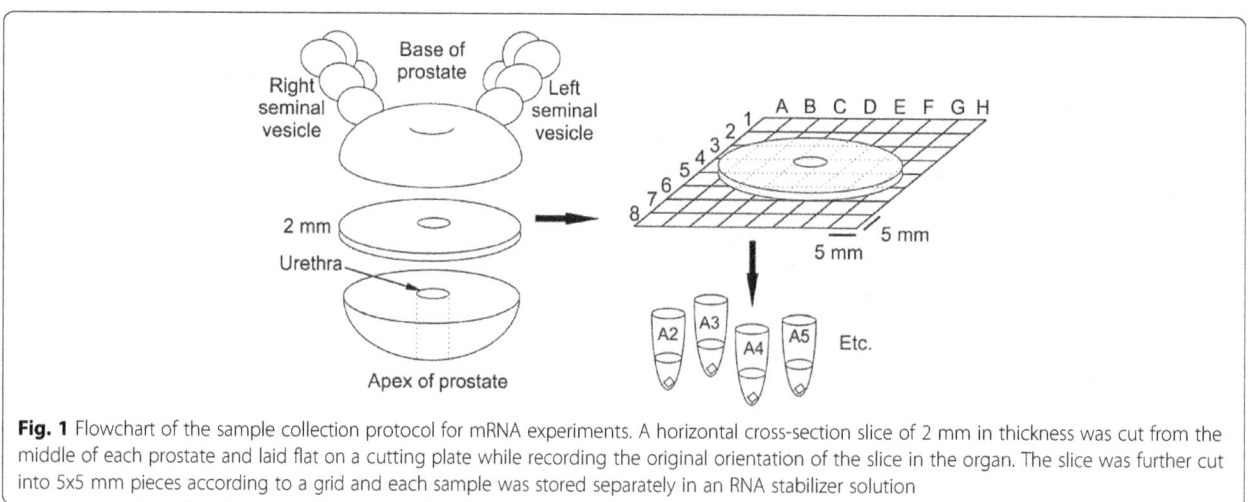

Fig. 1 Flowchart of the sample collection protocol for mRNA experiments. A horizontal cross-section slice of 2 mm in thickness was cut from the middle of each prostate and laid flat on a cutting plate while recording the original orientation of the slice in the organ. The slice was further cut into 5x5 mm pieces according to a grid and each sample was stored separately in an RNA stabilizer solution

Real-time PCR for *PCA3* and *TMPRSS2-ERG* mRNAs

RNA extraction and reverse transcription were performed with RNeasy Mini kit (Qiagen, Germany) and High Capacity cDNA Archive kit (Applied Biosystems, USA) according to manufacturer's instructions and as described previously [10]. Artificial internal standard RNA was added to each sample at the beginning of RNA extraction process, after cell lysis [11].

Quantitative real-time PCR assays using a closed-tube concept [12] and time-resolved fluorometry-based detection were performed as described previously [9, 10] to measure *PCA3* and *TMPRSS2-ERG* mRNA levels in each tissue piece. Levels of *KLK3* (kallikrein-related peptidase 3, gene encoding PSA) mRNA and internal standard RNA were also measured for control and normalization purposes [11–14]. The oligonucleotide sequences are presented in Table 1. External DNA standards (Table 2) were used to form a standard curve and the lowest dilutions equal the limits of detection for the particular assays.

Immunohistochemistry

For immunohistochemistry (IHC) experiments, sections of 3–4 μm were cut from the FFPE tissue macro blocks immediately from the superior and inferior side of the HE-stained sections. The sections were pretreated in xylene and ethanol, and the heat-induced antigen retrieval was performed in a microwave oven using Target Retrieval Solution (Dako) followed by cooling at RT. Staining was performed by incubating the slides for one hour at RT in a humid chamber with rabbit monoclonal ERG antibody (clone EPR3864; Epitomics) that was used in 1:250 dilution. EnVision™ + Dual Link System-HRP (Dako) was used as the secondary antibody with a 30-min incubation at RT. The staining was visualized by incubation in DAB+ Chromogen solution (Dako) for 10 min at RT. After counterstaining with hematoxylin, dehydration, and treatment by xylene, the slides were analysed by an experienced uropathologist. The vascular endothelial cells served as

Table 1 Sequences of the primers and probes used in this study

Oligonucleotide	Sequence (5'- > 3')	GenBank database sequence number	Position in sequence
KLK3			
5' primer	TGA ACC AGA GGA GTT CTT GAC	X05332	523–543
3' primer	CCC AGA ATC ACC CGA GCA G	X05332	667–685
reporter probe	CCT TCT GAG GGT GAA CTT GCG C	X05332	596–617
quencher probe	AAT CAC CCT CAG AAG G	X05332	600–601, 604–617
mmPSA			
5' primer	TGA ACC AGA GGA GTT CTT GCA	X05332	523–543
3' primer	CCC AGA ATC ACC CGA GCG A	X05332	667–685
reporter probe	CCT TCT GAG GGT GAT TGC GCA C	X05332	594–601, 604–617
quencher probe	AAT CAC CCT CAG AAG G	X05332	600–601, 604–617
PCA3			
5' primer	GGT GGG AAG GAC CTG ATG ATA C	AF103907	95–116
3' primer	GGG CGA GGC TCA TCG AT	AF103907	505–521
reporter probe	AGA AAT GCC CGG CCG CCA TC	AF103907	478–497
quencher probe	CCG GGC ATT TCT	AF103907	478–489
TMPRSS2-ERG III			
5' primer	TAG GCG CGA GCT AAG CAG GAG	NM_005656.3	4–24
3' primer	GTA GGC ACA CTC AAA CAA CGA CTG G	NM_004449.4	338–362
reporter probe	AGC GCG GCA GGA AGC CTT ATC AGT T	NM_005656.3 and NM_004449.4	57–64 and 310–326
quencher probe	TTC CTG CCG CGC T	NM_005656.3 and NM_004449.4	57–64 and 310–314
TMPRSS2-ERG VI			
5' primer	CGG CAG GTC ATA TTG AAC ATT CC	NM_005656.3	73–95
3' primer	GCA CAC TCA AAC AAC GAC TGG	NM_004449.4	338–358
reporter probe	CTT TGA ACT CAG AAG CCT TAT CAG TTG TGA	NM_005656.3 and NM_004449.4	139–149 and 312–330
quencher probe	GGC TTC TGA GTT CAA AG	NM_005656.3 and NM_004449.4	139–149 and 312–317

Lanthanide chelates were attached to the 5′ ends of the reporter probes via an amino group to enable signal measurement with time-resolved fluorescence and phosphate groups to the 3′ ends to prevent them from functioning as starting points for DNA synthesis. Quencher molecules were attached to the 3′ ends of the quencher probes. The oligonucleotide sequences have been previously published for *KLK3* [12, 13], mmPSA [11–13], *PCA3* [10, 20], *TMPRSS2-ERG* III [9, 21, 22], and *TMPRSS2-ERG* VI [9] assays

Table 2 Dilutions of external DNA standards used in the real-time PCR assays

Target RNA	Range (molecules per mL of template)		Total number of points on standard curve
	Lowest concentration	Highest concentration	
KLK3	2.5×10^3	2×10^{11}	8
PCA3	1.3×10^3	2.5×10^{11}	7
TMPRSS2-ERG III	5×10^3	5×10^7	4
TMPRSS2-ERG VI	2×10^4	2×10^8	4

positive controls for the staining with ERG antibody and cells of the benign glands as the negative control.

Data analysis

The specific locations of tissue were translated to match samples used for mRNA measurements by dividing the digital images of HE-stained tissue slides into equal amount of regions. Thus, potential shrinkage of the tissue was accounted for on average. Each sample piece was given coordinates on two axis (one giving values from A to K, and the other giving values from 1 to 10). Samples were classified into four categories based on morphology-based examination of the immediately adjacent HE-stained tissue. Sample was deemed as a carcinoma sample if one or both studied HE sections revealed adenocarcinoma at the same location, and PIN if one or both studied HE sections revealed PIN lesion. If both studied HE sections contained only histologically benign tissue in that area but the sample immediately next to the sample was classified as carcinoma or PIN sample, the sample was classified as "histologically benign tissue immediately adjacent to a carcinoma/PIN sample" (HBAC). If HE sections showed only histologically benign tissue in the sample and the samples next to it, sample was marked as histologically benign area (HB).

Samples were considered to contain measurable amounts of target mRNAs only when three PCR replicates gave a rise in fluorescence signals. Copy numbers were calculated as previously described [10], taking into account the potential RNA loss in extraction by using an internal RNA standard. For TMPRSS2-ERG mRNAs, samples that produced signal in only one or two out of the three PCR replicates were considered as samples where TMPRSS2-ERG mRNA expression was detectable but not quantifiable. Limits of detection for the real-time PCR assays are presented

Mann–Whitney U test was used to study associations between mRNA and protein expression of the target genes and the histology of the tissue (SPSS 20.0, IBM).

Results

Patient and tumour characteristics

The essential clinicopathological characteristics of the five cases are presented in Table 3. All cases were clinically

and pathologically organ confined. Two patients (B and D) had 5-alpha-reductase inhibitor therapy and one patient (E) had a combination therapy of 5-alpha-reductase inhibitor and α_1 receptor antagonist prior to surgery. No positive margins were detected and all patients achieved serum PSA of <0.1 ng/mL postoperatively. Using ultrasensitive PSA measurement, two patients had detectable postoperative serum PSA (0.004 and 0.026 ng/mL). During the follow-up of 8–11 months, none of the patients had experienced clinical or biochemical recurrences. Patients D and E had clearly one index tumour, patients A and C had two or more carcinoma foci (between 6 and 18 mm), and patient B had two small, well-differentiated carcinoma foci (both <10 mm).

KLK3 mRNA expression

KLK3 mRNA levels were measured from all samples for control purposes. There were no statistically significant differences in KLK3 mRNA levels between carcinoma, PIN, HBAC, or HB samples (data not shown).

PCA3 mRNA expression

All five prostates showed PCA3 mRNA expression. It was universally expressed in prostates A and B and in 80–96 % of samples of prostates C, D, and E. When all samples from the five prostates were combined, the median expression level was highest (9.54×10^5 mRNA copies/µg total RNA) in the samples that were classified as carcinoma samples, second highest in PIN samples, third highest in samples adjacent to carcinoma or PIN samples, and lowest in HB samples (2.62×10^5 mRNA

Table 3 Characteristics of the five patients included in the study

Patient	Age	PSA (ng/mL)		Gleason sum	Tumour volume (%)
		preoperative	postoperative		
A	67	4.5	<0.003	3 + 4	10
B	59	9.2	<0.003	3 + 3	2
C	59	8.5	<0.003	3 + 4	5
D	67	16	0.026	4 + 3	8
E	66	18	0.004	4 + 3	15

Tumour volume in the whole prostate was estimated based on the macro sections taken every 5 mm and covering the whole organ

copies/μg total RNA (Fig. 2). The statistically significant difference in median *PCA3* mRNA values between carcinoma samples and HB samples was 3.6-fold ($p < 0.001$). The difference between carcinoma samples and samples adjacent to carcinoma or PIN was 3.1-fold ($p < 0.001$).

When the five studied prostate cross-sections were looked at individually, the same trend of statistically significantly higher *PCA3* mRNA expression in carcinoma areas persisted only for prostate C, where the difference between medians of carcinoma and HB samples was 20-fold ($p < 0.003$), and for prostate D with a 5.2-fold difference ($p < 0.001$).

TMPRSS2-ERG mRNA expression

TMPRSS2-ERG III mRNA was detected in 3 out of 5 prostates (B, C, and E) and *TMPRSS2-ERG* VI mRNA in 2 out of 5 prostates (prostates C and E). The samples containing detectable *TMPRSS2-ERG* expression and their location in relation to carcinoma areas are depicted in Fig. 3. Reliably quantifiable expression of *TMPRSS2-ERG* III or VI mRNAs was found in four histologically benign samples, two of which were HBAC samples. The third sample was located next to a PIN lesion and the fourth resided in an area that was regarded as histologically benign. In addition, detectable but not quantifiable expression of these mRNAs was found in one carcinoma focus of prostate C, one carcinoma sample of prostate E, in four HBAC samples, and in five HB samples. One of the HB samples was adjacent to a PIN area. None of the

individual samples showed simultaneous expression of both *TMPRSS2-ERG* mRNA isoforms.

ERG protein expression

IHC experiments detected positive ERG staining only in prostate C (Fig. 4). Based on the morphological analysis, all ERG positive areas contained carcinoma tissue. *TMPRSS2-ERG* mRNA was detectable in one out of the four individual tissue samples matching the ERG positive areas and the other three samples were located adjacent to *TMPRSS2-ERG* mRNA positive samples. One of the samples contained *TMPRSS2-ERG* III mRNA and the others *TMPRSS2-ERG* VI mRNA, but the amounts were not quantifiable in any of them. Areas in the same and other prostates containing either quantifiable or only detectable expression of *TMPRSS2-ERG* mRNAs were negative for ERG in IHC.

Discussion

Field effect is a recognized phenomenon in several cancers, including prostate cancer. It suggests that larger areas of the tissue than just the histologically identifiable tumour regions are changed on the molecular level. We studied the extent and location of the mRNA expression of two suggested prostate cancer markers, *TMPRSS2-ERG* fusion gene and *PCA3*, in a systematic way in cross-sections of cancerous prostates containing both histologically benign and carcinoma areas.

In addition to overexpression in tumours, increased expression of *PCA3* has been described also in areas adjacent to carcinoma foci and the phenomenon was explained by a carcinogenic field effect [3]. The thus far reported findings of *TMPRSS2-ERG* in BPH (benign prostatic hyperplasia) tissue, or in a benign area from a cancerous prostate, have sometimes been speculated to result from small carcinoma foci that resided in sampled tissues and were unnoticed despite microscopic examination [5, 7]. Also the possibility of the samples containing precancerous tissue has been proposed [6, 7]. Our previous study, showing that 44 % of the histologically benign sampled areas of cancerous prostates contained *TMPRSS2-ERG* mRNA transcripts in contrast to none of the seven benign tissues of cancer-free prostates [9], led us to hypothesize on *TMPRSS2-ERG* expression not being limited to carcinoma foci in cancerous prostates.

The fusion gene mRNAs were detectable in two carcinoma samples in this study, and also in 13 histologically benign samples. However, eight of the *TMPRSS2-ERG* positive histologically benign samples resided immediately next to samples classified as carcinoma or PIN. Due to the sample collection set-up, those samples could also contain cancer cells originating from the adjacent sample areas as the protocol of matching tissue morphology with the location of samples used for mRNA measurements was not

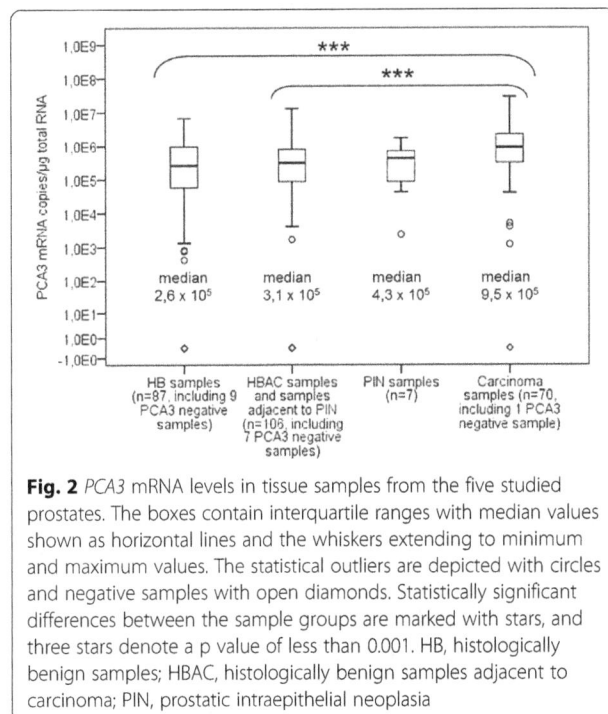

Fig. 2 *PCA3* mRNA levels in tissue samples from the five studied prostates. The boxes contain interquartile ranges with median values shown as horizontal lines and the whiskers extending to minimum and maximum values. The statistical outliers are depicted with circles and negative samples with open diamonds. Statistically significant differences between the sample groups are marked with stars, and three stars denote a p value of less than 0.001. HB, histologically benign samples; HBAC, histologically benign samples adjacent to carcinoma; PIN, prostatic intraepithelial neoplasia

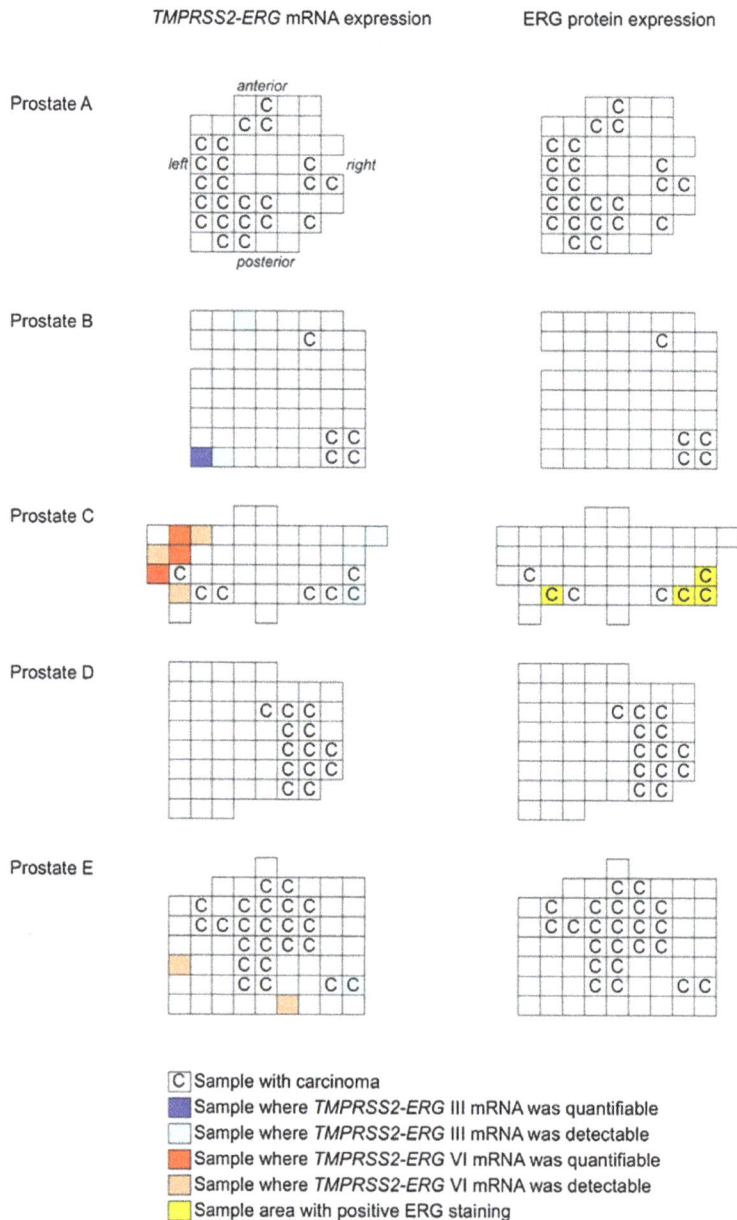

Fig. 3 Location of detected *TMPRSS2-ERG* mRNA expression and ERG protein expression in relation to carcinoma areas. Morphologically determined carcinoma areas are marked with C in the five prostates. Dark blue boxes denote samples with quantifiable *TMPRSS2-ERG* III mRNA expression, and light blue boxes represent samples with detectable but not quantifiable *TMPRSS2-ERG* III mRNA expression. Red boxes denote samples with quantifiable *TMPRSS2-ERG* VI mRNA expression and light orange boxes represent detectable but not quantifiable *TMPRSS2-ERG* VI mRNA expression. Yellow boxes denote ERG protein expression. *TMPRSS2-ERG* mRNAs were found in prostates B, C, and E and ERG protein expression only in prostate C. None of the samples showed simultaneous expression of both *TMPRSS2-ERG* mRNA variants

able to fully account for site-specific tissue shrinkage caused by the fixation of the tissue. Yet we detected *TMPRSS2-ERG* expression in five samples without evidence of carcinoma foci in the immediate vicinity. In contrary to our previous study [9], none of the individual samples in this limited cohort showed simultaneous expression of both studied *TMPRSS2-ERG* isoforms. The detection rate in cancerous samples was also higher, 66 %, in

the previous study, which could potentially be due to the sampling protocol which was more laborious and time-consuming in this study, potentially leading to RNA degradation and thus lower detection rates.

The tissue regions that were positively stained in ERG IHC matched the locations of carcinoma lesions, and either contained detectable *TMPRSS2-ERG* mRNA or were located adjacent to samples that did. However, all

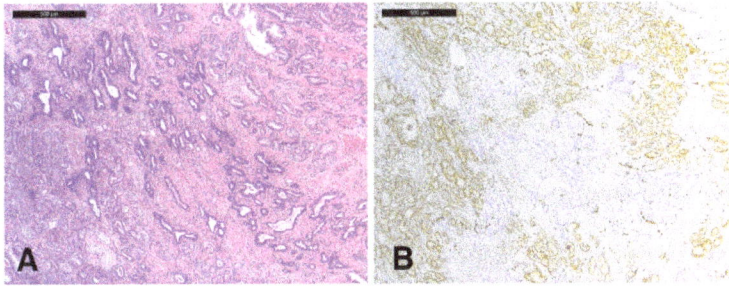

Fig. 4 Histology of prostate C showing (**a**) HE staining and (**b**) immunohistochemical ERG staining from the same area. The nuclei of malignant glands stain positively for ERG suggesting that ERG is overexpressed due to *TMPRSS2-ERG* fusion. Scale bar 500 μm

TMPRSS2-ERG mRNA positive areas did not stain positively for ERG even within a specific prostate, suggesting that the mRNA assays can reveal additional suspicious areas compared to IHC methods alone. This could be due to the IHC-negative areas not producing such amounts or forms of ERG protein that the antibody recognizes, even though previous reports of it have demonstrated correct identification of all the samples with the *TMPRSS2-ERG* rearrangement [15]. The rearrangement variant type did not seem to play a role in identifying ERG protein expression.

PCA3 is a non-coding gene that does not produce a functional protein, so its expression was studied only on the mRNA level. *PCA3* is reported to be 10–100-fold overexpressed in prostate tumours [16, 17], but in our previous studies, we have seen values of this magnitude only when carcinomas were compared to prostates without clinical prostate cancer [9] and a 5.8-fold increase of *PCA3* expression in tumours was observed when they were compared to benign areas of cancerous prostates [8]. In this cross-section study, we detected a three times higher expression in the carcinoma samples than in the histologically benign areas next to malignant tumours or at locations further away. It would therefore seem that the increase in *PCA3* mRNA expression is not limited to the carcinoma foci in a cancerous prostate, but rather that there is a more global field change.

The set-up of this study is admittedly of a preliminary and experimental nature and due to the small size of the cohort, the conclusions can only be suggestive. The fact that only approximately half of prostate cancer cases are *TMPRSS2-ERG* positive [18] contributed to the even smaller number of *TMPRSS2-ERG* positive cases in our study. Additionally, we only studied one section of each prostate here in order to ensure the reliability of the routine pathological diagnostic procedure. This, however, could limit the conclusions drawn considering that prostate cancer, as also was seen in these specimens, is often a multifocal disease. The neoadjuvant therapy administered to three of the patients could also have had an effect on

the results. However, despite these limitations, we find the set-up of this study novel and of interest. Clark and colleagues conducted a similar type of study using prostate cross-section slices and obtaining samples from cancerous and nonmalignant areas of the prostate, deemed as such based on the morphology of the slices above and below [5]. They, however, only looked at two matched samples from each prostatectomy specimen instead of the more systematic approach adopted here, which comprised a systematic and quantitative examination of mRNA levels throughout the tissue slice.

Utilizing these findings for diagnostic purposes would entail qRT-PCR assays performed on biopsies or tissue material obtained from transurethral resection of the prostate (TURP), where a finding of *TMPRSS2-ERG* mRNAs or high *PCA3* expression would indicate an increased risk of having or developing prostate cancer. While the routine formalin fixation may hamper the use of qRT-PCR assays, the recently introduced, alternative non-crosslinking fixatives such as PAXgene (Preanalytix) could be used for such purposes [19]. To our knowledge, there have been no reports of the fusion gene detected in tissues of men without any prostatic disorders, which supports the potential to use the fusion gene for risk analyses. However, there have been findings of *TMPRSS2-ERG* in the tissue of 6–8 % men with BPH but without history or suspicion of prostate cancer [5, 7]. This is suggested to be due to the fusion gene being a sign of early changes in the gland, but not always leading to malignancy, and naturally means that a positive *TMPRSS2-ERG* mRNA test result does not require the presence of a current prostate carcinoma.

Conclusions

Our systematic study, despite its highly preliminary nature, shows that even though it is rare, it is possible to detect *TMPRSS2-ERG* transcripts in cancerous prostates in areas other than the carcinoma regions. If validated with larger cohorts and biopsy or TURP material, this could bring a new additive to assessment of risk of prostate cancer especially in men with negative biopsies.

Abbreviations

BPH: Benign prostatic hyperplasia; cDNA: Complementary DNA; ERG: ETV-related gene; FFPE: Formalin-fixed, paraffin-embedded; HB: Histologically benign; HBAC: Histologically benign tissue immediately adjacent to a carcinoma/PIN sample; HE: Hematoxylin-eosin; IHC: Immunohistochemistry; KLK3: Kallikrein-related peptidase 3; mRNA: Messenger RNA; PCA3: Prostate cancer antigen 3; PCR: Polymerase chain reaction; PIN: Prostatic intraepithelial neoplasia; PSA: Prostate specific antigen; qRT-PCR: quantitative reverse-transcription PCR; TMPRSS2: Transmembrane protease serine 2; TURP: Transurethral resection of the prostate.

Competing interests

The authors declare that they have no competing interests.

Authors' contributions

RMV participated in the study design and coordination, sample collection, and immunohistochemistry experiments; performed qRT-PCR assays and their data analysis; performed statistical analysis of the data; and drafted the manuscript. NTO participated in the sample collection; performed immunohistochemistry experiments, qRT-PCR assays, and their data analyses; and critically revised the manuscript for important intellectual content. PJB provided the clinical data; participated in the data interpretation; and critically revised the manuscript for important intellectual content. PT participated in the study design and coordination; performed the sample collection, histological examination of the tissue sections, and digital imaging; participated in the data interpretation; and critically revised the manuscript for important intellectual content. KP conceived the study; participated in the study design and coordination; participated in the data analysis and interpretation; and critically revised the manuscript for important intellectual content. All authors read and approved the final manuscript.

Authors information

Riina-Minna Väänänen is the corresponding author. Pekka Taimen and Kim Pettersson have a joint senior authorship.

Acknowledgments

The authors would like to thank Krista Bergendahl and Sinikka Collanus for excellent technical assistance.

Author details

[1]Department of Biotechnology, University of Turku, Turku, Finland.
[2]Department of Urology, Turku University Hospital, Turku, Finland.
[3]Department of Pathology, University of Turku and Turku University Hospital, Turku, Finland.

References

1. Slaughter DP, Southwick HW, Smejkal W. Field cancerization in oral stratified squamous epithelium; clinical implications of multicentric origin. Cancer. 1953;6:963–8.
2. Ogden GR1, Cowpe JG, Green MW. Evidence of field change in oral cancer. Br J Oral Maxillofac Surg. 1990;28:390–2.
3. Popa I, Fradet Y, Beaudry G, Hovington H, Beaudry G, Têtu B. Identification of PCA3 (DD3) in prostatic carcinoma by in situ hybridization. Mod Pathol. 2007;20:1121–7.
4. Nonn L, Ananthanarayanan V, Gann PH. Evidence for field cancerization of the prostate. Prostate. 2009;69:1470–9.
5. Clark J, Merson S, Jhavar S, Flohr P, Edwards S, Foster CS, et al. Diversity of TMPRSS2-ERG fusion transcripts in the human prostate. Oncogene. 2007;26:2667–73.
6. Furusato B, Gao CL, Ravindranath L, Chen Y, Cullen J, McLeod DG, et al. Mapping of TMPRSS2-ERG fusions in the context of multi-focal prostate cancer. Mod Pathol. 2008;21:67–75.
7. Robert G, Jannink S, Smit F, Aalders T, Hessels D, Cremers R, et al. Rational basis for the combination of PCA3 and TMPRSS2: ERG gene fusion for prostate cancer diagnosis. Prostate. 2013;73:113–20.
8. Väänänen RM, Lilja H, Cronin A, Kauko L, Rissanen M, Kauko O, et al. Association of transcript levels of 10 established or candidate-biomarker gene targets with cancerous versus non-cancerous prostate tissue from radical prostatectomy specimens. Clin Biochem. 2013;46:670–4.
9. Väänänen RM, Lilja H, Kauko L, Helo P, Kekki H, Cronin AM, et al. Cancer-associated Changes in the Expression of TMPRSS2-ERG, PCA3, and SPINK1 in Histologically Benign Tissue From Cancerous vs Noncancerous Prostatectomy Specimens. Urology. 2014;83:511. e1-7.
10. Väänänen RM, Rissanen M, Kauko O, Junnila S, Väisänen V, Nurmi J, et al. Quantitative real-time RT-PCR assay for PCA3. Clin Biochem. 2008;41:103–8.
11. Nurmi J, Lilja H, Ylikoski A. Time-resolved fluorometry in end-point and real-time PCR quantification of nucleic acids. Luminescence. 2000;15:381–8.
12. Nurmi J, Wikman T, Karp M, Lövgren T. High-performance real-time quantitative RT-PCR using lanthanide probes and a dual-temperature hybridization assay. Anal Chem. 2002;74:3525–32.
13. Nurmi J, Ylikoski A, Soukka T, Karp M, Lövgren T. A new label technology for the detection of specific polymerase chain reaction products in a closed tube. Nucleic Acids Res. 2000;28, E28.
14. Rissanen M, Helo P, Väänänen RM, Wahlroos V, Lilja H, Nurmi M, et al. Novel homogenous time-resolved fluorometric RT-PCR assays for quantification of PSA and hK2 mRNAs in blood. Clin Biochem. 2007;40:111–8.
15. van Leenders GJ, Boormans JL, Vissers CJ, Hoogland AM, Bressers AA, Furusato B, et al. Antibody EPR3864 is specific for ERG genomic fusions in prostate cancer: implications for pathological practice. Mod Pathol. 2011;24:1128–38.
16. Bussemakers MJ, van Bokhoven A, Verhaegh GW, Smit FP, Karthaus HF, Schalken JA, et al. DD3: a new prostate-specific gene, highly overexpressed in prostate cancer. Cancer Res. 1999;59:5975–9.
17. Hessels D, Klein Gunnewiek JM, van Oort I, Karthaus HF, van Leenders GJ, van Balken B, et al. DD3 (PCA3)-based molecular urine analysis for the diagnosis of prostate cancer. Eur Urol. 2003;44:8–15.
18. Tomlins SA, Bjartell A, Chinnaiyan AM, Jenster G, Nam RK, Rubin MA, et al. ETS gene fusions in prostate cancer: from discovery to daily clinical practice. Eur Urol. 2009;56:275–86.
19. Staff S, Kujala P, Karhu R, Rökman A, Ilvesaro J, Kares S, et al. Preservation of nucleic acids and tissue morphology in paraffin-embedded clinical samples: comparison of five molecular fixatives. J Clin Pathol. 2013;66:807–10.
20. de Kok JB, Verhaegh GW, Roelofs RW, Hessels D, Kiemeney LA, Aalders TW, et al. DD3 (PCA3), a very sensitive and specific marker to detect prostate tumors. Cancer Res. 2002;62:2695–8.
21. Tomlins SA, Rhodes DR, Perner S, Dhanasekaran SM, Mehra R, Sun XW, et al. Recurrent fusion of TMPRSS2 and ETS transcription factor genes in prostate cancer. Science. 2005;310:644–8.
22. Cerveira N, Ribeiro FR, Peixoto A, Costa V, Henrique R, Jerónimo C, et al. TMPRSS2-ERG gene fusion causing ERG overexpression precedes chromosome copy number changes in prostate carcinomas and paired HGPIN lesions. Neoplasia. 2006;8:826–32.

13

Tramadol for premature ejaculation

Marrissa Martyn-St James[1]*, Katy Cooper[1], Eva Kaltenthaler[1], Kath Dickinson[1], Anna Cantrell[1], Kevan Wylie[2], Leila Frodsham[3] and Catherine Hood[4]

Abstract

Background: Tramadol is a centrally acting analgesic prescribed off-label for the treatment of premature ejaculation (PE). However, tramadol may cause addiction and difficulty in breathing and the beneficial effect of tramadol in PE is yet not supported by a high level of evidence. The purpose of this study was to systematically review the evidence from randomised controlled trials (RCT) for tramadol in the management of PE.

Methods: We searched bibliographic databases including MEDLINE to August 2014 for RCTs. The primary outcome was intra-vaginal ejaculatory latency time (IELT). Methodological quality of RCTs was assessed. Between-group differences in IELT and other outcomes were pooled across RCTs in a meta-analysis. Statistical and clinical between-trial heterogeneity was assessed.

Results: A total of eight RCTs that evaluated tramadol against a comparator were included. The majority of RCTs were of unclear methodological quality due to limited reporting. Pooled evidence (four RCTs, 721 participants), suggests that tramadol is significantly more effective than placebo at increasing IELT over eight to 12 weeks (p = 0.0007). However, a high level of statistical heterogeneity is evident (I-squared = 74%). Single RCT evidence indicates that tramadol is significantly more effective than paroxetine taken on-demand, sildenafil, lidocaine gel, or behavioural therapy on IELT in men with PE. Tramadol is associated with significantly more adverse events including: erectile dysfunction, constipation, nausea, headache, somnolence, dry mouth, dizziness, pruritus, and vomiting, than placebo or behavioural therapy over eight to 12 weeks of treatment. However, addiction problems or breathing difficulties reported by patients for PE is not assessed in the current evidence base.

Conclusions: Tramadol appears effective in the treatment of PE. However, these findings should be interpreted with caution given the observed levels of between-trial heterogeneity and the reporting quality of the available evidence. The variability across placebo-controlled trials in terms of the tramadol dose evaluated and the treatment duration does not permit any assessment of a safe and effective minimum daily dose. The long-term effects and side effects, including addiction potential, for men with PE have not been evaluated in the current evidence base.

Keywords: Premature ejaculation, Tramadol, Systematic review, Meta-analysis, Efficacy, Safety

Background

Premature ejaculation (PE) is commonly defined by a short ejaculatory latency, a perceived lack of ejaculatory control; both related to self-efficacy; and distress and interpersonal difficulty [1]. PE can be either lifelong (primary), present since first sexual experiences, or acquired (secondary), beginning later [2]. The recently updated International Society of Sexual Medicine's Guidelines for the Diagnosis and Treatment of Premature Ejaculation (PE) propose that PE is a male sexual dysfunction characterised by ejaculation within about one minute of vaginal penetration (lifelong PE) or a reduction in latency time to ≤3 minutes (secondary PE), the inability to delay ejaculation, and negative personal consequences [3].

* Correspondence: m.martyn-stjames@sheffield.ac.uk
[1]School for Health and Related Research (ScHARR), University of Sheffield, Regent Court, 30 Regent Street, Sheffield S1 4DA, UK
Full list of author information is available at the end of the article

The treatment of PE should attempt to alleviate concern about the condition as well as increase sexual satisfaction for the patient and the partner [4]. Available treatment pathways for the condition are varied and treatments may include both behavioural and/or pharmacological interventions. Tramadol is a centrally acting analgesic agent that combines opioid receptor activation and re-uptake inhibition of serotonin and noradrenaline, prescribed off-label for the treatment of PE. Dapoxetine (a selective serotonin re-uptake inhibitor) is currently the only approved oral drug to treat PE. In May 2009, the US Food and Drug Administration released a warning letter about tramadol's potential to cause addiction and difficulty in breathing [5]. Tramadol has previously been evaluated by three systematic reviews [6-8], two of which have pooled data in a meta-analysis [7,8]. The search methodology and inclusion criteria vary across these reviews. Of the two reviews including a meta-analysis, one [7] pooled data across different study types (observational studies and RCTs) using a mean difference [7]. One review pooled IELT effect estimates across studies using a standardised mean difference [8]. The European Association of Urology guidelines for the management of PE summarise that tramadol has shown a moderate beneficial effect with a similar efficacy as dapoxetine. However, that the beneficial effect of tramadol in PE is yet not supported by a high level of evidence [9].

The aim of this study was to systematically review the evidence base for tramadol in the management of PE, by summarising evidence from randomised controlled trials (RCTs) and reporting a mean difference meta-analysis of RCT IELT data. The review addressed the question "in men with premature ejaculation, what is the clinical effectiveness of tramadol as compared with a non-active comparators or other treatments, evaluated in randomised controlled trials". The review is registered on PROSPERO 2013:CRD42013005289. Available from http://www.crd.york.ac.uk/PROSPERO/display_record.asp?ID=CRD42013005289.

Methods

The review was undertaken in accordance with the general principles recommended in the Preferred Reporting Items for Systematic Reviews and Meta-Analyses (PRISMA) statement [10].

Searches

The following databases were searched from inception to 5 August 2014 for published and unpublished research evidence: MEDLINE; Embase; Cumulative Index to Nursing and Allied Health Literature (CINAHL); The Cochrane Library including the Cochrane Systematic Reviews Database (CDSR), Cochrane Controlled Trials

Register (CCRT), Database of Abstracts of Reviews of Effects (DARE) and the Health Technology Assessment (HTA) database; ISI Web of Science (WoS), including Science Citation Index, and the Conference Proceedings Citation Index-Science. Full search terms are reported elsewhere [11]. The U.S. Food and Drug Administration (FDA) website and the European Medicines Agency (EMA) website were also searched. Existing systematic reviews were also checked for eligible studies. All citations were imported into Reference Manager Software and any duplicates deleted. The MEDLINE search strategy is presented as an Additional file 1.

Study selection

Searches were screened for potentially relevant studies by one reviewer and a subset checked by a second reviewer (and a check for consistency undertaken). Full texts were screened by two reviewers. Details of studies identified for inclusion were extracted using a data extraction sheet.

Eligible studies

RCTs in adult men with PE that evaluated tramadol were eligible for inclusion. Randomised crossover design studies were excluded to avoid double counting of participants in the meta-analysis. Theses and dissertations were not included. Non-English publications were included where sufficient data could be extracted from an English-language abstract or tables.

Outcomes

The primary outcome was intra-vaginal ejaculatory latency time (IELT). Other outcomes included sexual satisfaction, control over ejaculation, relationship satisfaction, self-esteem, quality of life, treatment acceptability and adverse events.

Data extraction

One reviewer performed data extraction of each included study. All numerical data were then checked by a second reviewer.

Methodological quality of studies

Methodological quality of RCTs was assessed using the Cochrane Collaboration risk of bias assessment criteria [12]. We classified RCTs as being at overall 'low' or 'high' risk of bias if they were rated as such for each of three key domains - allocation concealment, blinding of outcome assessment and completeness of outcome data (attrition <30%).

Data synthesis

Where possible, between-group differences for direct comparisons (e.g., tramadol vs. placebo) were pooled across trials in a pairwise meta-analysis using Cochrane RevMan software (version 5.2) (RevMan 2012 [13]). Continous variables were analysed as a mean difference (MD) and dichotomous variables as a risk ratio (RR). No subgroup or sensitivity analyses were planned. For comparisons where there was little apparent clinical heterogeneity and the I^2 value (I^2 statistic [14]) was 40% or less, a fixed-effect model was applied. Random-effects models were applied where I^2 value was >40%. Between-group effect estimates were considered significant at $p < 0.05$. Where >5 RCT comparisons were available, publication bias was assessed by visual inspection of funnel plots.

Ethical approval and consent from patients

The project was not primary research involving humans or animals but was a secondary analysis of human subject data available in the public domain.

Results

Search results

The searches identified 2,331 citations (as part of a wider project assessing a variety of treatments for PE [11]). Of these, 2,319 citations were excluded as titles/abstracts. Twelve full-text articles were obtained as potentially relevant. The study selection process is fully detailed in the PRISMA flow diagram in Figure 1. A total of seven RCTs that evaluated tramadol against a comparator (placebo, another agent, or behavioural therapy) and one RCT that evaluated different tramadol doses (eight RCTs in total) were identified.

Details of the included RCTs, the comparator(s), outcomes assessed and the risk of bias assessment are detailed in Table 1.

Risk of bias assessment of RCTs

The majority of RCTs were considered at overall unclear risk of bias mainly due to lack of reporting of information

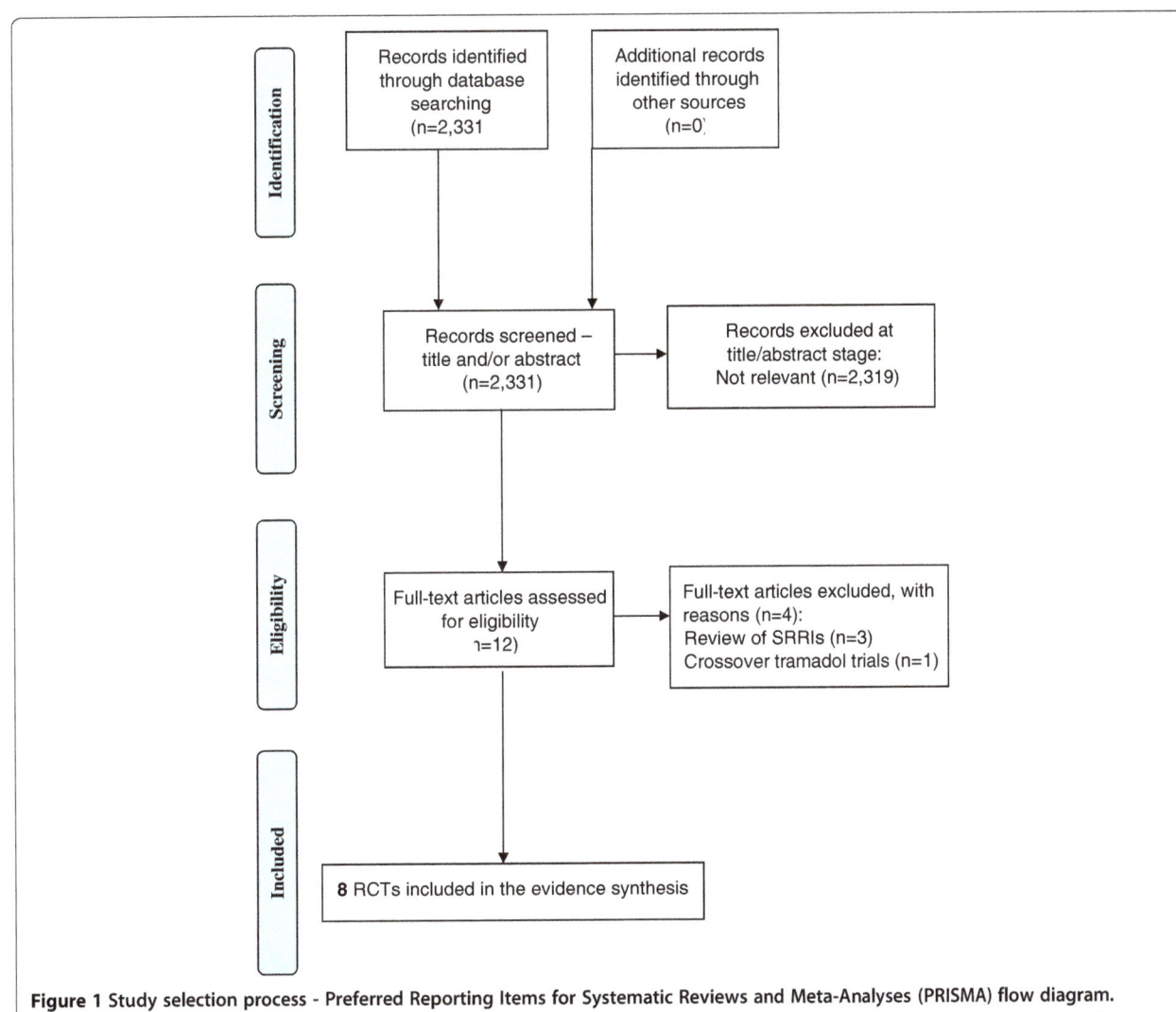

Figure 1 Study selection process - Preferred Reporting Items for Systematic Reviews and Meta-Analyses (PRISMA) flow diagram.

Table 1 RCT characteristics, efficacy and safety outcomes, and risk of bias assessment

RCT (country) duration	PE definition, Lifelong/ acquired PE, erectile dysfuntion	Treatment, comparator, numbers analysed/randomised (%) When taken	Efficacy outcomes and results	Adverse events	Risk of bias assessment
Alghobary 2010 [15] (Egypt) 6 weeks	DSM-IV-TR All lifelong PE ED, NR	- Tramadol 50 mg 2 to 3 h PC, 17/17 (100%) - Paroxetine 20 mg/d, 18/18 (100%)	IELT (Stopwatch): see Figure 3. Arabic Index of Premature Ejaculation (AIPE): significant improvement in scores at 6 weeks with both tramadol and paroxetine. Difference between groups not significant. Tramadol group had less rigid erections than paroxetine group	The drugs were generally tolerated and no serious side-effects encountered apart from mild headache and gastric upset with paroxetine and mainly gastric upset with tramadol and no withdrawn cases recorded.	Unclear risk - allocation method and blinded outcome assessment not reported
Bar-Or 2012 [18] (11 EU countries) 12 weeks	DSM-IV-TR All lifelong PE ED, excluded	- Tramadol 62 mg, 206/232 (89%) - Tramadol 89 mg, 198/217 (91%) - Placebo, 200/228 (88%) 2 to 8 h PC	IELT (Stopwatch): see Figure 3. Premature Ejaculation Profile (PEP): Mean change for all 4 measures significantly higher in both tramadol groups than placebo Female partner PEP scores: more had improvement (>= 1 category) for tramadol than placebo on all 4 measures	Any adverse event: Tramadol 62 mg: 12% Tramadol 89 mg: 16% Placebo: 7% No difference was observed in the incidence of withdrawal by treatment group (0.0% placebo, 1.0% 62 mg tramadol, 1.6% 89 mg tramadol). There were no serious AEs.	Unclear risk - allocation method and blinded outcome assessment not reported
Eassa 2013 [20] (Egypt) 24 weeks	PE def, NR All lifelong PE ED, excluded	- Tramadol 25 mg, 100/100 (100%) - Tramadol 50 mg, 100/100 (100%) - Tramadol 100 mg 100/100 (100%) 2 to 3 h PC	IELT (Stopwatch): see Figure 3	Tramadol 25 mg - somnolence (100%); pruritus (100%) Tramadol 50 mg - somnolence (100%); pruritus (100%); dizziness (18%); headache (16%); dry mouth (13%) Tramadol 100 mg - somnolence (100%); pruritus (100%); dizziness (38%); headache (30%); dry mouth (20%); nausea (20%); vomiting (17%)	Unclear risk - allocation method and blinded outcome assessment not reported
Gameel 2013 [16] (Egypt) 4 weeks	IELT of <2 min in >75% of episodes All had PE for >1 year ED, excluded	- Tramadol 50 mg 2 h PC + inert lubricating gel 15 min PC, 29/30 (97%) - Sildenafil 50 mg 1 h PC + inert lubricating gel 15 min PC, 30/30 (100%) - Paroxetine 20 mg 4 h PC + inert lubricating gel 15 min PC, 28/30 (93%) - Lidocaine gel 15 min PC + oral multivitamin 1-4 h PC, 30/30 (100%) - Placebo (oral multivitamin 1-4 h PC + inert lubricating gel 15 min PC), 27/30 (90%)	IELT (stopwatch): see Figure 3. Sexual satisfaction (0 to 5 point scale: Tramadol and paroxetine were associated with comparable drug-induced improvements in sexual satisfaction, but tramadol was associated with significantly better sexual satisfaction scores than was the local anaesthetic.	Greater sleep disturbance, dry mouth, nausea, dizziness, fatigue, vomiting, sweating, and headache were reported with tramadol, sildenafil and paroxetine. All side effects were reported as being tolerable.	Unclear risk - allocation method and blinded outcome assessment not reported
Kahn 2013 [21] (India) 8 weeks	DSM-IV TR 41/60 (68%) lifelong PE ED, excluded	- Tramadol 100 mg/d, 4 weeks then 2 or 8 h PC, 4 weeks; 30/30 (100%) - Placebo/ d, 4 weeks then 2 or 8 h PC, 4 weeks; 30/30 (100%)	IELT (stopwatch): Week 8 tramadol daily 202.5 s, 2 or 8 h PC, 238.2 s (p < 0.001 vs baseline); placebo daily 94.8 s (p = 0.632 vs baseline) placebo 2 or 8 h PC 96.6 s (p = 0.611 vs baseline). Coital frequency tramadol daily 4.32/week (p = 0.005) tramadol 2 or 8 h PC 4.86/week (p = 0.005). Coital frequency placebo daily 2.88/week (p = 0.875) placebo 2 or 8 h PC 3.23/week (p = 0.752).	The overall AE rate was 9.8% (6.7%, and 12.4% for placebo and 100 mg tramadol respectively) ED occurred in 3.33% of men (n = 1). Vertigo was observed in 3.33% of patients (n = 2); dizziness, headache, drowsiness, and common cold were observed in 6.67% of patients (n = 2 each). There were no serious AEs.	Unclear risk - allocation method and blinded outcome assessment not reported

Table 1 RCT characteristics, efficacy and safety outcomes, and risk of bias assessment *(Continued)*

Kaynar 2012 [17] (Turkey) 8 weeks	IELT ≤2 min during 90% intercourse episodes All lifelong PE ED, excluded	- Tramadol 25 mg, 30/30 (100%) - Placebo, 30/30 (100%) 2 h PC	IELT (stopwatch): see Figure 3. Ability of ejaculation control (AEC): Tramadol: Mean increase 2.0 Placebo: Mean increase 0.57 Tramadol better than placebo (p < 0.001) Sexual satisfaction scores (SSS) Tramadol: Mean increase 1.80 (SD 0.98). Placebo: Mean increase 0.53 (SD 0.92) Tramadol better than placebo (p < 0.001)	Any adverse event: Tramadol: 27% Placebo: 0% Mild nausea/headache: Tramadol: 20% Mild somnolence: Tramadol: (6.5%)	Unclear risk - allocation method and blinded outcome assessment not reported
Safarinejad 2006 [19] (Iran) 8 weeks	IELT ≤2 min during 90% coitus All lifelong PE ED, excluded	- Tramadol 50 mg, 29/32 (91%) - Placebo, 28/32 (88%) 2 h PC	IELT (stopwatch): see Figure 3. IIEF: intercourse satisfaction: Tramadol: mean change 4 Placebo: mean change −1 Between-groups p < 0.05	Any adverse event: Tramadol: 28% Placebo: 16% (mainly nausea)	Unclear risk - blinded outcome assessment not reported
Xiong 2011 [22] (China) 12 weeks	IELT ≤2 min All lifelong PE ED, NR	- Tramadol 50 mg 2 h PC with behavioural therapy (not reported which) (n = 36) - Behavioural therapy alone (n = 36);	IELT (stopwatch): see Figure 3. IIEF Tramadol + BT: mean change 4 BT alone: mean change 2 Between-groups p < 0.05	Any adverse event: Tramadol: 28% Placebo: 0% Tramadol: nausea (11.1%), vomiting (2.8%), dry mouth (5.6%), dizziness (8.3%).	Unclear risk - allocation method and blinded outcome assessment not reported (unable to assess fully – body text of article in Chinese)

/d, daily; DSM, Diagnostic and Statistical Manual of Mental Disorders; ED, erectile dysfunction; IELT, intra-vaginal ejaculatory latency time; IIEF, International Index of Erectile Dysfunction; NR, not reported; PC, pre-coitus; PE, premature ejaculation.

to inform the risk of bias assessment. Three RCTs were described as single-blind and were considered at high risk of performance bias [15-17]. One RCT was considered to be at overall high risk of bias as randomisation to study groups was according to patients' presentation sequence at clinic, suggesting a non-random component in the sequence generation [17]. A summary of the risk of bias assessment for each included RCT is presented in Figure 2.

Characteristics of RCTs

RCT details of the treatments, efficacy and safety outcomes, and the risk of bias assessment are presented in Table 1. Where reported, the definition of PE was varied and was defined according to: DSM-IV (Diagnostic and Statistical Manual of Mental Disorders) criteria [15,18], an IELT of two minutes or less [16,17,19], or was not reported [20]. The majority of RCTs recruited samples comprising men with lifelong PE and without erectile dysfunction.

Tramadol was prescribed across all RCTs, on-demand one to four hours prior to sexual intercourse. Prescribed doses varied and range from 25 mg [17,20] to 100 mg [20,21]. Comparators included placebo [17-19,21], selective serotonin re-uptake inhibitors (SSRI) [15,16], phosphodiesterase-5 (PDE5) inhibitors [16], anaesthetic gel [16] and behavioural therapy [22]. One RCT evaluated three tramadol doses only (no placebo) [20]. Treatment duration ranged from four weeks to six months. The majority of included RCTs were 8 weeks duration. Only one trial was undertaken in the EU (across 11 EU countries) [18]. The remainder were undertaken in Egypt [15,16,20], Turkey [17], India [21], Iran [19] and China [22].

Outcome data reported by RCTs

IELT was assessed by all of the included RCTs (Table 1, Figure 3, Figure 4). Where reported, the assessment method was by stopwatch. The reporting of other efficacy outcomes was much more varied, both in the assessment method and the outcome data available (Table 1). Across the majority of RCTs, outcome data for adverse event reporting was disparate in terms of limited reporting of types of adverse events and patient numbers.

Data synthesis

IELT as a mean outcome with a variance estimate was available for all but two RCTs [21,23]. One reported significant changes in IELT at week eight in the tramadol group ($p < 0.001$) [23]. P-values for the between-group difference compared with placebo, or the change in the placebo group, were not reported. One RCT reported significant changes in IELT at week eight with tramadol daily ($p < 0.001$) or on-demand ($p < 0.001$), but not placebo ($p = 0.632$ and 0.611). P-values for the between-group difference were not reported.

Tramadol vs. placebo: Meta-analysis of mean IELT change (minutes) at 8 or 12 week follow-up, based on -four RCT study group comparisons from -three RCTs ($n = 721$), displayed high heterogeneity ($I^2 = 74\%$). The pooled mean difference (MD) in IELT was 1.24 minutes, favouring tramadol [MD (random effects) 95% confidence interval [CI], 0.52 to 1.95; $p = 0.009$]. The between-group difference in end of study values at four weeks based on one RCT ($n = 56$) was 4.50 minutes (95% CI 3.75 to 5.25; $p < 0.00001$), in favour of tramadol. The forest plot for these analyses is presented in Figure 2.

Significant improvements on measures of the Premature Ejaculation Profile (PEP) ($p < 0.05$ for all) with tramadol compared with placebo were reported by one RCT [18]. Significant between-group differences on the International

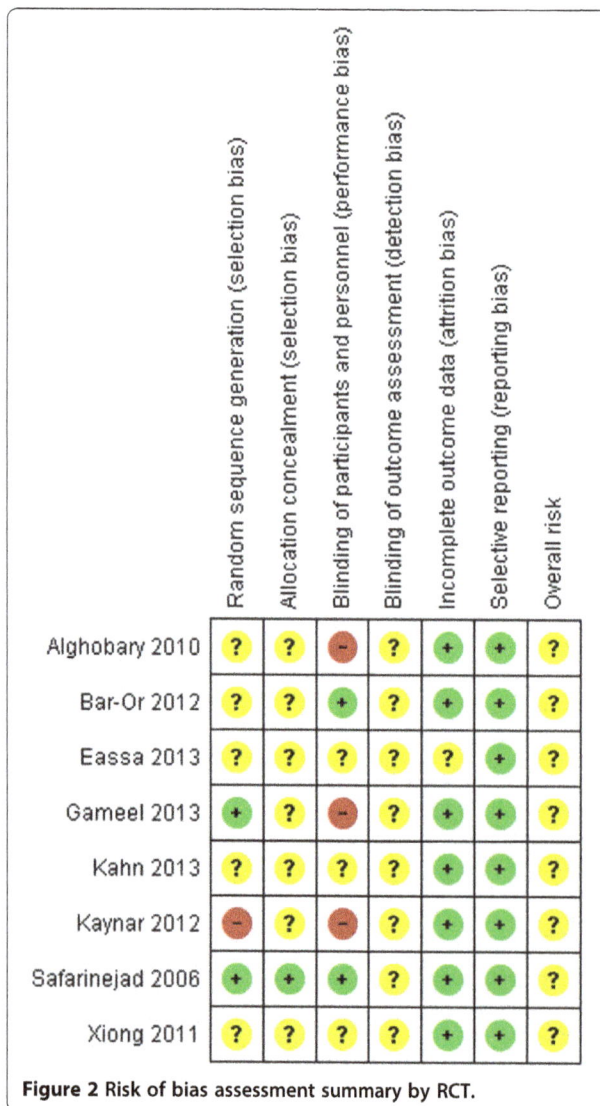

Figure 2 Risk of bias assessment summary by RCT.

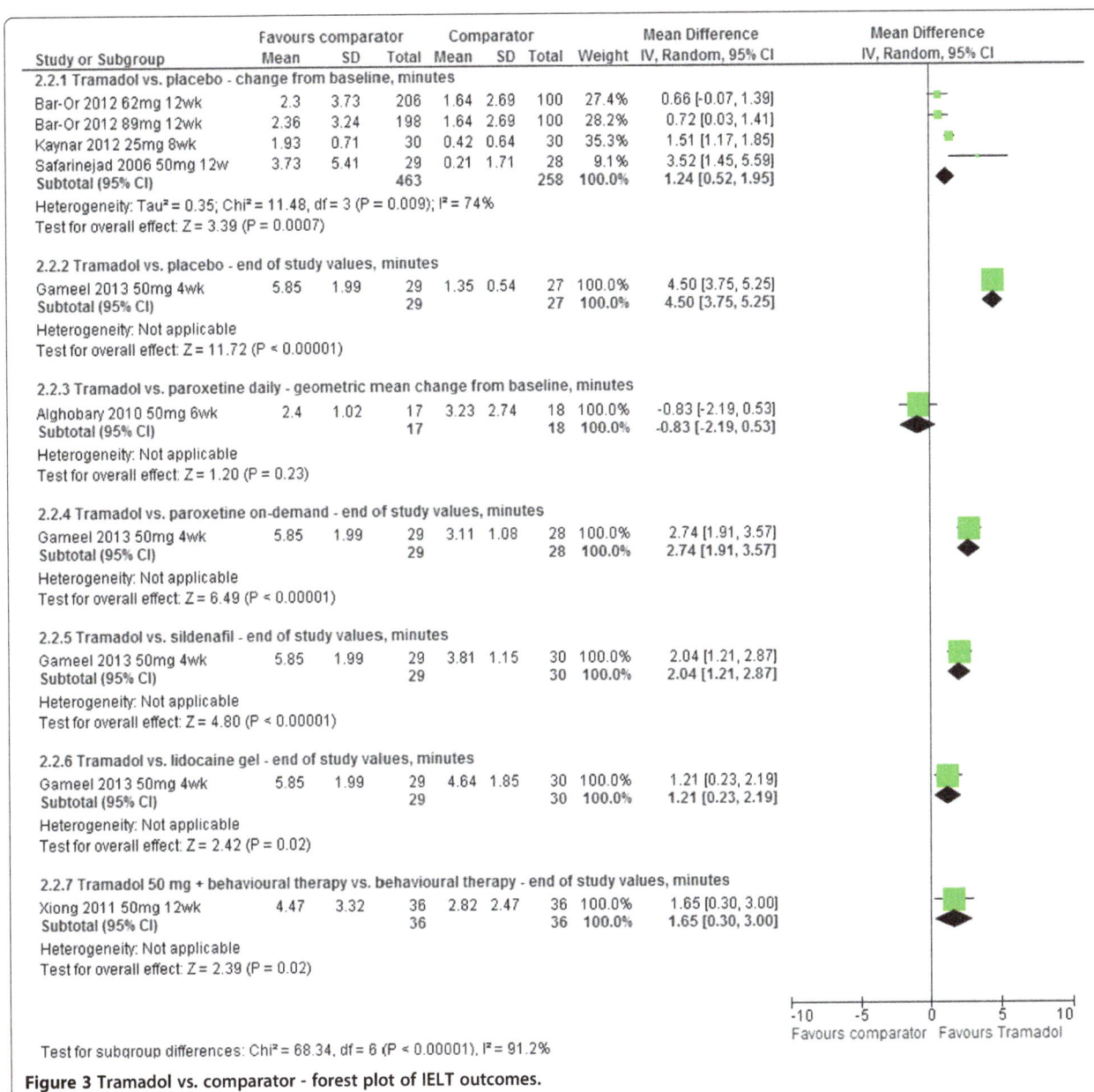

Figure 3 Tramadol vs. comparator - forest plot of IELT outcomes.

Index of Erectile Function (IIEF) mean number of coitus per week and mean intercourse satisfaction favouring tramadol (p < 0.05) were reported by one RCT [19] A statistically significant increase in weekly coitus associated with tramadol daily (p = 0.005) or on-demand (p = 0.005) was reported by one RCT (p-values for placebo p = 0.875 and 0.752 respectively) [21]. One RCT reported significant improvements on ability of ejaculation control and sexual satisfaction scores (instrument not reported) for tramadol over placebo (p < 0.001 for both) [17]. One RCT reported a significant between-group difference of p < 0.05 on the IIEF intercourse satisfaction score in favour of tramadol [17].

Where reported, adverse events associated with tramadol included: erectile dysfunction, constipation, nausea,

headache, somnolence, dry mouth, dizziness, pruritus (itching), and vomiting. Meta-analysis of numbers experiencing adverse events at 8 or 12 week follow-up displayed low heterogeneity ($I^2 = 0\%$). The pooled relative risk (RR) across five RCTs (583 participants) was 2.27 [RR (fixed effect) 95% confidence interval [CI], 1.45 to 3.57; p = 0.0004] in favour of placebo (lower risk). The forest plot for this analysis is presented in Figure 4.

Tramadol vs. paroxetine (SSRI): The between-group difference in geometric mean IELT (minutes) at 6 weeks, based on one RCT (n = 70) comparing tramadol with paroxetine taken daily, was −0.83 [95% CI, −1.80 to 0.14; p = 0.09]. The between-group difference in end of study mean IELT (minutes) at four weeks based on one RCT

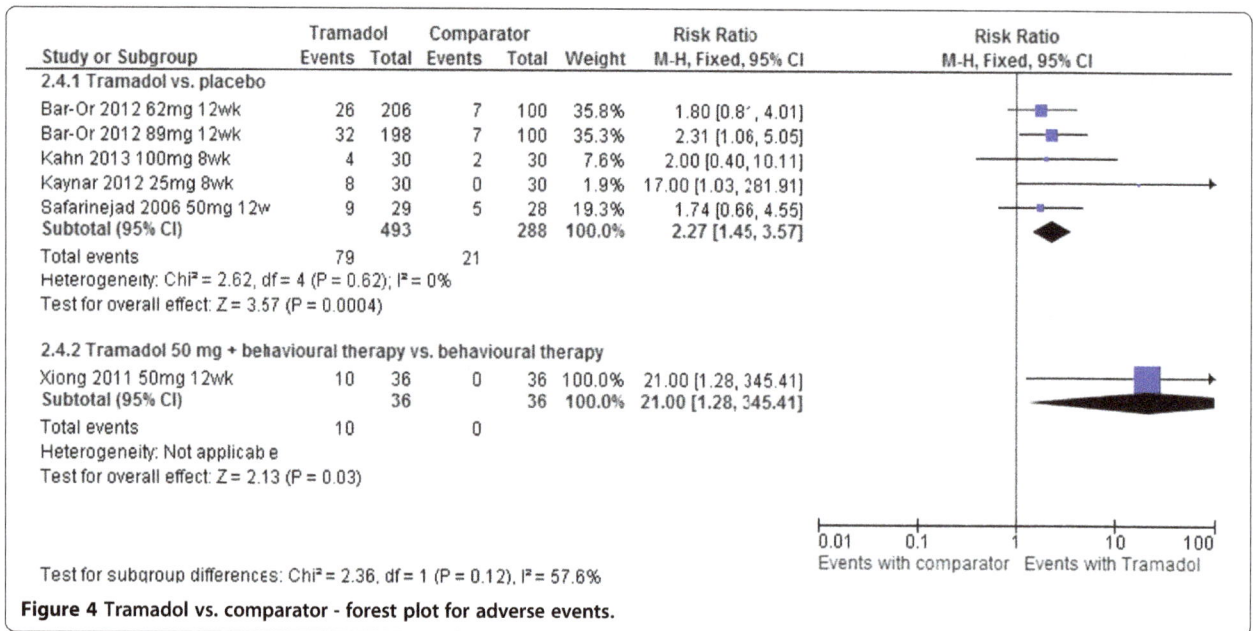

Figure 4 Tramadol vs. comparator - forest plot for adverse events.

(n = 57) was 2.74 (95% CI 1.91 to 3.57); p < 0.00001, in favour of tramadol compared with paroxetine taken on-demand (Figure 2).

One RCT [15] reported that paroxetine daily improved the Arabic Index of Premature Ejaculation score at 6 weeks (p < 0.05) and 12 weeks (p < 0.05) whereas tramadol improved AIPE at 6 weeks but not at 12 weeks. One RCT reported that both tramadol and paroxetine on-demand were associated with comparable improvements in sexual satisfaction (p > 0.05) [16].

One RCT reported that mild headache and gastric upset were associated with paroxetine daily and mainly gastric upset with tramadol [15] One RCT reported that sleep disturbance, dry mouth, nausea, dizziness, fatigue, vomiting, sweating, and headache were reported with tramadol, sildenafil and paroxetine on-demand, but that all side effects were tolerable [16].

Tramadol vs. sildenafil (PDE5 inhibitor): The between-group difference in end of study mean IELT (minutes) at four weeks based on one RCT (n = 59) was 2.01 (95% CI 1.21 to 2.87); p < 0.00001, in favour of tramadol (Figure 2).

Tramadol with behavioural therapy vs. behavioural therapy alone: The between-group difference in mean IELT (minutes) at 12 weeks, based on one RCT (n = 72), was 1.65, significantly favouring tramadol combined with behavioural therapy [95% CI, 0.30 to 3.00; p = 0.02]. The forest plot for this analysis is presented in Figure 2. The same RCT reported a between-group difference at 8 weeks of P < 0.05 on the International Index of Erectile Function (IIEF) favouring the tramadol group [22]. The between-group difference in numbers of participants experiencing adverse events at 12 weeks was 21.00 [RR (random effects) 95% confidence interval [CI], 1.28 to

345.410; p = 0.03] in favour of behavioural therapy alone (lower risk). The forest plot for this analysis is presented in Figure 4.

Tramadol vs. lidocaine gel: The between-group difference in end of study mean IELT (minutes) at four weeks based on one RCT (n = 59) was 1.21 (95% CI 0.23 to 2.17); p = 0.02, in favour of tramadol (Figure 2). The same RCT reported that tramadol was associated with significantly better sexual satisfaction scores than was the local anaesthetic (p < 0.05) [16].

Tramadol 25 mg, 50 mg, or 100 mg: One RCT (n = 300) evaluated three different doses of tramadol. The between-group differences in mean IELT (minutes) at 24 weeks were: 10.65 in favour of tramadol 50 mg *vs.* 25 mg [95% CI, 9.76 to 10.76; p < 0.00001]; 23.32 in favour of tramadol 100 mg *vs.* 25 mg [95% CI, 22.59 to 24.05; p < 0.00001]; and 13.06 in favour of tramadol 100 mg *vs.* 50 mg [95% CI, 12.33 to 13.79; p < 0.00001]. The forest plot for this analysis is presented in Figure 5. The same RCT [20], reported that all patients in the trial experienced one or more adverse events (all experienced somnolence and pruritus).

Discussion

Pooled evidence across four RCT study groups (721 participants), suggests that tramadol is significantly more effective than placebo at increasing IELT over eight to 12 weeks. However, a high level of between-trial statistical heterogeneity is evident. The largest between-group effect size (3.52 min) was notable for one RCT [19]. Three clinical studies by the same investigator have been retracted in the past three years. However, excluding this RCT from the analysis did not significantly alter the

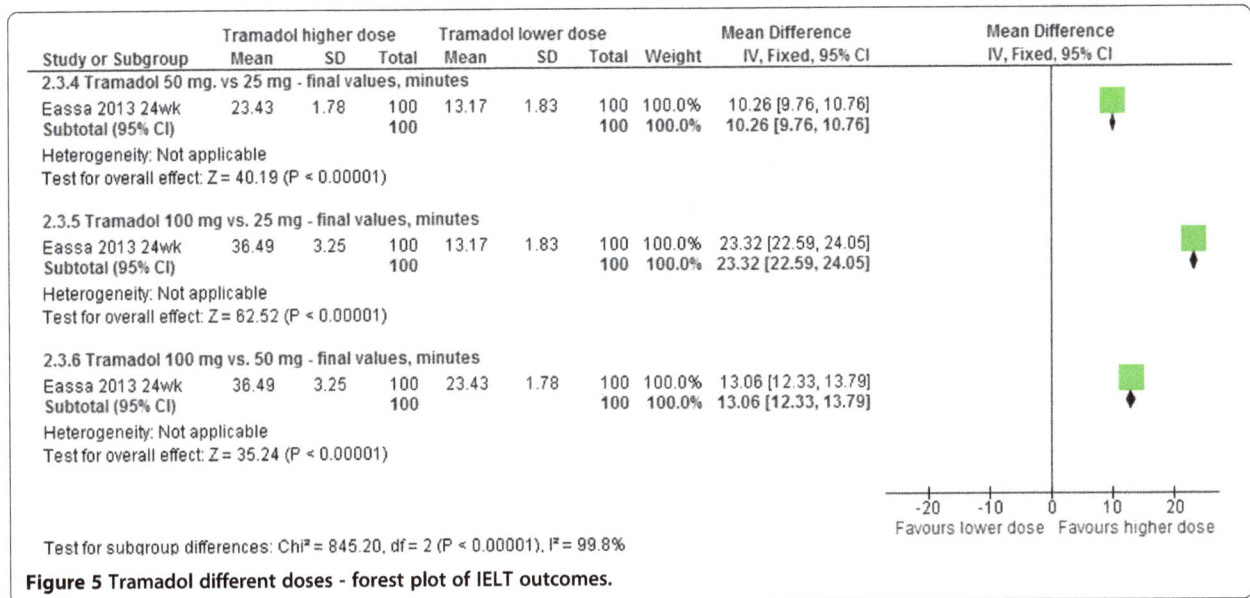

Study or Subgroup	Tramadol higher dose			Tramadol lower dose			Weight	Mean Difference IV, Fixed, 95% CI	Mean Difference IV, Fixed, 95% CI
	Mean	SD	Total	Mean	SD	Total			
2.3.4 Tramadol 50 mg. vs 25 mg - final values, minutes									
Eassa 2013 24wk	23.43	1.78	100	13.17	1.83	100	100.0%	10.26 [9.76, 10.76]	
Subtotal (95% CI)			100			100	100.0%	10.26 [9.76, 10.76]	
Heterogeneity: Not applicable									
Test for overall effect: Z = 40.19 (P < 0.00001)									
2.3.5 Tramadol 100 mg vs 25 mg - final values, minutes									
Eassa 2013 24wk	36.49	3.25	100	13.17	1.83	100	100.0%	23.32 [22.59, 24.05]	
Subtotal (95% CI)			100			100	100.0%	23.32 [22.59, 24.05]	
Heterogeneity: Not applicable									
Test for overall effect: Z = 62.52 (P < 0.00001)									
2.3.6 Tramadol 100 mg vs 50 mg - final values, minutes									
Eassa 2013 24wk	36.49	3.25	100	23.43	1.78	100	100.0%	13.06 [12.33, 13.79]	
Subtotal (95% CI)			100			100	100.0%	13.06 [12.33, 13.79]	
Heterogeneity: Not applicable									
Test for overall effect: Z = 35.24 (P < 0.00001)									

Test for subgroup differences: Chi² = 845.20, df = 2 (P < 0.00001), I² = 99.8%

Figure 5 Tramadol different doses - forest plot of IELT outcomes.

overall effect size (1.02 min) or reduce the between-trial heterogeneity (I-squared = 71%).

The placebo-controlled RCTs prescribed tramadol doses from 25 mg to 89 mg. Reporting of the methodological quality across these RCTs was limited. Blinded outcome assessment was not reported by any of the RCTs, which may have contributed to detection bias. Allocation concealment was not reported by five of RCTs, which may have contributed to selection bias [16-18,20-22]. One of the RCTs randomised participants according to their presentation sequence at clinic, which may have also contributed to selection bias [17]. As such, these results should be interpreted with caution.

The evidence from one RCT (70 participants) suggests that there is no difference in IELT between tramadol taken two to three hours prior to sexual intercourse and paroxetine daily [15]. Conversely, evidence from another RCT (59 participants) indicates that tramadol is significantly more effective than paroxetine taken on-demand at increasing IELT [16]. However, concealment of allocation and blinded outcome assessment were not reported by either RCT, and treatment duration was relatively short (six and four weeks respectively). As such, these results should be interpreted with caution. One of these RCTs also did not include a placebo group comparison [15]. Commonly used SSRIs in the management of PE including paroxetine (20 to 40 mg/d), are prescribed daily [9]. SSRIs such as paroxetine are absorbed slowly [24]. The half-lives of fluoxetine, paroxetine and sertraline range from 16 to 96 hours [25]. The pharmacokinetic properties of paroxetine may also account for the diverse results for the effects of tramadol compared with paroxetine on IELT.

Single RCT evidence also suggests that tramadol is significantly more effective than sildenafil, lidocaine gel, or

behavioural therapy on IELT in men with PE. However, reporting of the methodological quality is limited in terms of concealment of group allocation and blinding of the outcome assessment across all RCTs included by this review.

Various assessment methods in terms of ejaculation control, patient/partners sexual satisfaction, anxiety and other patient-reported outcomes have been used across RCTs to measure the effectiveness of tramadol. Across placebo-controlled RCTs, tramadol was reported as significantly more effective than placebo for various patient-reported outcomes. Pooled evidence across trials (817 participants) suggests that tramadol is associated with significantly more adverse events including: erectile dysfunction, constipation, nausea, headache, somnolence, dry mouth, dizziness, pruritus (itching), and vomiting, than placebo or behavioural therapy over eight to 12 weeks of treatment. Addiction to tramadol by patients treated with tramadol for PE was not assessed in the current evidence base. Likewise, patient acceptability of treatment was not reported. However, one RCT reported 100% follow-up of all patients prescribed 25 mg, 50 mg or 100 mg of tramadol over 24 weeks [20]. All participants at all doses (100%) reported somnolence. The trial was considered of unclear methodological quality.

With the exception of one RCT [18], all of the included RCTs were conduction in non-EU countries, five being conducted in Middle East and Arab State countries [15-17,19,20]. In a population-based stopwatch study, Waldinger et al. [26] observed the largest difference in IELT observed between Turkey and participants from the United Kingdom and the United States. Because characteristics of PE may differ culturally, the observations from this review might not be gene-ralizable across men from EU countries.

The risk of bias assessment indicates the majority of RCTs of tramadol in the treatment of PE are of unclear risk of detection bias, mainly due to limited reporting re-garding blinding of the outcome assessment. Key aspects of best practice in RCT design to minimise bias include a robust randomisation method, concealment of treat-ment group allocation, and, where possible, blinding of participants and trial personnel, and blinded outcome assessment; all of which should be clearly stated in the RCT report [27].

Although our database search strategy was compre-hensive, the possibility of a publication bias cannot be discounted. Insufficient numbers of RCT comparisons were available for any meaningful assessment of funnel plot symmetry to be undertaken. Nonetheless, although the RCTs identified for inclusion were of unclear meth-odological quality, it could be considered unlikely that any additional unpublished data for the effects of trama-dol compared with placebo would contribute signifi-cantly to the overall findings of this review.

The RCTs evaluating tramadol identified for inclusion evaluated treatments over four to 12 weeks and none re-ported a long-term follow-up on efficacy and safety out-comes, including addiction potential. However, more important is a requirement for clearer evaluations of the relationship between treatment-related increases in IELT, ejaculatory control and sexual satisfaction associated with tramadol. Adverse event data suggest that tramadol is associated with a number of adverse events, but that these appear tolerable. However, the long-term use of tramadol for the treatment of PE in terms of a safety profile including addiction potential is unclear from the current evidence base.

The results observed by this review for the effective-ness of tramadol in treatment of PE are comparable with other reviews [6-8]. However, where meta-analyses have previously been undertaken, methodological errors are evident [7,8]. This review has pooled data across RCTs, where appropriate, in a meta-analysis using a mean dif-ference to summarise IELT outcomes and has avoided double-counting of participants in the analysis.

The European Association of Urology 2014 Guidelines on male sexual dysfunction recommend that pharmaco-logical treatment options include 'on demand' dapoxe-tine, daily use of a longer acting selective serotonin reuptake inhibitor (SSRI) [off-label use], daily use of clo-mipramine (off-label use), 'on demand' topical local an-aesthetic agents (off-label use) and 'on demand' tramadol (off-label use) [9]. Given that tramadol has been exten-sively evaluated against placebo for the treatment of PE in the current evidence base, with limited head-to-head comparisons between tramadol and other treatments

(paroxetine, sildenafil and lidocaine gel), further direct comparisons between tramadol and other SSRIs includ-ing dapoxetine, other PDE5 inhibitors, and other top-ical anaesthetics should now be investigated. Whilst the observed increases in IELT were statistically significant in favour of tramadol, it is difficult to quantify how ac-ceptable and meaningful these changes are for men with PE, without being able to evaluate the relationship between IELT, ejaculation control, and sexual satisfac-tion from the current RCT evidence base for tramadol. The trade-off between IELT and other effectiveness out-comes versus adverse effects and addiction potential should also be further evaluated.

Conclusion
Tramadol appears more effective than placebo or behav-ioural therapy in the treatment of PE. However, these findings should be interpreted with caution given the observed levels of between-study heterogeneity and the methodological quality of the available evidence.

Abbreviations
DSM: Diagnostic and Statistical Manual of Mental Disorders; EU: European Union; IIEF: International Index of Erectile Function; IELT: Intra-vaginal ejaculatory latency time; PDE5: Phosphodiesterase-5; PE: Premature ejaculation; RCT: Randomised controlled trial; SSRI: Selective serotonin reuptake inhibitor.

Competing interests
The authors declare that they have no competing interests.

Authors' contributions
MMSJ and KC selected studies for inclusion and undertook quality assessment and data extraction. MMSJ undertook the meta-analysis and drafted the manuscript. KC, EK, KW, LF and CH commented on the manuscript. All authors read and approved the final manuscript.

Acknowledgements
KC and AC designed the search strategy and ran the electronic searches for the project. KW, LF and CH acted as clinical advisors.

Funding
This work was funded by NIHR Evaluation, Trials and Studies Coordinating Centre (NETSCC).
The views and opinions expressed therein are those of the authors and do not necessarily reflect those of the Health Technology Assessment Programme, NIHR, NHS or the Department of Health.

Author details
[1]School for Health and Related Research (ScHARR), University of Sheffield, Regent Court, 30 Regent Street, Sheffield S1 4DA, UK. [2]Porterbrook Clinic, Sexual Medicine, Sheffield, UK. [3]Institute of Psychosexual Medicine, London, UK. [4]St George's Hospital, London, UK.

References

1. McMahon CG, Althof S, Waldinger MD, Porst H, Dean J, Sharlip I, et al. An evidence-based definition of lifelong premature ejaculation: report of the International Society for Sexual Medicine Ad Hoc Committee for the Definition of Premature Ejaculation. BJU Int. 2008;102:338–50.

2. Godpodinoff ML. Premature ejaculation: clinical subgroups and etiology. J Sex Marital Ther. 1989;15:130–4.

3. Althof SE, McMahon CG, Waldinger MD, Serefoglu EC, Shindel AW, Adaikan PG, et al. An Update of the International Society of Sexual Medicine's Guidelines for the Diagnosis and Treatment of Premature Ejaculation (PE). Sex Med. 2014;11(6):1392–422.

4. Richardson D, Goldmeier D, Green J, Lamba H, Harris JRW. Recommendations for the management of premature ejaculation: BASHH Special Interest Group for Sexual Dysfunction. Int J STD AIDS. 2006;17:1–6.

5. U.S.Food and Drug Administration. Warning letter to William Weldon, CEO & Chairman of Johnson & Johnson, regarding Ultram-ER web advertisement. 19-5-2009. http://www.fda.gov/downloads/Drugs/.../UCM153130.pdf [Accessed 10-7-2014].

6. Wong BLK, Malde S. The use of tramadol "on-demand" for premature ejaculation: a systematic review. Urology. 2013;81:98–103.

7. Wu T, Yue X, Duan X, Luo D, Cheng Y, Tian Y, et al. Efficacy and safety of tramadol for premature ejaculation: a systematic review and meta-analysis. Urology. 2012;80:618–24.

8. Yang L, Qian S, Liu H, Liu L, Pu C, Han P, et al. Role of Tramadol in Premature Ejaculation: A Systematic Review and Meta-Analysis. Urol Int. 2013. [Epub ahead of print].

9. Hatzimouratidis K, Eardley I, Giuliano F, Hatzichristou D, Moncada I, Salonia AVY, et al. Guidelines on male sexual dysfunction: erectile dysfunction and premature ejaculation. Eur Urol. 2014;57:804–14.

10. Moher D, Liberati A, Tetzlaff J, Altman DG, The PRISMA Group. Preferred Reporting Items for Systematic Reviews and Meta-Analyses: The PRISMA Statement. PLoS Med. 2009;6:e1000097.

11. Cooper K, Martyn-St James M, Kaltenthaler E, Dickinosn K, Cantrell A. Interventions to treat premature ejaculation. Health Technol Assess. 2013. In Press.

12. Higgins JPT, Altman DG, Sterne JAC, on behalf of the Cochrane Statistical Methods Group and the Cochrane Bias Methods Group. Assessing risk of bias in included studies. In: Higgins JPT GS, editor. Cochrane Handbook for Systematic Reviews of Interventions Version 5.1.0 (updated March 2011). The Cochrane Collaboration; 2011. Available from www.cochrane-handbook.org.

13. The Nordic Cochrane Centre TCC. The Cochrane Collaboration Review Manager (RevMan). [5.2]. 2012.

14. Higgins JPTH, Thompson SG, Deeks JJ, Altman DG. Measuring inconsistency in meta-analyses. BMJ. 2003;327:557–60.

15. Alghobary M, El-Bayoumy Y, Mostafa Y, Mahmoud EHM, Amr M. Evaluation of tramadol on demand vs. daily paroxetine as a long-term treatment of lifelong premature ejaculation. J Sex Med. 2010;7:2860–7.

16. Gameel TA, Tawfik AM, Abou-Farha MO, Bastawisy MG, El-Bendary MA, El-Gamasy AE-N. On-demand use of tramadol, sildenafil, paroxetine and local anaesthetics for the management of premature ejaculation: a randomised placebo-controlled clinical trial. Arab J Urol. 2013;11:392–7.

17. Kaynar M, Kilic O, Yurdakul T. On-demand tramadol hydrochloride use in premature ejaculation treatment. Urology. 2012;79:145–9.

18. Bar-Or D, Salottolo KM, Orlando A, Winkler JV, Tramadol ODT, Study Group. A randomized double-blind, placebo-controlled multicenter study to evaluate the efficacy and safety of two doses of the tramadol orally disintegrating tablet for the treatment of premature ejaculation within less than 2 minutes. Eur Urol. 2012;61:736–43.

19. Safarinejad MR, Hosseini SY. Safety and efficacy of tramadol in the treatment of premature ejaculation: a double-blind, placebo-controlled, fixed-dose, randomized study. J Clin Psychopharmacol. 2006;26:27–31.

20. Eassa BI, El-Shazly MA. Safety and efficacy of tramadol hydrochloride on treatment of premature ejaculation. Asian J Androl. 2013;15:138–42.

21. Kahn AH, Deepa R. Tramadol use in premature ejaculation: daily versus sporadic treatment. Indian j psychol med. 2013;35:256–9.

22. Xiong GG, Wu FH, Chen SH, Yao WL. [Safety and efficacy of tramadol hydrochloride with behavioral modification in the treatment of premature ejaculation]. Zhonghua Nan Ke Xue. 2011;17:538–41.

23. Generali J, Cada DJ. Tramadol: Premature ejaculation. Hosp Pharm. 2006;41:1048–50.

24. Modi NB, Dresser MJ, Simon M, Lin D, Desai D, Gupta S. Single- and multiple-dose pharmacokinetics of dapoxetine hydrochloride, a novel agent for the treatment of premature ejaculation. J Clin Pharmacol. 2006;46 (3):301–9. ALZA Corporation, 1900 Charleston Road, Building M11-4A, Mountain View, CA 94043, USA.

25. Hiemke C, Hartter S. Pharmacokinetics of selective serotonin reuptake inhibitors. Pharmacol Ther. 2000;85:11–28.

26. Waldinger MD, Quinn P, Dilleen M, Mundayat R, Schweitzer DH, Boolell M. A multinational population survey of intravaginal ejaculation latency time. J Sex Med. 2005;2:492–7.

27. Schulz KF, Altman DG, Moher D. CONSORT 2010 Statement: updated guidelines for reporting parallel group randomised trials. BMJ. 2010;340:c332.

14

Changing paradigms in management of metastatic Castration Resistant Prostate Cancer (mCRPC)

Eva Gupta[1*], Troy Guthrie[2] and Winston Tan[1]

Abstract

Recently, the standard of care for metastatic Castration Resistant Prostate Cancer (mCRPC) has changed considerably. Persistent androgen receptor (AR) signaling has been identified as a target for novel therapies and reengages the fact that AR continues to be the primary target responsible for metastatic prostate cancer. Androgen receptor gene amplification and over expression have been found to result in a higher concentration of androgen receptors on tumor cells, making them extremely sensitive to low levels of circulating androgens. Additionally, prostate cancer cells are able to maintain dihydrotestosterone (DHT) concentration in excess of serum concentrations to support tumor growth. For many years ketoconazole was the only CYP17 inhibitor that was used to treat mCRPC. However, significant toxicities limit its use. Newly approved chemotherapeutic agents such as Abiraterone (an oral selective inhibitor of CYP17A), which blocks androgen biosynthesis both within and outside the prostate cancer cells), and enzalutamide (blocks AR signaling) have improved overall survival. There are also ongoing phase III trials for Orteronel (TAK- 700), ARN- 509 and Galeterone (TOK-001), which targets androgen signaling. In this review, we will present the rationale for the newly approved hormonal treatments, their indications and complications, and we will discuss ongoing trials that are being done to improve the efficacy of the approved agents. Finally, we will talk about the potential upcoming hormonal treatments for mCRPC.

Keywords: Castration resistant prostate cancer, CYP17 inhibition, Androgen deprivation therapy, Abiraterone, Enzalutamide, Ketoconazole, Orteronel, ARN-509, Galeterone (TOK-001)

Introduction

Prostate cancer is the most common cancer affecting men and represents the second leading cause of cancer related mortality in the western world [1]. In 1941, Huggins and Hodges et al. [2], demonstrated that androgen withdrawal led to regression of prostate cancer and alleviation of pain in these patients. This demonstrated the androgen dependence of normal prostate and prostate cancer cells for growth and survival.

The initial standard of care in many high-risk patients includes androgen deprivation therapy (ADT) [3,4] and radiation therapy. ADT can be achieved by either medical or surgical castration (bilateral orchidectomy) [5]. Castration reduces the serum testosterone to very low levels, which is known as the castration level. Until recently, medical castration was achieved by Gonadotropin-releasing hormone (GnRH) agonists. GnRH agonists inhibit the

pituitary release of luteinizing hormone, which is necessary for testicular androgen production. Degarelix is a GnRH antagonist, which lowers androgen levels but causes an unacceptably high rate (40%) of local injection site reactions and has not found much favor in clinical practice. Anti-androgens, such as flutamide and bicalutamide, can block the interaction of testosterone and DHT with its receptor. Combination GnRH agonists and androgen blockers has been called total androgen blockade (TAB) and was popular in the 1990's to treat metastatic prostate cancer. Despite total androgen blockade, prostate cancer is known to progress in 18 to 48 months and is referred to as castration resistant prostate cancer (CRPC). CRPC is characterized by elevated levels of prostate specific antigen PSA despite low levels of testosterone. Prostate cancer deaths are typically the result of metastatic castrate resistant prostate cancer (mCRPC), and historically, the median survival for men with mCRPC has been less than 2 years [6]. Randomized studies with TAB have failed to demonstrate improvement in overall survival (OS) [7]. This is

* Correspondence: gupta.eva@mayo.edu
[1]Mayo Clinic, 4500 San Pablo Rd S, Jacksonville 32224, FL, USA
Full list of author information is available at the end of the article

thought to occur due to multiple escape mechanisms that fuel tumor growth [8]. Previously this was thought to be a hormone refractory state, but recently it has been recognized that androgen receptor expression is never lost. In the castration resistant state, androgen receptor gene amplification [9,10], alterations in expression of coactivators, and androgen receptor gene over expression have been found to result in higher concentrations of androgen receptors on tumor cells, making them extremely sensitive to low levels of circulating androgens. Prostate cancer cells have also been found to be able to maintain dihydrotestosterone (DHT) concentrations in excess of serum concentrations to support growth and proliferation [11]. They may also synthesize DHT de-novo [12] or convert adrenal steroids to DHT, which has five fold greater affinity than testosterone for the androgen receptor. In addition, selective mutations in the androgen receptor when exposed to anti-androgens may be responsible for resistance. Metastatic CRPC is an invariably fatal disease. Chemotherapy including docetaxel [13] as first-line, cabazitaxel as second-line, and active cellular immunotherapy with sipuleucel-T [14] has also not been found to produce a major survival improvement in mCRPC.

Focus has now shifted to the inhibitors of steroid biosynthesis [15]. CYP17 is a cytochrome P450 enzyme [16] that catalyzes two key reactions involved in the production of sex steroids (Figure 1). The 17α-hydroxylase activity converts pregnenolone to 17α-hydroxypregnenolone, which is a major precursor of metabolism into mineralocorticoids, glucocorticoids and androgens Treatment with ketoconazole, which inhibits 17α-hydroxylase, leads to suppression of glucocorticoid and mineralocorticoid production and causes a secondary increase in pituitary ACTH. In addition to suppression of androgens, it has been shown to slow tumor activity. Ketoconazole is a non-steroidal imidazole anti-fungal agent with CYP17 inhibition that has been used off-label as second-line hormonal therapy for prostate cancer since the 1980s [17-20]. It is an inhibitor of testicular and adrenal androgen synthesis, and high doses have typically been used to suppress tumor activity. High dose ketoconazole (HDK) has been has shown to have PSA response, but no survival benefit has been shown [21]. It is also associated with potential and significant adverse events, including fatal hepatic dysfunction, adrenal insufficiency (bone fragility, hypotension, and hyperkalemia), nausea and vomiting, gynecomastia, QT prolongation, and potentially fatal drug interactions. In a trial to evaluate the efficacy of ketoconazole along with simultaneous anti-androgen withdrawal (AAWD) in 20 patients with CRPC, Small et al. found 55% had a greater than 50% fall in prostatic specific antigen (PSA) [22]. In another study of 50 patient [23], Small et al. demonstrated that patients who have progressive disease despite anti-androgen withdrawal also benefit from subsequent

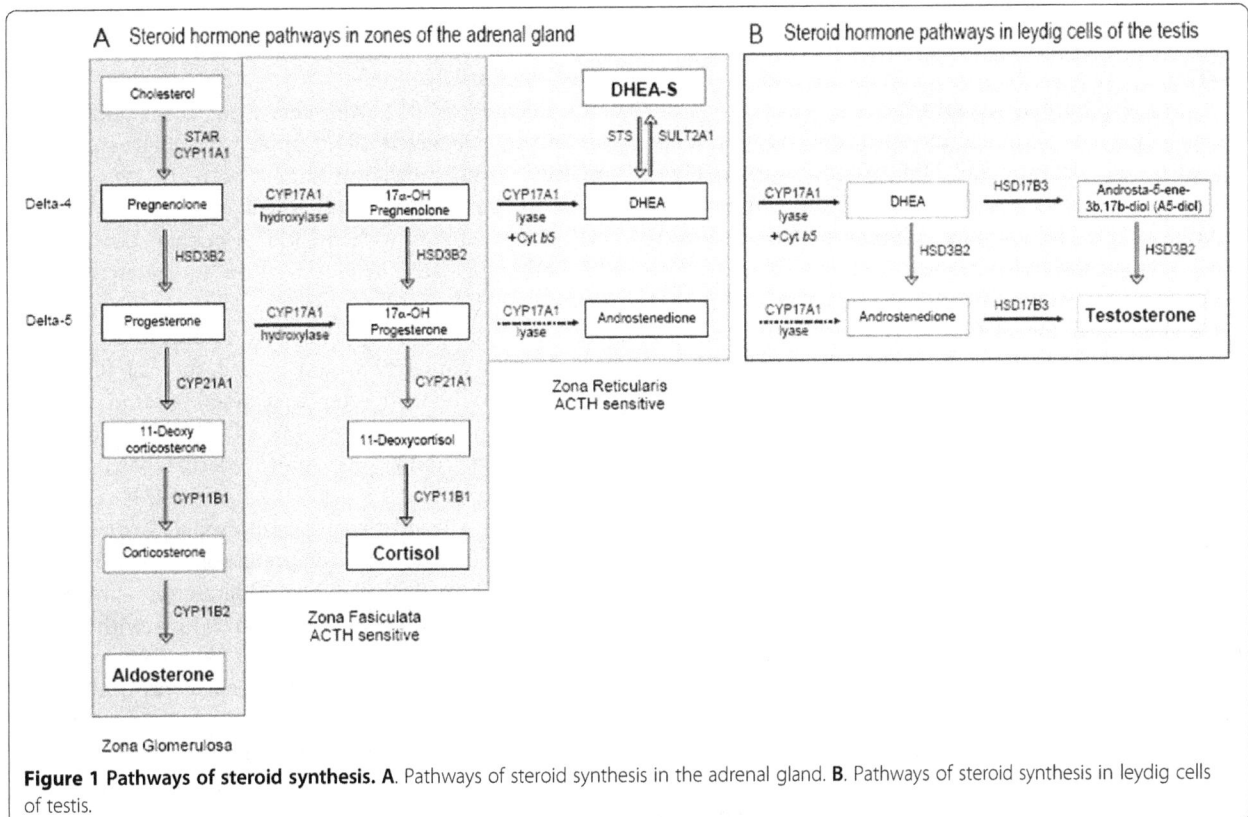

Figure 1 Pathways of steroid synthesis. A. Pathways of steroid synthesis in the adrenal gland. **B**. Pathways of steroid synthesis in leydig cells of testis.

ketoconazole therapy. In a larger phase III study of HDK therapy [24] the authors randomized 260 patients to AAWD alone (n = 132), or together with oral Ketoconazole (400 mg tid) and hydrocortisone (30 mg by mouth each morning, 10 mg by mouth. each evening; n = 128). PSA response (27% vs. 11%) and objective response (20% vs. 2%) were significantly more in the ketoconazole group compared to AAWD alone, although there was no difference in survival. Androgen levels have been shown to decline with Ketoconazole therapy, but the levels then climb at the time of progression. Progressive disease while on Ketoconazole has been postulated due to an escape from HDK induced androgen suppression, and it highlights the need for more effective agents.

In addition to blocking CYP17 activity, ketoconazole also inhibits other important metabolizing enzymes, such as CYP3A and CYP24A1, suggesting that concomitant ketoconazole administration may alter drug exposure or pharmacokinetic variability. This necessitates careful monitoring of adverse events and drug interactions. The responses observed after treatment with ketoconazole lead to the investigation of stronger and more selective CYP 17 inhibitors with a more favorable toxicity profile than ketoconazole [25].

The last several years, has seen new drug development on the rational of targeted approaches based on a better understanding of the disease process. These have created a changing paradigm in the hormonal treatment of advanced prostate cancer.

Review
New approved hormonal treatments
Recently two new hormonal therapy agents have been approved by the US Food and Drug Administration (FDA) for the treatment of patients with mCRPC: Abiraterone acetate (Zytiga) [26] and enzalutamide previously known as MDV3100 (now called Xtandi) [27].

Abiraterone (Zytiga) is an oral, selective and potent irreversible inhibitor of CYP17A, which is an enzyme that catalyzes both 17 alpha-hydroxylase and 17, 20-lyase reactions. It blocks androgen biosynthesis both within and outside of the prostate gland. It was first found to be efficacious in Phase I-II studies [28] of castrate-resistant prostate cancer. It was also tested in the treatment of patients with CRPC, who are either chemotherapy naive or have received prior therapy with docetaxel [29,30]. Abiraterone decreases the production of androgens by the adrenals, prostate, and also within the tumor cells. Evidence from phase I and phase II studies [31,32] demonstrated that Abiraterone suppresses the serum androgen levels and achieves PSA and clinical responses in chemotherapy naïve and docetaxel pretreated patients with mCRPC. Phase II and III studies have used a 1000 mg/day dose, although the maximum tolerated dose was 2000mg/day. Abiraterone was generally well tolerated. Hypokalemia (88%), hypertension (40%) and fluid overload (13%) were the most common adverse events noted.

A large randomized controlled phase III trial of 1195 patients (COU-AA-301) [33] comparing Abiraterone-prednisone vs. placebo-prednisone had to be terminated early (median survival 12.8 months) when the study met planned primary outcomes at the time of interim analysis. Patients with prior ketoconazole treatment for prostate cancer and a history of adrenal gland or pituitary disorders were excluded in this trial. The OS rate favored abiraterone (14.8 months vs. 10.9 months). Secondary end points, including time to PSA progression (10.2 vs. 6.6 months; P < 0.001), progression-free survival (5.6 months vs. 3.6 months; P < 0.001), pain palliation (44% vs. 2%), and PSA response rate (29% vs. 6%, P < 0.001) favored the treatment group. Mineralocorticoid-related adverse events, including fluid retention (31% vs. 22% placebo; P < 0.001) and hypokalemia (17% vs. 8% placebo), were more frequently reported in the Abiraterone acetate-prednisone group than in the placebo–prednisone group. There was a non-significant increase in grade 1–2 cardiac events in the treatment group (13% vs. 11% placebo). Seventy percent of patients in this trial had received one prior chemotherapy regimen, and 30% had been treated with two prior chemotherapeutic regimens. Abiraterone acetate is now considered standard of care for patients following chemotherapy. This study led to the approval of Abiraterone acetate for docetaxel pretreated CRPC in April 2011.

In December 2012, Abiraterone in combination with prednisone received FDA approval for treatment of mCRPC in chemotherapy naïve patients as well. In a phase III randomized controlled trial (COU-AA-302) [34], 1088 patients with mCRPC who had not received chemotherapy were assigned either to abiraterone and prednisone (N = 546) or placebo plus prednisone (N = 542). The primary endpoints were radiographic progression free survival (rPFS) and overall survival (OS). The study was unblinded after a planned interim analysis, which was performed after 43% of the expected deaths had occurred. Abiraterone improved rPFS (16.5 months vs. 8.3 months, HR 0.53; 95% CI 0.45-0.62; P < 0.001). It also showed a trend towards improved OS (median not reached, vs. 27.2 months for prednisone alone; HR 0.75; 95% CI, 0.61 to 0.93; P = 0.01). Abiraterone–prednisone showed superiority over prednisone alone with respect to time to initiation of cytotoxic chemotherapy (25.2 vs. 16.8 months, p-value <0.001) opiate use for cancer-related pain (not reached vs. 23.7 months, p-value <0.001), prostate-specific antigen progression (11.1 vs. 5.6 months, p-value <0.001), and decline in performance status (12.3 vs. 10.9 months, p-value 0.005).

Toxicity profile- the main adverse events of Abiraterone are related to excess mineralocorticoid, which includes fluid retention (33%) and hypokalemia (18%). This is due to the inhibition of 17 alpha hydroxylase, which causes a compensatory rise in ACTH. Abiraterone should be administered with prednisone daily and monthly potassium and blood pressure monitoring is essential during treatment. While co-administration of prednisone is manageable, long term use in earlier disease phases could be problematic due to the potential adverse events. These include diabetes, weight gain, Cushing syndrome and osteoporosis. Fatigue, joint swelling, edema, cough, vomiting, elevated liver enzymes, hyperglycemia and hypercholesterolemia have also been reported.

In a recent retrospective study, Peer et al. [35] found abiraterone to be superior to ketoconazole in the treatment of docetaxel refractory mCRPC. PSA response was 46% in the abiraterone group vs. 19% in the ketoconazole group (OR 4.3, P = 0.04), median biochemical progression free survival (PFS) 7 vs. 2 months (HR 1.54, P = 0.02), median radiological PFS 8 vs. 2.5 months (HR 1.8, P = 0.043), median OS 19 vs. 11 months (HR 0.53, P = 0.79) and treatment interruption due to severe adverse events 8% (n = 2) versus 31% (n = 8) (0R 0.6, P = 0.023).

Enzalutamide (Xtandi)

Enzalutamide (formerly MDV300) is an oral, second-generation androgen receptor antagonist that competitively inhibits androgen binding to the AR. In contrast to the first generation anti-androgens such as flutamide and bicalutamide, enzalutamide binds to the receptor with greater affinity [36]. In the setting of increased AR expression, bicalutamide is associated with AR recruitment to enhancer regions and aberrant recruitment of coactivators to these transcription complexes, leading to target gene activation rather than repression [37]. Enzalutamide does not display agonism in AR-overexpressing cells and this may explain its increased molecular efficacy. Enzalutamide may induce a conformational change in AR distinct from that induced by bicalutamide making it more efficacious in inhibiting the translocation of AR to the nucleus and its DNA interaction. In a phase I-II study [36], 140 men including 78% with mCRPC received doses ranging from 30-600mg daily. Half of the patients had previously received chemotherapy and three-fourths had received at least two lines of hormonal therapy. PSA responses were observed in 62% of the chemotherapy naïve patients and 51% in docetaxel treated patients [36]. 22% of the patients had a soft tissue response and 56% of the patients with bone disease had stabilized bone disease. The maximum tolerated dose was determined to be 240 mg daily. The median rPFS was 56 weeks and 24 weeks in the chemotherapy naïve and the chemotherapy pretreated group, respectively.

Enzalutamide was approved after the publication of a phase III [37], double-blind placebo-controlled randomized trial by Scher et el (AFFIRM TRIAL) in which 1199 men with mCRPC were randomized after chemotherapy to placebo vs. oral enzalutamide at a dose of 160 mg per day. The median OS was 18.4 months in the enzalutamide group versus 13.6 months in the placebo group (P < 0.001). The secondary endpoints including the PSA-level response rate (54% in the enzalutamide group vs. 2% in the placebo group), soft tissue response rate (29% vs. 4%), the time to PSA progression (8.3 months in the enzalutamide group vs. 3 months in the placebo group), rPFS (8.3 months in the enzalutamide group vs. 2.9 months in the placebo group), time to the first skeletal event (16.7 months in the enzalutamide group vs. 13.3 months in the placebo group) quality of life response rate (43% in the enzalutamide group vs. 18% in the placebo group) pain palliation achieved in (45% in the enzalutamide group vs. 7% in the placebo group) showed significant improvement in the enzalutamide group. The enzalutamide group had higher incidence of fatigue, hot flashes, musculoskeletal pain and headaches. Rates of hyperglycemia, weight gain and glucose intolerance were not different between the two groups. Cardiac disorders were seen in 6% of the patients receiving enzalutamide and 8% in the placebo group. Hypertension was seen in 6.6% in the enzalutamide group vs. 3.3% in the placebo group. Seizures were reported in 0.6% in the enzalutamide group vs. placebo.

The results of the large phase III randomized trial (PREVAIL trial) [38] were recently presented at the 2014 Genitourinary Cancer Symposium. This trial evaluated enzalutamide against placebo in chemotherapy naïve men with mCRPC. In the study, 1,717 chemotherapy naïve patients with mCRPC were assigned to receive 160 mg/day of enzalutamide vs. placebo in a double blind fashion. After a median follow-up of 20 months, interim analysis showed that enzalutamide significantly reduced the risk of death by 29% (HR 0.706, 95% CI 0.60-0.84, p <0.0001) and decreased the risk of radiographic progression by 81% (HR 0.186,95% CI 0.15-0.23, P < 0.0001). 59% of the patients in the enzalutamide group had a soft tissue response compared with 5% in the placebo arm. Enzalutamide also delayed the median time to chemotherapy initiation by 17 months as compared to placebo. The patients on the placebo arm needed to start cytotoxic chemotherapy after a median of 10.8 months due to disease progression. Median time to PSA progression was 2.8 months in the placebo group vs. 11.2 months in the enzalutamide group. The adverse effects included grade 1–2 fatigue (36% vs. 26%), back pain (27% vs. 22%) constipation (22% vs. 17%) and arthralgia (20% vs. 16%) in the enzalutamide vs. placebo group. The patients with a history of seizure disorders were excluded from the trial.

The results of the PREVAIL data will be submitted to the FDA for approval. If enzalutamide gets approval, there will be more choices available to treat chemotherapy naïve patients with mCRPC.

Toxicity profile- enzalutamide is reported to cause fatigue (11%), hot flashes (20%), headache (12%), nausea, diarrhea, constipation and musculoskeletal pain. Other reported adverse events include hyperglycemia, weight gain and glucose intolerance. Seizure was reported in 0.6% of the enzalutamide group at 360 to 600 mg doses. Thus the maximum tolerated dose (MTD) is 240 mg/day (Table 1).

New drugs under development

Orteronel (TAK 700) - is a non-steroidal, selective inhibitor of 17, 20 lyase, which is involved in androgenic steroid production. Selective inhibition improves its toxicity profile as compared to CYP17 inhibition. Orteronel causes less treatment related adverse events. In phase I and II studies [39], Orteronel given in twice daily doses of 100, 200,300,400 and 600 mg was well tolerated. The most common adverse events were gastrointestinal toxicity and grade 3 fatigue. At 12 weeks, the median DHEA-S and testosterone levels decreased from baseline in all the groups [39]. The mean number of circulating tumor cells decreased from 16.6 (per 7.5 ml blood) at baseline to 3.9 at 12 weeks.

The results of a large randomized, double blind, multicenter phase III study (ELM-PC4) was presented at the ASCO symposium in January 2014. The results showed that there was no improvement in OS with orteronel + prednisone vs. placebo in patients with mCRPC that progressed during or following chemotherapy. However there was improvement in rPFS over the control arm.

Currently the Radiation Therapy Oncology Group (RTOG) has a trial using TAK/orteronel in addition to conventional LHRH agonist to test if it will improve overall survival. The southwest oncology group (SWOG) is conducting a trial to compare overall survival in newly diagnosed metastatic prostate cancer patients who were randomly assigned to androgen deprivation therapy (ADT) + TAK-700 vs. ADT + bicalutamide.

ARN509- is a small molecule that is structurally similar to enzalutamide. It inhibits both AR nuclear translocation and AR binding to DNA [40]. In contrast to bicalutamide, it exhibits no agonist activity in prostate cancer cells that over express AR. In a phase I study [41] of men with mCRPC, it was shown to have an excellent safety profile at 240 mg/day. Preliminary results were reported by the Prostate Cancer Working Group in 2013 at the GU cancer symposium [42]. Among 46 men with mCRPC, 26 were treatment naïve and 21 had prior treatment with abiraterone. At 12 weeks, the PSA response was 88% in the treatment naïve and 29% in the prior-treatment group. The toxicity profile included fatigue (38%), nausea (29%) and pain (24%). Currently, a phase II multicenter study (NCT01171898) is evaluating the activity of ARN-509 in three different populations of men with mCRPC (high risk non-metastatic CRPC, metastatic treatment naïve CRPC and progressive disease after abiraterone acetate) and further phase III trials are planned.

Galeterone (TOK-001) - is another addition to the next generation androgen receptor antagonists and CYP17A1 inhibitors. It works by disrupting multiple androgen signaling pathways simultaneously and by down regulating the androgen receptor [43,44]. ARMOR 1 [45] was a multicenter dose escalation study of Galeterone for the treatment of chemotherapy naïve non-metastatic prostate cancer and mCRPC. The data from ARMOR 1 were presented at the 2012 AACR and 2012 ASCO meetings, showed that the drug is well tolerated. ARMOR2 is an ongoing phase II

Table 1 Newly approved hormonal agents for the treatment of mCRPC

Drug	Date of FDA approval and indication	Mechanism of action	Side effects
Abiraterone acetate (Zytiga)	December2012- (COU-AA-301) In combination with prednisone for treatment of patients in mCRPC [29] April 2012- (COU-AA-302) [30] Treatment of mCRPC in patients with have received prior chemotherapy containing Docetaxel	An androgen biosynthesis inhibitor of 17 alpha hydroxylase/C-17,20-lyase within prostate cancer cells and outside	Fatigue, joint swelling, edema, hot flashes, diarrhea, cough. Administration of prednisone is necessary to overcome hypertension, hypokalemia, fluid overload from mineralocorticoid excess induced by CYP17-inhibition
Enzalutamide (Xtandi) Previously known as MDV3100	August 2012- AFFIRM trial [34] Monotherapy for mCRPC who have previously received Docetaxel January 2014- PREVAIL trial [35] Survival benefit in chemotherapy naïve patients. Awaiting FDA approval.	Androgen receptor inhibitor- inhibits multiple steps in AR signaling	Fatigue, hot flashes, musculoskeletal pain, hyperglycemia, weight gain, Seizures in 0.6% of the patients.

multicenter trial to evaluate the efficacy and safety of Galeterone in the following populations - metastatic treatment naïve patients, non-metastatic treatment naïve patients, patients who have progressed on Abiraterone and patients who have progressed on Enzalutamide. The primary endpoints of the study are reduction in PSA levels and safety. The secondary endpoints include tumor response by the Response Evaluation Criteria in Solid Tumors (RECIST), AR modulation and levels of circulating tumor cells and markers of CYP17lyase inhibition (Table 2).

Treatment sequencing and combination therapy
The last decade has seen tremendous progress in prostate cancer research and has led to a better understanding of prostate cancer biology. This understanding has led to multiple new drugs that have been approved and have shown a survival benefit in patients with metastatic disease. With the approval of abiraterone and enzalutamide for castrate resistant prostate cancer in the post chemotherapy setting and abiraterone in the chemotherapy naïve state, there is an emerging theme of questions on how we use the new drugs sequentially. We would like to propose a schema that might help the clinician, but the ultimate answer would only be provided by randomized clinical trials. What we know based on the trials include the following:

Chemotherapy naïve
Sipuleucel-T- (Provenge) - immunotherapy
  Abiraterone
  Docetaxel

Post chemotherapy- docetaxel
Cabazitaxel- chemotherapy
  Abiraterone
  Enzalutamide

Symptomatic bone metastasis
Radium 223 (Xofigo)

What we do not know is to whom we should give chemotherapy first or if we should give chemotherapy after initial therapies have failed. Clinically, physicians are giving sipuleucel-T or abiraterone first followed by chemotherapy. For those with significant visceral disease and aggressive presentation most would start with docetaxel. If enzalutamide is approved in the chemotherapy naïve patients, which drug would become the first line of treatment, enzalutamide or abiraterone? We would need to do randomized trials of sequential treatments to answer these questions.

When the data of ECOG 3809 (randomized trial of chemotherapy- docetaxel for 6 cycles plus leuprolide and bicalutamide or hormone therapy alone) is published, should we start patients with metastatic disease with hormone therapy plus chemotherapy upfront? Although, it is good to have a plethora of treatment options today, there appears to be more questions than answers.

Conclusion
It is amazing that we have turned around in the past few years from calling progressive metastatic prostate cancer-hormone refractory to castrate resistant disease. We now realize that the optimal hormone suppression in the past was not adequate. With a variety of better androgen receptor blockers and targets, we are now at a point

Table 2 Newer agents under development for the treatment of mCRPC

Agent	Mechanism of action	Phase of development	Side effects	Ongoing trials
Orteronel (TAK-700)	Non-steroidal, selective inhibitor of 17, 20lyase, an enzyme required for androgen biosynthesis.	The results of Phase III trial (ELM-PC 4) did not show any survival benefit in chemotherapy naïve patients. An improvement in rPFS was seen.	Fatigue, GI toxicity	RTOG and SWOG- TAK + LHRH agonist to test whether improvement in OS or not
Galeterone (TOK-001)	Next generation AR antagonist and CYP17A1 inhibitor	ARMOR 1- phase I study showed the drug is well tolerated [42]	Fatigue, Nausea, Diarrhea	ARMOR 2 is underway in 4 distinct populations
				1. Metastatic and treatment naïve
				2. Non metastatic and treatment naïve
				3. Patients who have progressed on abiraterone
				4. Patients who have progressed on enzalutamide
ARN-509	Inhibits AR translocation and AR binding to DNA, does not exhibit agonist properties in the context of AR over-expression	Results from phase I studies showed that the drug is well tolerated and PSA decline at 12 weeks (>50% from the baseline) were observed in 46.7% of the patients. [38]	Fatigue, nausea, pain	Phase II study is underway in patients with mCRPC (NCT01171898)

where we can continue to improve the efficacy of these agents. Should we stop LHRH agents once we use these agents, what is the ideal testosterone level that we need to achieve, what level would correlate with response, are there markers that are better than testosterone and many more? Future research should be directed towards optimizing efficacy through less toxic combinations and should ultimately make a difference in improving the survival and quality of life of our patients.

Competing interests
The authors declare that they have no competing interests.

Authors' contributions
EG, TG and WT contributed equally to this article. All authors read and approved the final manuscript.

Author details
¹Mayo Clinic, 4500 San Pablo Rd S, Jacksonville 32224, FL, USA. ²Baptist Cancer Institute, Jacksonville, FL, USA.

References
1. Siegel R, Naishadham D, Jemal A: Cancer statistics, 2013. CA Cancer J Clin 2013, 63(1):11–30.
2. Huggins C, Hodges CV: Studies on prostatic cancer. I. The effect of castration, of estrogen and androgen injection on serum phosphatases in metastatic carcinoma of the prostate. CA Cancer J Clin 1972, 22(4):232–240.
3. Borgmann V, Hardt W, Schmidt-Gollwitzer M, Adenauer H, Nagel R: Sustained suppression of testosterone production by the luteinising-hormone releasing-hormone agonist buserelin in patients with advanced prostate carcinoma. A new therapeutic approach? Lancet 1982, 1(8281):1097–1099.
4. Sharifi N, Gulley JL, Dahut WL: Androgen deprivation therapy for prostate cancer. J Am Med Assoc 2005, 294(2):238–244.
5. Becker LE, Birzgalis EP: Orchiectomy in the management of adenocarcinoma of the prostate. Surg Gynecol Obstet 1966, 122(4):840–843.
6. Cookson MS, Roth BJ, Dahm P, Engstrom C, Freedland SJ, Hussain M, Lin DW, Lowrance WT, Murad MH, Oh WK, Penson DF, Kibel AS, Cookson MS, Roth BJ, Dahm P, Engstrom C, Freedland SJ, Hussain M, Lin DW, Lowrance WT, Murad MH, Oh WK, Penson DF, Kibel AS: Castration-resistant prostate cancer: AUA Guideline. J Urol 2013, 190(2):429–438.
7. Laufer M, Denmeade SR, Sinibaldi VJ, Carducci MA, Eisenberger MA: Complete androgen blockade for prostate cancer: what went wrong? J Urol 2000, 164(1):3–9.
8. Taplin ME, Bubley GJ, Shuster TD, Frantz ME, Spooner AE, Ogata GK, Keer HN, Balk SP: Mutation of the androgen-receptor gene in metastatic androgen-independent prostate cancer. N Engl J Med 1995, 332(21):1393–1398.
9. Cai C, He HH, Chen S, Coleman I, Wang H, Fang Z, Nelson PS, Liu XS, Brown M, Balk SP: Androgen receptor gene expression in prostate cancer is directly suppressed by the androgen receptor through recruitment of lysine-specific demethylase 1. Cancer Cell 2011, 20(4):457–471.
10. Watson PA, Chen YF, Balbas MD, Wongvipat J, Socci ND, Viale A, Kim K, Sawyers CL: Constitutively active androgen receptor splice variants expressed in castration-resistant prostate cancer require full-length androgen receptor. Proc Natl Acad Sci U S A 2010, 107(39):16759–16765.
11. Montgomery RB, Mostaghel EA, Vessella R, Hess DL, Kalhorn TF, Higano CS, True LD, Nelson PS: Maintenance of intratumoral androgens in metastatic prostate cancer: a mechanism for castration-resistant tumor growth. Cancer Res 2008, 68(11):4447–4454.
12. Locke JA, Guns ES, Lubik AA, Adomat HH, Hendy SC, Wood CA, Ettinger SL, Gleave ME, Nelson CC: Androgen levels increase by intratumoral de novo steroidogenesis during progression of castration-resistant prostate cancer. Cancer Res 2008, 68(15):6407–6415.
13. Petrylak DP, Tangen CM, Hussain MH, Lara PN Jr, Jones JA, Taplin ME, Burch PA, Berry D, Moinpour C, Kohli M, Benson MC, Small EJ, Raghavan D, Crawford ED: Docetaxel and estramustine compared with mitoxantrone and prednisone for advanced refractory prostate cancer. N Engl J Med 2004, 351(15):1513–1520.
14. Kantoff PW, Higano CS, Shore ND, Berger ER, Small EJ, Penson DF, Redfern CH, Ferrari AC, Dreicer R, Sims RB, Xu Y, Frohlich MW, Schellhammer PF, IMPACT Study Investigators: Sipuleucel-T immunotherapy for castration-resistant prostate cancer. N Engl J Med 2010, 363(5):411–422.
15. Reid AH, Attard G, Barrie E, de Bono JS: CYP17 inhibition as a hormonal strategy for prostate cancer. Nat Clin Pract Urol 2008, 5(11):610–620.
16. De Coster R, Wouters W, Bruynseels J: P450-dependent enzymes as targets for prostate cancer therapy. J Steroid Biochem Mol Biol 1996, 56(1–6 Spec No):133–143.
17. De Coster R, Mahler C, Denis L, Coene MC, Caers I, Amery W, Haelterman C, Beerens D: Effects of high-dose ketoconazole and dexamethasone on ACTH-stimulated adrenal steroidogenesis in orchiectomized prostatic cancer patients. Acta Endocrinol 1987, 115(2):265–271.
18. Eichenberger T, Trachtenberg J: Effects of high-dose ketoconazole on patients who have androgen-independent prostatic cancer. Can J Surg 1989, 32(5):349–352.
19. Pont A: Long-term experience with high dose ketoconazole therapy in patients with stage D2 prostatic carcinoma. J Urol 1987, 137(5):902–904.
20. Witjes FJ, Debruyne FM, Fernandez del Moral P, Geboers AD: Ketoconazole high dose in management of hormonally pretreated patients with progressive metastatic prostate cancer. Dutch South-Eastern Urological Cooperative Group. Urology 1989, 33(5):411–415.
21. Keizman D, Huang P, Carducci MA, Eisenberger MA: Contemporary experience with ketoconazole in patients with metastatic castration-resistant prostate cancer: clinical factors associated with PSA response and disease progression. Prostate 2012, 72(4):461–467.
22. Small EJ, Baron A, Bok R: Simultaneous antiandrogen withdrawal and treatment with ketoconazole and hydrocortisone in patients with advanced prostate carcinoma. Cancer 1997, 80(9):1755–1759.
23. Small EJ, Baron AD, Fippin L, Apodaca D: Ketoconazole retains activity in advanced prostate cancer patients with progression despite flutamide withdrawal. J Urol 1997, 157(4):1204–1207.
24. Small EJ, Halabi S, Dawson NA, Stadler WM, Rini BI, Picus J, Gable P, Torti FM, Kaplan E, Vogelzang NJ: Antiandrogen withdrawal alone or in combination with ketoconazole in androgen-independent prostate cancer patients: a phase III trial (CALGB 9583). J Clin Oncol 2004, 22(6):1025–1033.
25. Chen Y, Clegg NJ, Scher HI: Anti-androgens and androgen-depleting therapies in prostate cancer: new agents for an established target. Lancet Oncol 2009, 10(10):981–991.
26. Abiraterone Acetate. http://www.fda.gov/drugs/informationondrugs/approveddrugs/ucm331628.htm.
27. Enzalutamide (XTANDI Capsules). 2012. http://www.fda.gov/drugs/informationondrugs/approveddrugs/ucm317997.htm.
28. Attard G, Reid AH, A'Hern R, Parker C, Oommen NB, Folkerd E, Messiou C, Molife LR, Maier G, Thompson E, Olmos D, Sinha R, Lee G, Dowsett M, Kaye SB, Dearnaley D, Kheoh T, Molina A, de Bono JS: Selective inhibition of CYP17 with abiraterone acetate is highly active in the treatment of castration-resistant prostate cancer. J Clin Oncol 2009, 27(23):3742–3748.
29. Danila DC, Morris MJ, de Bono JS, Ryan CJ, Denmeade SR, Smith MR, Taplin ME, Bubley GJ, Kheoh T, Haqq C, Molina A, Anand A, Koscuiszka M, Larson SM, Schwartz LH, Fleisher M, Scher HI: Phase II multicenter study of abiraterone acetate plus prednisone therapy in patients with docetaxel-treated castration-resistant prostate cancer. J Clin Oncol 2010, 28(9):1496–1501.
30. Reid AH, Attard G, Danila DC, Oommen NB, Olmos D, Fong PC, Molife LR, Hunt J, Messiou C, Parker C, Dearnaley D, Swennenhuis JF, Terstappen LW, Lee G, Kheoh T, Molina A, Ryan CJ, Small E, Scher HI, de Bono JS: Significant and sustained antitumor activity in post-docetaxel, castration-resistant prostate cancer with the CYP17 inhibitor abiraterone acetate. J Clin Oncol 2010, 28(9):1489–1495.
31. Attard G, Reid AH, Yap TA, Raynaud F, Dowsett M, Settatree S, Barrett M, Parker C, Martins V, Folkerd E, Clark J, Cooper CS, Kaye SB, Dearnaley D, Lee G, de Bono JS: Phase I clinical trial of a selective inhibitor of CYP17, abiraterone acetate, confirms that castration-resistant prostate cancer commonly remains hormone driven. J Clin Oncol 2008, 26(28):4563–4571.

32. Ryan CJ, Shah S, Efstathiou E, Smith MR, Taplin ME, Bubley GJ, Logothetis CJ, Kheoh T, Kilian C, Haqq CM, Molina A, Small EJ: **Phase II study of abiraterone acetate in chemotherapy-naive metastatic castration-resistant prostate cancer displaying bone flare discordant with serologic response.** *Clin Cancer Res* 2011, **17**(14):4854–4861.

33. de Bono JS, Logothetis CJ, Molina A, Fizazi K, North S, Chu L, Chi KN, Jones RJ, Goodman OB Jr, Saad F, Staffurth JN, Mainwaring P, Harland S, Flaig TW, Hutson TE, Cheng T, Patterson H, Hainsworth JD, Ryan CJ, Sternberg CN, Ellard SL, Fléchon A, Saleh M, Scholz M, Efstathiou E, Zivi A, Bianchini D, Loriot Y, Chieffo N, Kheoh T, *et al*: **Abiraterone and increased survival in metastatic prostate cancer.** *N Engl J Med* 2011, **364**(21):1995–2005.

34. Ryan CJ, Smith MR, de Bono JS, Molina A, Logothetis CJ, de Souza P, Fizazi K, Mainwaring P, Piulats JM, Ng S, Carles J, Mulders PF, Basch E, Small EJ, Saad F, Schrijvers D, Van Poppel H, Mukherjee SD, Suttmann H, Gerritsen WR, Flaig TW, George DJ, Yu EY, Efstathiou E, Pantuck A, Winquist E, Higano CS, Taplin ME, Park Y, Kheoh T, *et al*: **Abiraterone in metastatic prostate cancer without previous chemotherapy.** *N Engl J Med* 2013, **368**(2):138–148.

35. Peer A, Gottfried M, Sinibaldi V, Carducci MA, Eisenberger MA, Sella A, Leibowitz-Amit R, Berger R, Keizman D: **Comparison of abiraterone acetate versus ketoconazole in patients with metastatic castration resistant prostate cancer refractory to docetaxel.** *Prostate* 2014, **74**(4):433–440.

36. Scher HI, Beer TM, Higano CS, Anand A, Taplin ME, Efstathiou E, Rathkopf D, Shelkey J, Yu EY, Alumkal J, Hung D, Hirmand M, Seely L, Morris MJ, Danila DC, Humm J, Larson S, Fleisher M, Sawyers CL, Prostate Cancer Foundation/Department of Defense Prostate Cancer Clinical Trials Consortium: **Antitumour activity of MDV3100 in castration-resistant prostate cancer: a phase 1–2 study.** *Lancet* 2010, **375**(9724):1437–1446.

37. Scher HI, Fizazi K, Saad F, Taplin ME, Sternberg CN, Miller K, de Wit R, Mulders P, Chi KN, Shore ND, Armstrong AJ, Flaig TW, Fléchon A, Mainwaring P, Fleming M, Hainsworth JD, Hirmand M, Selby B, Seely L, de Bono JS, AFFIRM Investigators: **Increased survival with enzalutamide in prostate cancer after chemotherapy.** *N Engl J Med* 2012, **367**(13):1187–1197.

38. Beer TM, Armstrong AJ, Sternberg CN, Higano CS, Iversen P, Loriot Y, Rathkopf DE, Bhattacharya S, Carles J, De Bono JS, Evans CP, Joshua AM, Kim C-S, Kimura G, Mainwaring PN, Mansbach HH, Miller K, Noonberg SB, Venner PM, Tombal B: **Enzalutamide in men with chemotherapy-naive metastatic prostate cancer (mCRPC): Results of phase III PREVAIL study.** *J Clin Oncol* 2014, **32**(4 Suppl):LBA1.

39. Agus WMS DB, Shevrin DH, Hart L, MacVicar GR, Hamid O, Hainsworth JD, Gross ME, Wang J, de Leon L, MacLean D, Dreicer R: **Safety, efficacy, and pharmacodynamics of the investigational agent TAK-700 in metastatic castration-resistant prostate cancer (mCRPC): Updated data from a phase I/II study.** *J Clin Oncol* 2011, **29**(15_suppl):4531.

40. Clegg NJ, Wongvipat J, Joseph JD, Tran C, Ouk S, Dilhas A, Chen Y, Grillot K, Bischoff ED, Cai L, Aparicio A, Dorow S, Arora V, Shao G, Qian J, Zhao H, Yang G, Cao C, Sensintaffar J, Wasielewska T, Herbert MR, Bonnefous C, Darimont B, Scher HI, Smith-Jones P, Klang M, Smith ND, De Stanchina E, Wu N, Ouerfelli O, *et al*: **ARN-509: a novel antiandrogen for prostate cancer treatment.** *Cancer Res* 2012, **72**(6):1494–1503.

41. Rathkopf DE, Morris MJ, Fox JJ, Danila DC, Slovin SF, Hager JH, Rix PJ, Chow Maneval E, Chen I, Gonen M, Fleisher M, Larson SM, Sawyers CL, Scher HI: **Phase I Study of ARN-509, a Novel Antiandrogen, in the Treatment of Castration-Resistant Prostate Cancer.** *J Clin Oncol* 2013, **31**(28):3525–3530.

42. Smith MR: **ARN-509 in men with high-risk nonmetastatic castration-resistant prostate cancer (CRPC).** *J Clin Oncol* 2013, **31**(6 Suppl):7.

43. Vasaitis T, Belosay A, Schayowitz A, Khandelwal A, Chopra P, Gediya LK, Guo Z, Fang HB, Njar VC, Brodie AM: **Androgen receptor inactivation contributes to antitumor efficacy of 17{alpha}-hydroxylase/17,20-lyase inhibitor 3beta-hydroxy-17-(1H-benzimidazole-1-yl)androsta-5,16-diene in prostate cancer.** *Mol Cancer Ther* 2008, **7**(8):2348–2357.

44. Purushottamachar P, Godbole AM, Gediya LK, Martin MS, Vasaitis TS, Kwegyir-Afful AK, Ramalingam S, Ates-Alagoz Z, Njar VC: **Systematic structure modifications of multitarget prostate cancer drug candidate galeterone to produce novel androgen receptor down-regulating agents as an approach to treatment of advanced prostate cancer.** *J Med Chem* 2013, **56**(12):4880–4898.

45. Taplin M, Chu F, Morrison J, Pili R, Rettig M, Stephenson J, Vogelzang N, Montgomery R: **ARMOR1: safety of galeterone (TOK-001) in a phase 1 clinical trial in chemotherapy naïve patients with castration resistant prostate cancer (CRPC).** *Cancer Res* 2012, **72**(8 Supplement):CT-07.

15

Prevalence of human papillomavirus in penile malignant tumors: viral genotyping and clinical aspects

Isaura Danielli Borges de Sousa[1], Flávia Castello Branco Vidal[1,2]*, João Paulo Castello Branco Vidal[3], George Castro Figueira de Mello[4], Maria do Desterro Soares Brandão Nascimento[1] and Luciane Maria Oliveira Brito[1,5]

Abstract

Background: The human papillomavirus (HPV) prevalence in males has been reported to be between 3.6% and 84%, depending specially on the socioeconomic status. HPV infection has been related as a risk factor for penile cancer. This is a rare tumor, and other risk factors include lack of personal hygiene and men who have not undergone circumcision. Penile cancer is less than 1% of cancers in men in the United States, however, is much more common in some parts of Asia, Africa, and South America, where it accounts for up to 10% of cancers in men. This study aimed to determine the prevalence of HPV-DNA in penile cancers in São Luís, Brazil and to correlate the virus presence to histopathological factors.

Methods: Tumor paraffin samples of 76 patients with penile carcinoma were tested in order to establish the prevalence and distribution of genotypic HPV using PCR/Nested and automated sequencing. To evaluate the association between HPV types and other clinical and morphological variables, a nonparametric ANOVA was performed using a Kruskal Wallis test, and statistical significance was determined to a value of $p < 0.05$.

Results: The average age of patients at the time of diagnosis was 66 years ± 17.10. Regarding location, 65.79% of the tumors were located in the glans, and the most common types were vegetative (34.21%) and squamous (98.68%). Most of the lesions ranged in size from 2.1 to 5.0 cm, presenting Jackson I stage and Broders II degree. It was observed that 32 patients had at least one invaded and/or infiltrated structure. Lymph node involvement was observed in 19.76% of the patients, and 21.05% showed an inflammatory process. In the molecular evaluation, HPV infection was observed in 63.15% of the lesions, and the most common type was HPV 16.

Conclusions: From the statistical analysis, it can be verified that the variables were not associated with infection by the HPV virus. Although penile cancer can result from various risk factors that act in synergy, an HPV virus infection is important for the development of such neoplasm.

Keywords: Papillomavirus Infections, Penile Neoplasms, Association, Men's health

* Correspondence: flavidal@hotmail.com
[1]Tumors and DNA Bank of Maranhão, Federal University of Maranhão (UFMA), São Luís, Brazil
[2]Department of Morphology, Federal University of Maranhão (UFMA), São Luís, Brazil
Full list of author information is available at the end of the article

Background

The human papillomavirus (HPV) is a DNA-virus from the Papoviridae family - genre Papillomavirus, with more than 100 types currently recognized, 20 of which can infect the genital tract; the man is the main disseminator [1,2].

Penile infection by HPV may be clinical, subclinical or latent. In clinical presentation, the diagnosis is simpler, because it is determined from a good clinical examination to uncover existing lesions. In subclinical and latent forms, other methods, such as peniscopy, are necessary to aid in detection, as it is not possible to detect changes (i.e., diagnosis) with the naked eye. In men, there is a higher frequency of the subclinical form [2].

Penile cancer mainly affects men over 50 years old, but approximately 19% of patients are 40 years of age or younger, and 7% are below the age of 30 [3]. The major risk factors of the disease are associated with hygiene, phimosis, smegma retention, inflammation process, and HPV infection [4].

The prevalence of the virus in males has been reported to be between 3.6% and 84%, depending on socioeconomic status [5,6]. Penile cancer represents 0.4% to 0.6% of all malignant tumors in developed countries, such as the United States and European countries, and more than 10% of all malignant tumors in developing countries, such as those in Asia, Africa and South America [3,4].

According to Nardi et al. [7] the highest incidence rates of penile carcinoma were found in Maranhão. Maranhão is a city situated in the Northeast of Brazil. Favorito et al. [8] observed a predominance of reports of penile cancer in the North and Northeast (53.02%), which are regions with lower human development indexes. The understanding of HPV prevalence and knowledge of the viral subtype distribution constitute important epidemiological information that can assist the development of local or regional public policies to prevent HPV and of new vaccines.

The aims of this study were to detect and perform HPV genotyping in biological specimens of penile tumors and to determine the existing associations between viral presence and histopathological clinical aspects.

Methods

Enrollment

This was a retrospective study performed in paraffined penile tumors collected at two public reference hospitals in Maranhão. A total of 76 samples were included in the study from patients diagnosed with penile cancer between the years 2001 and 2011. Patient information as well as the histopathological characteristics of the tumors obtained from medical records. As the samples consisted in paraffined tumours, there was no written informed consent from the patients. The patient identity was not disclosed in this research. This work was approved by the Ethics in Research Committee of the University Hospital of the Federal University of Maranhão (HU/UFMA).

Inclusion criteria

Paraffin blocks and histological slides of penile tumors as a result of biopsy or surgical treatment, with or without lymphadenectomy at any follow-up in the archives of the Pathology Services.

Exclusion criteria

Histological slides and/or paraffined blocks not found in the archives of the Pathology Services of referral hospitals and reports did not provide complete information.

HPV analysis

The samples were reviewed by the pathologist, and blocks with tumor representativeness (over 50% of the total area of the fragment) were selected. After microtomy, sections suffered a process of deparaffinization. The sections were stored at 4°C, awaiting DNA extraction.

The extraction of the genomic DNA from the samples was performed using the QIAamp DNA FFPE Tissue Purification Kit (QIAGEN®) according to the extraction protocol suggested by the manufacturer.

The Nested PCR reactions were performed by using primers PGMY09 and PGMY11 for the first round, and primers GP + 5 and GP + 6 for the second round [9].

The sequencing reactions were performed in the Laboratory of Genetics of the National Cancer Institute (INCA) with ET Dye Terminator Cycle Sequencing kit (GE Healthcare, UK) according to the manufacturer's suggested protocol.

Statistical analysis

All data were collected and prospectively input in an EpiInfo 3.4.3 and Microsoft Office 2007® were used for the statistical analysis.

To evaluate the association between HPV types and other clinical and morphological variables, a nonparametric ANOVA was performed using the Kruskal Wallis test with a statistical significance level of 5% probability ($p < 0.05$).

Results and discussion

Tumor biopsies of penile cancer were evaluated in 76 patients aged 26 to 97 years with a mean of 60.7 years and standard deviation of ±17.10, presenting a higher prevalence in the over 66 age group. The clinical representation and pathologic characteristics distribution is shown on Table 1.

These results correspond with those obtained in the literature [10-14]. The average age of the patients at diagnosis predominates in advanced age (>50 years), which suggests that men seek health services very late in

Table 1 Age, clinical presentation and pathologic characteristics from 76 patients diagnosed with penile cancer

Age at diagnosis	N	%
Average age	60.6 ± 17.10	-
26-45	16	21.05
46-55	12	15.79
56-65	16	21.05
66-97	32	42.11
Lesion area		
Glans add other regions	50	65.79
Foreskin	08	10.53
Corpus	03	3.95
Non evaluable	15	19.74
Predominant morphology		
Ulceration	17	22.37
Vegetating	26	34.21
Ulceration and Vegetating	17	22.37
Nodule and Vegetating	01	1.32
Non evaluable	16	21.05
Size of the lesion (cm)		
≤0,5	00	00
06-2,0	20	26.32
2,1-5,0	40	52.63
≥5,1	14	18.42
Non evaluable	02	2.63
Staging of Jackson 1966		
Stage I	33	43.42
Stage II	16	21.05
Stage III	11	14.48
Stage IV	16	21.05
Broders' Classification		
Grade I	26	34.21
Grade II	36	47.37
Grade III	06	7.89
Non evaluable	08	10.53
Invasion		
Present	18	23.69
Absent	58	76.31
Infiltration		
Corpus add other regions	24	31.58
Perineural	01	1.32
Urethra	03	3.95
Stroma	03	3.95
Urethra and Stroma	01	1.32
Absent	44	57.89

Table 1 Age, clinical presentation and pathologic characteristics from 76 patients diagnosed with penile cancer (Continued)

Lymph node involvement		
Present	15	19.73
Absent	61	80.27
Lymphatic embolization		
Present	04	5.26
Absent	72	94.74
Inflammatory process		
Present	16	21.05
Absent	60	78.95

life [15]. Younger individuals are also affected, but in smaller percentages [7].

Regarding the location of the lesions, the glans, in an isolated form or associated with other regions, was the most affected structure as in the research by Delgado et al. [10], Wanick et al. [11] and Favorito et al. [8].

Studies have shown that the lesions on the glans are directly linked to poor hygiene. This occurs due to the formation of a mass, called smegma, followed by likely irritation of the site and onset of injury, facilitating various infections and future neoplasia if left untreated [10].

Regarding the clinical morphology, the predominantly found lesion was the vegetating type followed by ulceration. The occurrence of both types of lesions in the same patient was observed in 22.37% of the cases. In a study performed in Spain, researchers observed that the vegetative lesion was also more present, in 66% of the cases [12]. On the other hand, in another research conducted in Rio de Janeiro [10], a larger number of lesions was detected in the form of ulcerations, nearly 55.88% of the studied cases.

The dimensions of the lesions were similar to those observed in the Wanick et al. results [10], with a larger number of cases: 52.63% of the cases, with size between 2.1 and 5.0 cm.

Unlike other studies, the moderately differentiated tumors (grade II) identified in this work, according to

Table 2 HPV prevalence and distribution according to oncogenic risk in 76 patients diagnosed with penile cancer

HPV	n	%
HPV +	48	63.15
HPV -	28	36.85
Oncogenic risk		
High risk	17	35.42
Low risk	6	12.50
Indeterminate	25	52.08

Table 3 Association of clinical presentation and pathologic characteristics data with HPV infection patients with penile cancer

	HPV +	HPV -	p-values*
Lesion area			0.543
Glans add other regions	31	19	
Foreskin	4	4	
Corpus	2	1	
Non evaluable	11	4	
Predominant morphology			0.377
Ulceration	11	06	
Vegetating	17	09	
Ulceration and Vegetating	09	07	
Nodule and Vegetating	01	00	
Non evaluable	10	06	
Size of the lesion (cm)			0.352
06-2,0	13	07	
2,1-5,0	23	17	
≥5,1	11	03	
Non evaluable	01	01	
Histologic type			0.285
Squamous	47	28	
Adenocarcinoma	01	00	
Staging of Jackson 1966			0.381
Stage I	21	12	
Stage II	07	09	
Stage III	07	04	
Stage IV	13	03	
Broders' Classification			0.352
Grade I	20	06	
Grade II	21	15	
Grade III	02	04	
Non evaluable	05	03	
Invasion			0.578
Present	10	08	
Absent	38	20	
Infiltration			0.535
Corpus add other regions	15	9	
Perineural	0	1	
Urethra	3	0	
Stroma	3	0	
Urethra and Stroma	1	0	
Absent	26	18	

Table 3 Association of clinical presentation and pathologic characteristics data with HPV infection patients with penile cancer (Continued)

	HPV +	HPV -	p-values*
Lymph node involvement			0.285
Present	09	06	
Absent	39	22	
Lymphatic embolization			0.285
Present	04	00	
Absent	44	28	
Inflammatory process			0.285
Present	10	06	
Absent	38	22	

*Estimated by univariate logistic regression analysis;
P = Statistical significance; 95% CI = 95% confidence interval.

Broder's classification, were the most prevalent. Fonseca et al. [13] identified a greater number of cases classified as well differentiated (grade I). However, Scheiner et al. [14] observed higher incidence of grade III (undifferentiated) tumors, which can be explained by the greater presence of stage III and IV patients.

The findings indicated that invasion was present in 23.68%, and infiltration occurred in at least one of the structures, with the highest prevalence in the corpus cavernosum. Koifman et al. [15] reported the presence of invasion of the spongiosum or cavernous corpus in 41.3% of the patients.

Regarding lymph node involvement, a percentage of 19.73% was observed. According to Sacoto et al. [12], patients with more advanced disease and positive lymph nodes at the time of diagnosis had a worse survival rate than those with localized stages.

The DNA of the HPV was detected in 63.15% (48/76) of the samples. The oncogenic risk distribution is shown on Table 2. This percentage is within the range reported in the literature, which shows that the rate of HPV infection in penile malignant tumors may vary from 20 to over 75% of cases [16]. According to a systematic review of the prevalence of HPV in invasive tumors of the penis, 48% of the samples presented HPV infection [17]. A Belgian study by D'Hauwers et al. [18], which had the same number of patients as in this study, revealed that 70.9% of the tumors had the HPV virus. However, a survey conducted in Vietnam demonstrated that only 23% of tumors had HPV infection [19]. A study conducted in Brazil showed that 75% of invasive penile tumors were infected by HPV [14]. These variations may be due to different techniques used for viral detection, regional differences or histological type of the analyzed tumor.

In our study, among the high-risk viral types present were the 16, 18, 45 and 69 types. The HPV of type 11 was the only low oncogenic risk found. Type 16 was the most prevalent, found in 10 cases, followed by type 11 of low risk with 6 cases, type 18 with 4 cases, type 69 with two cases and type 45 with 1 case. The automated sequencing technique was not effective for viral genotyping, because in more than 50% of the samples it was not possible to achieve. This may be due to the presence of co-infections in these samples, which prevents the device from detecting the virus, as described by Gharizadeh et al. (2005) and Verteramo et al. (2009) [20,21]. The most common viral type found in this study was HPV 16, high-risk type. This virus type was also the most found in other studies such as those developed by Do et al. [19] (89%), D'Hauwers et al. [18] (48.3%) and Heidman et al. [16] in (52%).

As shown in Table 3, no association was found (p < 0.05) between infection with HPV virus and clinical and histopathological and clinical variables, as was the case in the research by Do et al. [19], Fonseca et al. [22] and Scheiner et al. [14].

Infections by HPV are strongly associated with the development of penile cancer; however, the role of viruses in the etiology is not very clear [21]. Although the etiology is still unknown, approximately 40% of all penile tumors are related to HPV infection [22].

Conclusion
HPV DNA was found in 48 of the 76 analyzed samples (63,15%). The high-risk type HPV 16 was observed in 21.28% (10/48) of the lesions followed by low-risk type HPV 11 in 12.76% (6/48) and high-risk types HPV 18 in 8.51% (4/48), HPV 69 in 4.25% (2/48) and HPV 45 in 2.13% (1/48). In 51.06% of the cases, genotyping was indeterminate, suggestive of co-infection.

The average age of the patients in the study was 60.6 years old. Prevalent lesions were larger than 2 cm, in the glans region, in general vegetating, and with Broder grade II (moderately differentiated). The clinical and histopathological variables did not tend to have an association with infection by the HPV virus.

Abbreviations
HPV: Human papillomavirus; HU/UFMA: University Hospital of the Federal University of Maranhão; INCA: National Cancer Institute.

Competing interests
The authors declare that they have no competing interests.

Authors' contributions
IDBS, FCBV and JPCBV performed the experiments under the supervision of MDSBN and LMOB. GCFM was the pathologist responsible for penile cancer identification. All the authors analyzed and interpreted the data. IDBS and FCBV wrote the manuscript draft, which was read and edited by all the authors. All authors read and approved the final version of the manuscript.

Acknowledgments
This study was supported by grants from the Coordination of Improvement of Higher Education Personnel (CAPES), Ministério da Saúde, Brasil, and Fundação de Amparo à Pesquisa e ao Desenvolvimento Científico e Tecnológico do Estado do Maranhão (FAPEMA).

Author details
[1]Tumors and DNA Bank of Maranhão, Federal University of Maranhão (UFMA), São Luís, Brazil. [2]Department of Morphology, Federal University of Maranhão (UFMA), São Luís, Brazil. [3]José Alencar Gomes da Silva National Cancer Institute, Department of Genetics, Rio de Janeiro, Brazil. [4]Maranhão State Institute of Oncology Aldenora Bello (IMOAB), São Luis, MA, Brazil. [5]Department of Medicine III, Federal University of Maranhão (UFMA), São Luís, Brazil.

References
1. Leto MGP, Júnior GFS, Porro AM, Tomimori J. Infecção pelo papilomavírus humano: etiopatogenia, biologia molecular e manifestações clínicas. An Bras Dermatol. 2011;86(2):11.
2. Rosenblatt C, Lucon AM, Pereyra EAG, Pinnotti JA, Arap S. Papilomavírus humano em homens – "triar ou não triar" – Uma revisão. einstein. 2004;2(3):212–6.
3. Pow-Sang M, Astigueta J. HPV infection and the risk of penile cancer. J Andrological Sci. 2009;16:1–6.
4. Mosconi AM, Roila F, Gatta G, Theodore C. Cancer of the penis. Crit Rev Oncol Hematol. 2005;53(2):165–77.
5. Chaves JHB, Vieira TKB, Ramos JS, Bezerra AFS. Peniscopia no rastreamento das lesões induzidas pelo papilomavirus humano. Revista Brasileira de Clinica Medica. 2011;9(1):30–5.
6. Spiess PE, Horenblas S, Pagliaro LC, Biagioli MC, Crook J, Clark PE, et al. Current concepts in penile cancer. J Natl Compr Canc Netw. 2013;11(5):617–24.
7. Nardi AC, Glina S, Favorito LA. I estudo epidemiológico sobre câncer de pênis no Brasil. Int Braz J Urol. 2007;33 Suppl 1:1–7.
8. Favorito LA, Nardi AC, Ronalsa M, Zequi SC, Sampaio FJB, Glina S. Epidemiologic study on penile cancer in Brazil. Int Braz J Urol. 2008;34(5):587–91.
9. Gravitt PE, Peyton CL, Alessi TQ, Wheeler CM, Coutlee F, Hildesheim A, et al. Improved amplification of genital human papillomaviruses. J Clin Microbiol. 2000;38(1):357–61.
10. Delgado MS, Martíneza FA, Márquez GP, Gonzáleza BB, Cosanoa AZ, Armadaa RL. Cáncer de pene. una revisión de 18 casos. Actas Urol Esp. 2003;27(10):797–802.
11. Wanick FBF, Teichner TC, Silva R, Magnanini MMF, Azevedo LMS. Carcinoma epidermoide do pênis: estudo clínico-patológico de 34 casos. An Bras Dermatol. 2011;86(6):1082–91.
12. Sacoto CDP, Marco SL, Solchaga GM, Alba AB, Moreno JLP, Cruz JFJ. Cáncer de pene. Nuestra experiencia en 15 años. Actas Urol Esp. 2009;33(2):143–8.
13. Fonseca AG, Pinto JASA, Marques MC, Drosdoski FS, Neto LORF. Estudo epidemiológico do câncer de pênis no Estado do Pará. Brasil Revista Pan-Amazônica de Saúde. 2010;1(2):85–90.
14. Scheiner MA, Campos MM, Ornellas AA, Chin EW, Ornellas MH, Andrada-Serpa MJ. Human papillomavirus and penile cancers in Rio de Janeiro, Brazil: HPV typing and clinical features. Int Braz J Urol. 2008;34(4):467–74.
15. Koifman L, Vides AJ, Koifman N, Carvalho JP, Ornellas AA. Epidemiological aspects of penile cancer in Rio de Janeiro: evaluation of 230 cases. Int Braz J Urol. 2011;37(2):231–40.
16. Heideman DA, Waterboer T, Pawlita M, Delis-van Diemen P, Nindl I, Leijte JA, et al. Human papillomavirus-16 is the predominant type etiologically involved in penile squamous cell carcinoma. J Clin Oncol. 2007;25(29):4550–6.
17. Backes DM, Kurman RJ, Pimenta JM, Smith JS. Systematic review of human papillomavirus prevalence in invasive penile cancer. Cancer Causes Control. 2009;20(4):449–57.
18. D'Hauwers KW, Depuydt CE, Bogers JJ, Noel JC, Delvenne P, Marbaix E, et al. Human papillomavirus, lichen sclerosus and penile cancer: a study in Belgium. Vaccine. 2012;30(46):6573–7.

19. Do HT, Koriyama C, Khan NA, Higashi M, Kato T, Le NT, et al. The etiologic role of human papillomavirus in penile cancers: a study in Vietnam. Br J Cancer. 2013;108(1):229–33.
20. Gharizadeh B, Oggionni M, Zheng B, Akom E, Pourmand N, Ahmadian A, et al. Type-specific multiple sequencing primers: a novel strategy for reliable and rapid genotyping of human papillomaviruses by pyrosequencing technology. J Mol Diagn. 2005;7(2):198–205.
21. Verteramo R, Pierangeli A, Mancini E, Calzolari E, Bucci M, Osborn J, et al. Human Papillomaviruses and genital co-infections in gynaecological outpatients. BMC Infect Dis. 2009;9:16.
22. Fonseca AG, Soares FA, Burbano RR, Silvestre RV, Pinto LO. Human Papilloma Virus: prevalence, distribution and predictive value to lymphatic metastasis in penile carcinoma. Int Braz J Urol. 2013;39(4):542–50.

16

Photodynamic diagnosis of shed prostate cancer cells in voided urine treated with 5-aminolevulinic acid

Yasushi Nakai, Satoshi Anai, Masaomi Kuwada, Makito Miyake, Yoshitomo Chihara, Nobumichi Tanaka, Akihide Hirayama, Katsunori Yoshida, Yoshihiko Hirao and Kiyohide Fujimoto*

Abstract

Background: Past attempts at detecting prostate cancer (PCa) cells in voided urine by traditional cytology have been impeded by undesirably low sensitivities but high specificities. To improve the sensitivities, we evaluate the feasibility and clinical utility of photodynamic diagnosis (PDD) of prostate cancer by using 5-aminolevulinic acid (5-ALA) to examine shed prostate cancer cells in voided urine samples.

Methods: One hundred thirty-eight patients with an abnormal digital rectal exam (DRE) and/or abnormal prostate-specific antigen (PSA) levels were recruited between April 2009 and December 2010. Voided urine specimens were collected before prostate biopsy. Urine specimens were treated with 5-ALA and imaged by fluorescence microscopy and reported as protoporphyrin IX (PPIX) positive (presence of cells demonstrating simultaneous PPIX fluorescence) or PPIX negative (lack of cells demonstrating fluorescence).

Results: Of the 138 patients, PCa was detected on needle biopsy in 81 patients (58.7%); of these 81 patients with PCa, 60 were PPIX-positive (sensitivity: 74.1%). Although 57 patients did not harbor PCa by conventional diagnostic procedures, 17 of these at-risk patients were found to be PPIX-positive (specificity: 70.2%). PPIX–PDD was more sensitive compared with DRE and transrectal ultrasound and more specific compared with PSA and PSA density. The incidence of PPIX–PDD positivity did not increase with increasing total PSA levels, tumor stage or Gleason score.

Conclusions: To our knowledge, this is the first successful demonstration of PPIX in urine sediments treated with 5-ALA used to detect PCa in a noninvasive yet highly sensitive manner. However, further studies are warranted to determine the role of PPIX–PDD for PCa detection.

Keywords: 5-aminolevulinic acid, Prostate cancer, Photodynamic diagnosis, Urine cytology

Background

Detection of prostate cancer (PCa) primarily relies on an abnormal digital rectal examination (DRE) and/or increased prostate specific antigen (PSA) levels. Despite its widespread use, PSA has marginal specificity, and 65%–70% males with elevated PSA levels within 4–10 ng/ml generally reveal a negative biopsy result [1]. Therefore, PSA is not the ideal screening tool for prostate cancer. To improve PSA specificity, various analyses have been introduced such as PSA density, PSA velocity, and free/total PSA; however, these methods have not appreciably improved the cancer detection rates. In addition, because of sampling errors or sampling inefficiencies associated with transrectal ultrasound-guided biopsy of the prostate, some PCa may be missed (false negative). Therefore, there is a clear need for clinically useful biomarkers that would allow earlier detection of clinically significant PCa. For this reason, there is currently considerable interest in novel noninvasive biomarkers (e.g., urine- or serum-based assays) to assist in the diagnosis of PCa [2]. Nevertheless, to date, no routinely used tumor biomarker has replaced PSA.

* Correspondence: kiyokun@naramed-u.ac.jp
Department of Urology, Nara Medical University, 840 Shijo-cho, Kashihara-shi, Nara 634-8522, Japan

Upon prostatic massage, prostate cells (including PCa cells) may be dislodged and displaced into the urethra and urine. However, unlike bladder cancer, wherein voided urinary cytology has proven useful in cancer detection and surveillance, past attempts at detecting PCa cells in voided urine by traditional cytology have been impeded by undesirably low sensitivities but high specificities [3-5]. The low sensitivity was presumably attributed to the scant number of prostate cells present in the voided urine and the difficulty in differentiating the malignant prostatic cells from the other shed cells and debris. Thus, based on recent technological advancements, we revisited the cytology-based approach to PCa detection in voided urine samples and investigated the use of photodynamic diagnosis (PDD). For example, in bladder cancer, several investigators have used photodynamic agents such as 5-aminolevulinic acid (5-ALA) to induce protoporphyrin IX (PPIX) accumulation in malignant tissue, which then enables it to be differentiated from benign tissue [6-9]. In the heme biosynthetic pathway, 5-ALA is a precursor in the heme biosynthesis pathway and is metabolized to fluorescent PPIX before being converted to photoinactive heme. PPIX, which temporarily accumulates in the cancer cells after exogenous application of 5-ALA, is the endogenous photosensitizer needed for PDD [10]. Selective PPIX accumulation in malignant tissue provides an intense color contrast between the red fluorescence of malignant lesions and the nonfluorescence of normal tissue.

Previously, Zaak et al. reported the results of a small feasibility study (n = 18), in which prostate tissue samples were analyzed after exposure to 5-ALA for the presence of prostate tumor(s). Briefly, prostate tissue samples from 16 patients who had undergone 5-ALA fluorescence microscopy revealed selective PPIX accumulation in the PCa cells, and only weak PPIX fluorescence could be detected in the benign epithelial cells. The two patients who were not treated with 5-ALA revealed no PPIX fluorescence within the prostate [11]. In this study, our aim was different from those of previous investigators. We evaluated the feasibility and clinical utility of PDD for PCa by using 5-ALA-induced PPIX to examine shed PCa cells in voided urine samples. The use of a fluorescence biomarker for the diagnosis of cancers is an intriguing and still fledgling concept for improving the detection accuracy of PCa.

Methods

Patients

After receiving approval from the Nara Medical University Hospital Institutional Review Board, 138 patients with an abnormal DRE and/or abnormal PSA levels were recruited between April 2009 and December 2010. All patients provided written informed consent and were subsequently enrolled in this prospective feasibility study. Patients with a past history of urothelial carcinoma were not eligible for this study. For all the patients, before transrectal ultrasound needle-guided biopsy of the prostate, an "attentive" (approximately 30 s) DRE was performed, and the first 50 ml of voided urine was collected. Thereafter, the patients underwent prostate needle biopsies at Nara Medical University Hospital. Biopsies were performed by adjusting the number of cores sampled (6–12) according to the age of the patient and the prostatic volume. The medical records of our patients were reviewed for demographics, clinical, and pathological information (e.g., tumor grade, Gleason score, and tumor stage) as well as outcome. The clinicopathological characteristics of this cohort are listed in Table 1. All voided urine specimens were stored at 4°C until processed, which typically occurred within 2 h of collection.

Sample preparations and 5-ALA treatment

Urine specimens were centrifuged at 800 g for 5 min. The supernatant was decanted, and the pellets were suspended in phosphate-buffered saline (PBS) buffer, from which two samples were collected. One sample was treated with 1-mM 5-ALA (Sigma-Aldrich Co. Saint Louis, MO, USA), diluted with PBS, and then incubated at 37°C for 2 h. The solution was centrifuged at $5000\,g$

Table 1 Characteristic of the study population

	Males with positive biopsy (n = 81)	Males with negative biopsy (n = 57)		Total (n = 138)
	Median (range)	Median (range)	p-value	Median (range)
Age (years)	72 (51-86)	67 (55-81)	0.002	70 (51-86)
PSA (ng/ml)	9.7 (3.8-690)	7.4 (1.4-24.1)	0.002	8.3 (1.4-690)
Free PSA (ng/ml)	1.5 (0.46-95)	1.2 (0.15-3.3)	0.008	1.4 (0.15-95)
%fPSA (%)	15 (3-38)	17 (2-39)	0.679	15 (3-39)
PV (cm³)	28.7 (11.5-95.2)	34.0 (16.2-111)	0.002	30.4 (11.5-111)
TZV (cm³)	13.3 (3.7-45)	16.9 (2.9-78)	0.04	15.2 (2.9-78)
PSAD (ng/ml/cm³)	0.39 (0.07-46.6)	0.20 (0.06-1.0)	<0.001	0.27 (0.06-46.6)

Abbreviation: SD standard deviation, PSA prostate-specific antigen, %fPSA percent-free PSA, PV prostate volume, TZV transition zone volume, PSAD PSA density.

for 5 min, the supernatant was decanted, and 60 µl of PBS was added to suspend the cells. Next, the cells were applied to a charged-surface microscope slide (Figure 1). The second aliquot of shed cells within the urine was similarly processed, except that it was not treated with 5-ALA. Furthermore, a minute amount of material was removed from the second aliquot in which RNA was extracted from the cells by using the RNeasy Mini kit (Qiagen, Hilden, Germany) as per the manufacturer's instructions. A High-Capacity cDNA Reverse Transcription kit (Life Technologies, Palo Alto, CA) was used for the conversion cDNA. Primer sets for PSA (fp- 5′ TGAC CAAGTTCATGCTGTGT3′ and rp- 5′ TCCTTGGAGG CCATGTGGGCCAT 3′) were used to perform quantitative reverse transcription polymerase chain reaction (RT-PCR). Further, the relative fold changes in mRNA levels were calculated after normalization to glyceraldehyde 3-phosphate dehydrogenase (GAPDH).

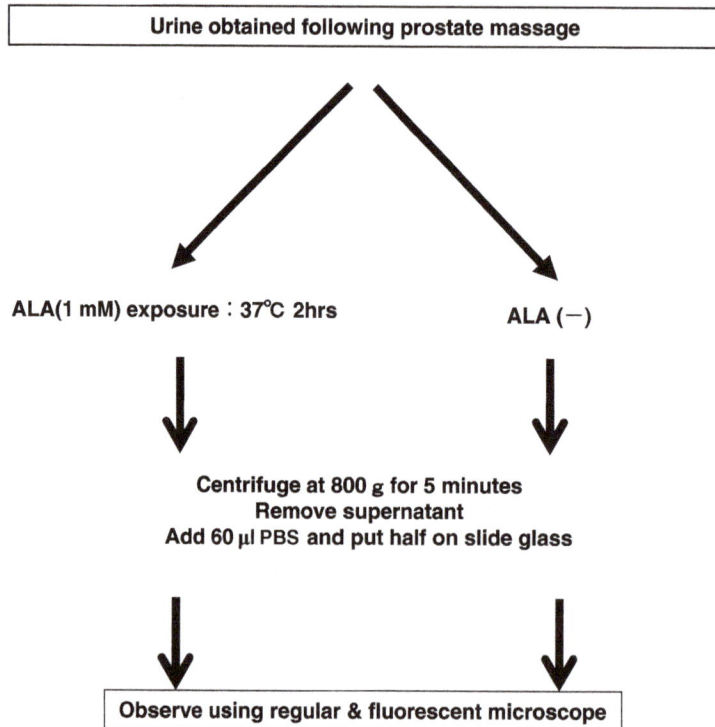

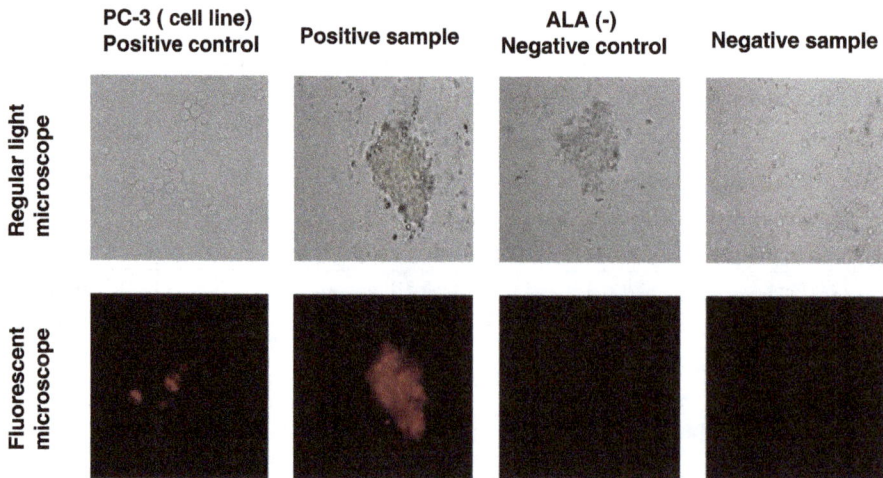

Figure 1 Workflow of the procedure and representative PPIX–PDD staining. DRE, digital rectal examination; ALA, aminolevulinic acid; RPM, revolutions per minute; PBS, phosphate buffered saline.

Photodynamic detection of PPIX in shed prostate cells

5-ALA-treated (and 5-ALA-untreated) urine cytospin slides were investigated for PPIX fluorescence at 100× magnification by fluorescent microscopy with the appropriate fluorescence filter sets (excitation filter, 380–420 nm; emission filter, 590 nm; Nikon Eclipse 400; Nikon Instruments Inc., Melville, NY, USA). The slides were evaluated for the following: (i) PPIX positivity, presence of cells demonstrating simultaneous fluorescence of PPIX and (ii) PPIX negativity, lack of cells demonstrating fluorescence.

Statistical analysis

The Mann–Whitney test was used to analyze the differences between the patients with or without PCa. We used the Chi-square test for trend to analyze whether the incidence of PPIX–PDD positivity was associated with cancer, PSA, Gleason score, and tumor stage. Multivariate logistic regression analysis was used to evaluate the demographic features, key clinical features [e.g., DRE, total PSA, %fPSA, PSA density (PSAD), and transrectal ultrasonography (TRUS)], and the PPIX–PDD results in order to determine their ability to independently predict PCa on prostate biopsy. Differences were considered statistically significant at p values <0.05.

Results

In this study, 81/138 (58.7%) patients revealed PCa on needle biopsy (Table 1). The median age of the patients without PCa was 67 (range 55–81) years, and the median age of patients with PCa was 72 (range 51–86) years (p = 0.002). The median PSA of the patients without PCa was 7.4 (range 1.4-24.1) ng/ml, and the median PSA of the patients with PCa was 9.7 (range 3.8-690) ng/ml (p = 0.002). Furthermore, the median free PSA (1.5 vs. 1.2 ng/ml, p = 0.008) and PSAD (0.39 vs. 0.20 ng/ml/cm^3, $p < 0.001$) values differed significantly between the patients with and without PCa, respectively. In addition, prostate volume (34.0 *vs.* 28.7 ml, p = 0.002) and transition zone volume (16.9 *vs.* 13.3 ml, p = 0.04) were significantly higher in the patients with PCa than in those without PCa.

The typical fluorescence of urine sediments placed on a cytospin slide from a patient with PCa was compared to its corresponding unstained urine sediments (Figure 1). These cells were found to express PSA by RT-PCR and were thus considered to be prostate cells (data not shown). The human prostate cancer cell line PC-3 was used as a positive control. Table 2 compares the PPIX–PDD results with the other clinical parameters (e.g., DRE, PSA, %fPSA, PSAD, and prostate volume) associated with PCa detection. Of the 81 patients with biopsy-proven PCa, 60 were determined positive for PPIX–PDD (sensitivity: 74.1%). PPIX–PDD was more sensitive compared with DRE and TRUS and more specific compared with

Table 2 Sensitivity and specificity of ALA, DRE, PSA, %sPSA, PSAD and TRUS

	Sensitivity	Specificity
ALA	74.1%	70.2%
DRE	44.4%	91.2%
PSAD (cut-off 0.15)	93.8%	29.8%
%fPSA (cut-off 20%)	78.7%	26.3%
PSA (cut-off 4ng/ml)	60.1%	50.0%
TRUS	34.6%	96.5%

Abbreviation: ALA aminolevulinic acid, *DRE* digital rectal examination, *TRUS* transrectal ultrasinography, *PSAD* PSA density, *%fPSA* percent free PSA.

PSA and PSAD. Although 57 patients did not harbor PCa by conventional diagnostic procedures, 17 of these at-risk patients were determined positive for PPIX–PDD (specificity: 70.2%). These patients have been under close surveillance to evaluate if their positive PPIX–PDD results will convert to clinical PCa.

The diagnostic accuracy of PPIX–PDD in the males with positive biopsy at different total PSA levels was 2/2 (100%) patients for PSA levels within 0–4 ng/ml, 28/39 (71.8%) for PSA levels within 4–10 ng/ml, 11/15 (73.3%) for PSA levels within 10–20 ng/ml, and 19/25 (76.0%) for PSA levels >20 ng/ml. The diagnostic accuracy at different tumor stages was 34/45 (75.6%) for tumor stage cT1, 22/32 (68.8%) for cT2, and 4/4 (100%) for cT3. The incidence of PPIX–PDD positivity did not increase with increase in the total PSA levels (p = 0.25) and tumor stage (p = 0.87). Furthermore, the diagnostic accuracy of PPIX–PDD in the males with positive biopsies was 15/24 (62.5%) for Gleason score (GS) 6, 26/34 (76.4%) for GS 7, and 19/23 (82.6%) for GS 8–10. The incidence of PPIX–PDD positivity increased with increasing GS, but the increase was not significant (p = 0.11) (Table 3).

In addition, on multivariate analysis, we evaluated the demographic features, key clinical features (e.g., DRE, total PSA, %fPSA, PSAD, and TRUS), and PPIX–PDD results to determine their ability to independently predict PCa on prostate biopsy (Table 4). Multivariate analysis indicated that ALA (HR, 8.00; 95% CI, 2.50–25.59; $p < 0.001$) and PSAD (HR, 28.43; 95% CI, 8.12–99.58; $p < 0.001$) were independent diagnostic factors for PCa.

Discussion

In this study, we demonstrated the feasibility of PPIX–PDD and 5- ALA in noninvasive detection of PCa cells extracorporeally in voided urine sediments. The use of voided urine samples in an attempt to diagnosis PCa is gaining widespread attention. For example, investigators are using RT-PCR to identify the prostate cancer antigen 3 (PCA-3) [12] and glutathione S-transferase P1[12] gene [13] in voided urine samples. Particularly, the sensitivity

Table 3 Diagnostic accuracy of PDD according to total PSA, grade (Gleason) and stage

	Males with positive biopsy (n=81)	Males with positive PDD (n=60)	Sensitivity	p-value*
0-4	2	2	100%	
4-10	39	28	71.8%	
10-20	15	11	73.3%	
20-	25	19	76.0%	0.25
Gleason score				
6	24	15	62.5%	
7	34	26	76.4%	
8-10	23	19	82.6	0.11
Clinical stage				
cT1	45	34	75.6%	
cT2	32	22	68.8%	
cT3	4	4	100%	
cT4	-	-	-	0.87

*Chi-square test for trend.

and specificity of PCA-3 have been reported to be 54% and 74%, respectively, for the entire cohort and 53% and 71%, respectively, for PSA within 4–10 ng/ml. In the present study, the sensitivity and specificity of PPIX–PDD were 74.1% and 70.2% in the entire cohort and 70.0% and 67.6% in the gray zone cases, which were superior to those reported for PCA-3. Interestingly, the positivity rate of PPIX–PDD did not increase with increasing total PSA or tumor stage. However, the positivity rate of PPIX–PDD did increase with increasing Gleason score though a non-significant trend ($p = 0.11$) was noted. These results showed a possibility that PCa detection with PPIX–PDD identified more clinically significant PCa compared with PCa detected by other reported methods. Stummer et al. reported that the fluorescence intensity of glioma by PPIX–PDD was associated with cellular density, tumor proliferation, and tumor angiogenesis [14]; these results supported our results

indicating that PPIX–PDD detected more aggressive clinically relevant cancers.

Although no reports regarding fluorescent cytology of shed PCa cells were found in the literature, several reports from the bladder cancer literature are available [15-17]; in these reports, voided urine after intravesical 5-ALA instillation was evaluated. Inoue et al. reported that regardless of the 5-ALA administration route (intravesical or oral), exposure to 5-ALA was well tolerated with only cystitis symptoms being reported [18]. Hence, in this extracorporeal model, shed prostate cells rather than patients were treated with 5-ALA.

Although the findings in the present study were quite compelling, the study had some limitations. First, we obtained limited pathological data on the patients with positive PPIX–PDD results and positive prostate biopsy results who proceeded to undergo radical prostatectomy. Second, with limited follow-up (mean follow-up, 27 months), we must cautiously interpret the false-positive PPIX–PDD results. It is possible that over time, these prostate biopsies will become positive. In this cohort, only 4 false positive patients had been performed repeated prostate needle biopsies after this study. 2 patients of them were diagnosed as prostate cancer. These false positive patients may need strict PSA follow-up or a saturation biopsy. Third, we didn't perform RT-PCR for every patient. We demonstrated RT-PCR in the first twenty patients. Then we evaluated the expression of PSA. We could confirm the existence of cells from prostate by that. In addition, these false-positive results may be attributed to autofluorescence. Tauber et al. reported that some biological materials had autofluorescence. To address this issue, the authors used bleaching fluorescence; however, the specificity of bleaching fluorescence was comparatively low [16]. In our study, we were able to subjectively estimate autofluorescence by examining the slide not treated with 5-ALA from each patient. Furthermore, cytological examinations are known to present interobserver variability. In the future, we hope to develop a more objective spectrophotometric method to quantify the intensity of PPIX fluorescence.

Table 4 Univariate and multivariate analysis of factors to predict PCa on prostate biopsy

	Univariate analysis			Multivariate analysis		
	OR	95% CI	p-value	OR	95% CI	p-value
ALA (positive/negative)	6.72	3.16-14.29	<0.001	8.00	2.50-25.59	<0.001
DRE (abnormal/normal)	8.00	2.89-22.15	<0.001	1.77	0.32-9.38	0.52
PSAD (>0.15/<0.15)	34.20	11.63-100.54	<0.001	28.43	8.12-99.58	<0.001
% fPSA (>20%/<20%)	1.57	0.71-3.53	0.27			
PSA (>20/>10, <20/<10)	2.37	1.43-3.95	0.001	1.97	0.81-4.80	0.14
TRUS (abnormal/normal)	13.50	3.06-59.66	0.001	7.35	0.52-104.58	0.14

Abbreviation: OR odds ratio, *ALA* aminolevulinic acid, *DRE* digital rectal examination, *PSAD* PSA density, *%fPSA* percent free PSA, *TRUS* transrectal uktrasonography.

Conclusions

To our knowledge, this is the first successful demonstration of PPIX in urine sediments treated with 5-ALA for detection of PCa in a noninvasive yet highly sensitive manner. The incidence of PPIX–PDD positivity increased with increasing Gleason score though a non-siginificant trend ($p = 0.11$) was noted. Further studies are warranted to determine the role of PPIX–PPD for PCa detection.

Abbreviations

ALA: Aminolevulinic acid; DRE: Digital rectal exam; GAPDH: Glyceraldehyde 3-phosphate dehydrogenase; GS: Gleason score; PBS: Phosphate-buffered saline; PDD: Photodynamic diagnosis; PCa: Prostate cancer; PCA-3: Prostate cancer antigen 3; PSA: Prostate-specific antigen; PSAD: PSA density; PPIX: Protoporphyrin IX; TRUS: Transrectal ultrasonography; RT-PCR: Reverse transcription polymerase chain reaction.

Competing interests

The authors declare that they have no competing interests.

Authors' contributions

YN and SA carried out the photodynamic detection and drafted the manuscript. SA also designed the experiments and interpreted the data. MK and MM helped with photodynamic detection and RT-PCR. YC provided valuable help with the experiments. NT contributed to the design and conception. AH revised this manuscript. KY and KF participated in study design. YH conceived of the study and participated in its design. All authors read and approved the final manuscript.

Acknowledgments

This work was supported by Department of Urology in Nara Medical University.

References

1. Draisma G, Etzioni R, Tsodikov A, Marriot A, Wever E, Gulati R, Feuer E, De Koning H: Lead time and overdiagnosis in prostate-specific antigen screening: importance of methods and context. *J Natl Cancer Inst* 2009, **101**:374–383.
2. Tanaka N, Fujimoto K, Chihara Y, Torimoto M, Hirao Y, Konishi N, Saito I: Prostatic volume and volume-adjusted prostate-specific antigen as predictive parameters for prostate cancer patients with intermediate PSA levels. *Prostate Cancer Prostatic Dis* 2007, **10**:274–278.
3. Sharifi R, Shaw M, Ray V, Rhee H, Nagubadi S, Guinan P: Evaluation of cytologic techniques for diagnosis of prostate cancer. *Urology* 1983, **4**:417–420.
4. Bologna M, Vicentini C, Festuccia C, Muzi P, Napolitano T, Biordi L, Miano L: Early diagnosis of prostatic carcinoma based on in vitro culture of viable tumor cells harvested by prostatic massage. *Eur Urol* 1988, **14**:474–476.
5. Garret M, Jassie M: Cytologic examination of post prostatic massage specimens as an aid in diagnosis of carcinoma of the prostate. *Acta Cytol* 1976, **20**:126–131.
6. Kriegmair M, Baumgartner R, Knuchel R, Idvall I, Ingvar C, Rydell R, Jocham D, Diddens H, Bown S, Gregory G, Montán S, Andersson-Engels S, Svanberg S: Detection of early bladder cancer by 5-aminolevulinic acid induced porphyrin fluorescence. *J Urol* 1996, **155**:105–109.
7. Filbeck T, Roessler W, Knuechel R, Straub M, Kiel HJ, Wieland WF: Clinical results of the transurethral resection and evaluation of superficial bladder carcinomas by means of fluorescence diagnosis after intravesical instillation of 5-aminolevulinic acid. *J Endourol* 1999, **13**:117–121.
8. König F, McGovern FJ, Larne R, Enquist H, Schomacker KT, Deutsch TF: Diagnosis of bladder carcinoma using protoporphyrin IX fluorescence induced 5-aminolaevulinic acid. *BJU Int* 1999, **83**:129–135.
9. Zaak D, Hungerhuber E, Schneede P, Stepp H, Frimberger D, Corvin S, Schmeller N, Kriegmair M, Hotstetter A, Knuechel R: Role of 5-aminolevulinic acid in the detection of urothelial premalignant lesions. *Cancer* 2002, **95**:1234–1238.
10. Steinbach P, Weingandt H, Baumgartner R, Kriegmair M, Hofstädter F, Knüchel R: Cellular fluorescence of the endogenous photosensitizer protoporphyrin IX following exposure to 5-aminolevulinic acid. *Photochem Photobiol* 1995, **62**:887–895.
11. Zaak D, Sroka R, Khoder W, Adam C, Tritschler S, Karl A, Reich O, Knuechel R, Baumgartner R, Tilki D, Popken G, Hofstetter A, Stief CG: Photodynamic diagnosis of prostate cancer using 5-aminolevulinic acid—first clinical experiences. *Urology* 2008, **72**:345–348.
12. Deras IL, Aubin SM, Blase A, Day JR, Koo S, Partin AW, Ellis WJ, Marks LS, Fradet Y, Rittenhouse H, Groskopf J: PCA3: a molecular urine assay for predicting prostate biopsy outcome. *J Urol* 2008, **179**:1587–1592.
13. Vener T, Derecho C, Jonathan B, Wang H, Rajpurohit Y, Skelton J, Mehrotra J, Varde S, Chowdary D, Stallings J, Leibovich B, Robin H, Pelzer A, Schäfer G, Auprich M, Mannweiler S, Amersdorfer P, Mazumder A: Development of a multiplexed urine assay for prostate cancer diagnosis. *Clin Chem* 2008, **54**:874–882.
14. Stummer W, Reulen HJ, Novotny A, Stepp H, Tonn JC: Fluorescence-guided resections of malignant gliomas–an overview. *Acta Neurochir Suppl* 2003, **88**:9–12.
15. Tauber S, Schneede P, Bernhard L, Liesmann F, Zaak D, Hofstetter A: Fluorescence cytology of the urinary bladder. *Urology* 2003, **61**:1067–1071.
16. Pytel A, Schmeller N: New aspect of photodynamic of bladder tumors: fluorescence cytology. *Urology* 2002, **59**:216–219.
17. Tauber S, Stepp H, Meier R, Bone A, Hofstetter A, Stief C: Integral spectrophotometric analysis of 5-aminolaevulinic acid-induced fluorescence cytology of the urinary bladder. *BJU Int* 2006, **97**:992–996.
18. Inoue K, Fukuhara H, Shimamoto T, Kamada M, Liyama T, Miyamura M, Kurabayashi A, Furihata M, Tanimura M, Watanabe H, Shuin T: Comparison between intravesical and oral administration of 5-aminolevulinic acid in the clinical benefit of photodynamic diagnosis for nonmuscle invasive bladder cancer. *Cancer* 2012, **118**:1062–1074.

17

The prevalence and outcomes of pT0 disease after neoadjuvant hormonal therapy and radical prostatectomy in high-risk prostate cancer

Jae Young Joung[1*], Jeong Eun Kim[1], Sung Han Kim[1], Ho Kyung Seo[1], Jinsoo Chung[1], Weon Seo Park[2], Eun Kyung Hong[2] and Kang Hyun Lee[1*]

Abstract

Background: To identify the prevalence and clinical outcomes of pT0 disease following neoadjuvant hormonal therapy (NHT) and radical prostatectomy (RP) in high-risk prostate cancer.

Methods: We retrospectively included 111 patients who had received NHT and RP for the treatment of high-risk prostate cancer. We classified the patients into two groups, the pT0 group and the non-pT0 group, depending on whether a residual tumor was observed.

Results: We identified 6 cases (5.4 %) with pT0 disease after reviewing the slides of all patients. There was no recurrence of disease in the pT0 group during a median follow-up of 59 months. Among the 105 patients in the non-pT0 group, biochemical recurrence (BCR) developed in 60 patients (57.1 %), with the median time to BCR being 14 months.

Conclusions: Among the 111 patients with high-risk prostate cancer, we found 6 cases that showed a complete pathological response after NHT and no recurrence of disease during the follow-up, meaning that the androgen deprivation therapy could potentially eradicate high-risk prostate cancer. This is one of the largest studies demonstrating the prevalence of pT0 disease and its outcomes after NHT among patients with high-risk prostate cancer.

Background

pT0 prostate cancer, also known as no residual tumor, undetectable tumor, or vanishing tumor, is not common in biopsy-proven cases of prostate cancer. In patients who have not received androgen deprivation therapy (ADT) prior to radical prostatectomy (RP), the incidence of pT0 disease is reported to be between 0.07 and 0.5 % [1, 2]. In reality, it is difficult for the surgeon to explain the final diagnosis of pT0 disease to patients, due to their concerns regarding unnecessary surgery for insignificant disease. Conversely, in patients with advanced stage disease such as high-risk disease or locally advanced disease, we suggest that a diagnosis of pT0 following ADT could indicate a complete pathological response or complete tumor eradication after neoadjuvant hormonal therapy

(NHT). pT0 disease is more common in patients who have received ADT, and has a wider prevalence than in patients who have not received ADT.

To date, the use of ADT prior to RP has been explored in multiple studies [3]. However, the use of ADT in a neoadjuvant setting prior to RP is not currently recommended due to the absence of clear evidence of a survival benefit of ADT for localized prostate cancer. Considering only high-risk disease or locally advanced disease, ADT followed by RP achieves long-term progression-free survival (PFS) and overall survival (OS) comparable to alternative strategies such as combined radiation therapy (RT) and ADT [4, 5].

At our institution, we perform ADT prior to RP in patients with locally advanced prostate cancer or high-risk disease at the surgeon's discretion. Notably, we have experienced pT0 disease following NHT and RP among these patients. We designed this study to confirm our hypothesis that pT0 disease following NHT and RP could show outstanding clinical outcomes in patients with high-risk

* Correspondence: urojy@ncc.re.kr; uroonoc@ncc.re.kr
[1]Center for Prostate Cancer, National Cancer Center, Goyang, South Korea
Full list of author information is available at the end of the article

disease. There exist rare reports in the literature that demonstrate the occurrence of pT0 disease in high-risk prostate cancer through subgroup analysis in a small number of patients [6, 7]. Here, we review our prostate cancer database to identify the prevalence of pT0 disease among patients with high-risk disease and the clinical outcomes of these patients during the follow-up. To the best of our knowledge, this is one of the largest studies to demonstrate the prevalence of pT0 disease after NHT in more than 100 patients belonging to the high-risk group.

Methods
Patient selection
Between May 2002 and June 2013 we retrospectively identified 120 patients who had received NHT and RP by reviewing the Korean National Cancer Center's prostate cancer database, in which the clinicopathological data and clinical outcomes were prospectively recorded. In each case, the combination of NHT and surgery was decided at the surgeon's discretion. Among these 120 patients, we selected 111 patients who had high-risk prostate cancer that was defined based on the D'Amico criteria as PSA ≥ 20 ng/ml, biopsy Gleason score (GS) ≥8, or clinical stage ≥ cT2c for the present study. After obtaining informed consent from each patient, NHT and RP were performed. NHT consisted of at least 3 months of luteinizing hormone-releasing hormone (LHRH) agonist therapy, and radical prostatectomy was performed with standard pelvic lymph node dissection. All of the patients were followed up with serum PSA evaluation every 3 months for the first year, biannually from the second to the fifth year, and annually thereafter. When biochemical recurrence (BCR) developed, radiological studies such as magnetic resonance imaging, computed tomography, or bone scanning were performed, if required. When the (PSA) nadir level did not decrease below 0.2 ng/ml following RP, adjuvant ADT or RT was given at the physician's discretion. Salvage RT or ADT was recommended for the patients who experienced local recurrence or distant metastasis.

For pathological diagnosis, all of the prostatectomy specimens were processed using complete transverse sections of the whole mounted prostatectomy specimens, from the apex to the base at 4-mm intervals. In addition to conventional hematoxylin & eosin (H&E) staining, we performed immunohistochemical staining in all the cases using several antibodies including PSA, PSMA, PSCA, AMACR, and p63. For the cases that were recorded as having pT0 disease in our database, two pathologists reviewed all the slides in each case in order to confirm the pT0 stage. This study was approved by the Institutional Review Board of the Korean National Cancer Center (NCCNCS05-049). Subject's informed consent was obtained and documented in accordance with local regulations, ICH-GCP requirements, and the ethical principles that have their origin in the principles of the Declaration of Helsinki.

Statistical analysis
For comparative analysis, we classified the patients into two groups, the pT0 group and the non-pT0 group depending on whether a residual tumor was observed. We compared the clinicopathological characteristics between the two groups using the Fisher's exact test for categorical variables, and the Wilcoxon rank-sum test for continuous variables. BCR definition that we currently use after RP is 2 consecutive values of 0.2 ng/ml or greater after surgery. Local recurrence was defined as a newly developed lesion identified around the area of prior prostatectomy in any of the imaging studies. Clinical outcomes of patients after treatment were determined based on BCR or clinical progression, including local recurrence, distant metastasis, and survival, by applying the Kaplan-Meier method. PFS was defined as the time to the first evidence of biochemical, local, or distant metastasis, or death in the absence of disease progression. Statistical significance was defined as $p < 0.05$. All analyses were performed using the SPSS software package (SPSS, Inc., Chicago, version 12.0 for Windows 2007).

Results
Among the 111 patients with high risk disease, we identified 6 cases (5.4 %) with pT0 disease in our study. After reviewing all the slides of these 6 cases, we did not find any apparent tumors, hence we finally confirmed the presence of pT0 disease. Microscopic findings in the prostate tissue after ADT included atrophy of the gland, basal cell prominence, vacuolated luminal cell layers, and squamous and transitional cell metaplasia of the non-tumor gland. The tumor glands usually showed smaller tumors within, pyknosis, empty glandular spaces, and vacuolization and degeneration of tumor cells with an inflammatory response. When pyknotic cells were positive for cytokeratin, PSA, or AMACR on immunohistochemical staining, they were considered to demonstrate the presence of a viable residual tumor.

Patient characteristics of the 6 cases of pT0 disease are presented in Table 1. Patient age was significantly different between the pT0 and the non-pT0 groups. The 6 patients with pT0 disease were older than the patients with non-pT0 disease ($p = 0.014$). Otherwise, no significant differences were observed in the clinical features including the baseline PSA level, biopsy GS, clinical stage, or number of positive biopsy cores (Table 2).

Regarding the pathological stage in the non-pT0 group, an organ-confined tumor (pT2) was found in 46 cases (43.8 %), locally-advanced disease including pT3 and pT4 were found in 46 cases (43.8 %), and pelvic lymph node (LN) metastasis was found in 13 cases (12.4 %). A positive

Table 1 Characteristics of patients with pT0 prostate cancer

Patient number	Age	PSA (ng/mL)) Baseline	PSA (ng/mL)) After NHT	Duration of NHT	Clinical stage	GS	Number of positive cores on biopsy	Maximal tumor length on biopsy (mm)	Duration of follow-up
1	66	24.6	<0.1	6 months	T2cNoMo	7	6	10.0	48
2	77	55.3	0.3	3 months	T3aN0M0	6	3	3.0	60
3	66	20.9	<0.1	6 months	T3aN0M0	7	3	21.0	80
4	76	6.18	<0.1	3 months	T2cNoMo	7	8	12.0	74
5	73	9.4	<0.1	12 months	T3aN0M0	7	8	5.0	57
6	74	19.38	<0.1	6 months	T3aN0M0	8	6	10.0	6

PSA prostate-specific antigen, *NHT* neoadjuvant hormonal therapy, *GS* Gleason score

surgical margin was observed in 28 patients (26.7 %) in the non-pT0 group including 7 patients (15.2 %) with stage pT2 and 15 patients (32.6 %) with stage pT3-pT4. ADT was added as an adjuvant treatment following RP in 18 patients (17.1 %), and there was no case that received adjuvant RT in this group. Patients in the pT0 group did not receive any additional treatment.

At the time of analysis, the median follow-up period was 54 months (range, 3 to 102 months) in all patients. In the pT0 group, all patients were alive and there was no

Table 2 Clinicopathological features between the two groups

	pT0 group (n = 6)	Non-pT0 group (n = 105)	P-value
Age, median (range)	73.5 (66–77)	66.0 (47–77)	0.014
PSA, median (range)	20.14 (6.18–55.30)	39.50 (4.16–261.80)	0.126
Biopsy GS (%)			0.447
2–6	1 (16.7)	19 (18.1)	
7	4 (66.7)	44 (41.9)	
8–10	1 (16.7)	42 (40.0)	
Clinical stage (%)			0.461
cT1c- cT2b	0 (0.0)	10 (9.5)	
cT2c	2 (33.3)	50 (47.6)	
cT3-cT4	4 (66.7)	45 (42.9)	
Median number of positive cores on biopsy (range)	6 (3–8)	6 (1–13)	0.599
Median maximum tumor length (range)	10.0 mm (3.0–21.0)	11.0 mm (0.5–25.0)	0.806
Median duration of NHT (range)	6 months (3–12)	3 months (3–30)	0.144
Median (PSA) nadir after NHT (range)	0.01 ng/ml (0.01–0.30)	0.20 ng/ml (0.01–23.70)	0.387
Pathological stage (%)			
pT0	6 (100.0)		
pT2		46 (43.8)	
pT3-pT4		46 (43.8)	
N1		13 (12.4)	
Positive resection margin		28 (26.7)	
In pT2		7 (15.2 %)	
In pT3-pT4		15 (32.6 %)	
In N1		6 (46.2 %)	
Seminal vesicle invasion		36 (34.3))	
Prostate volume, median (range)	22.0 gm (16.0–24.1)	24.9gm (7.5–50.0)	0.280
Tumor volume, % (range)	0	20 (1–90)	

PSA prostate-specific antigen, *NHT* neoadjuvant hormonal therapy, *GS* Gleason score, *NA* not available

recurrence of disease during the median follow-up of 59 months (range, 6 to 80 months). Among the 105 patients in the non-pT0 group, BCR developed in 60 patients (57.1 %), and the median time to BCR was 14 months (range, 5–56 months). Clinical progression occurred in 11 patients (10.5 %) including 9 patients (8.6 %) with local recurrence and 9 patients (8.6 %) with metastasis. 5-year PFS was 30.3 %, and 5-year clinical PFS and 5-year metastasis-free survival were 86.2 and 87.2 %, respectively. 6 patients (5.7 %) progressed to castration-resistant prostate cancer. Death occurred in 11 patients (10.5 %); prostate cancer-specific death in 3 cases (2.9 %) and death due to other causes in 8 cases (7.6 %). At 5 years, the overall survival (OS) and cancer-specific survival (CSS) were 91.5 and 97.7 %, respectively (Fig. 1).

Discussion

In patients with high-risk prostate cancer, we observed 6 cases (5.4 %) of pT0 disease that showed no tumor recurrence during the follow-up. Our results indicate that ADT can induce a complete pathological response, and can potentially eradicate advanced prostate cancer.

Regarding the issue of pT0 disease in surgical specimens, the majority of surgeons were initially concerned about unnecessary surgery or overtreatment in patients with no residual tumors. The occurrence of pT0 disease has been reported in many previous studies of prostatectomy series. The prevalence of pT0 disease was found to be between 0.2 and 1.3 % in the prostatectomy series, and it was more common in localized prostate cancer in the low-risk group and in small tumors such as those with less than 2 positive

cores on biopsy [1, 8–10]. In Korean patients, the likelihood of occurrence of pT0 disease was found to be related to the biopsy Gleason score, the number of positive cores on biopsy, the tumor length in a positive core, and prostate volume [10].

pT0 disease in prostatectomy specimens is more commonly detected in patients who receive ADT prior to surgery. Due to the effect of androgen deprivation, the prostate tumor shows glandular shrinkage including pyknosis, empty glandular spaces, and vacuolization and degeneration of tumor cells. In addition, ADT reduces the frequency of tumor extension to surgical margins [11].

The occurrence of pT0 disease following ADT has led to increased clinical interest in investigating the role of ADT, because patients with pT0 stage prostate cancer are expected to have an extremely favorable prognosis. NHT is initially intended to improve the surgical outcomes by minimizing the rate of positive surgical margins following RP. Early studies assessing the efficacy of NHT demonstrated a decrease in tumor volume and positive surgical margin rates, and an increase in the rate of pathologically organ-confined cancer [12, 13]. Many investigators have assessed the effect of combined NHT and RP on the survival outcomes in patients with prostate cancer, however, the effect of NHT adjunctive to RP has not been satisfactorily supported by existing evidence [3], which is different to the results seen with ADT prior to RT [14, 15]. Several guidelines have stated that there is no benefit to the administration of ADT prior to RP in localized cancer, based on the results of previous studies. Considering only

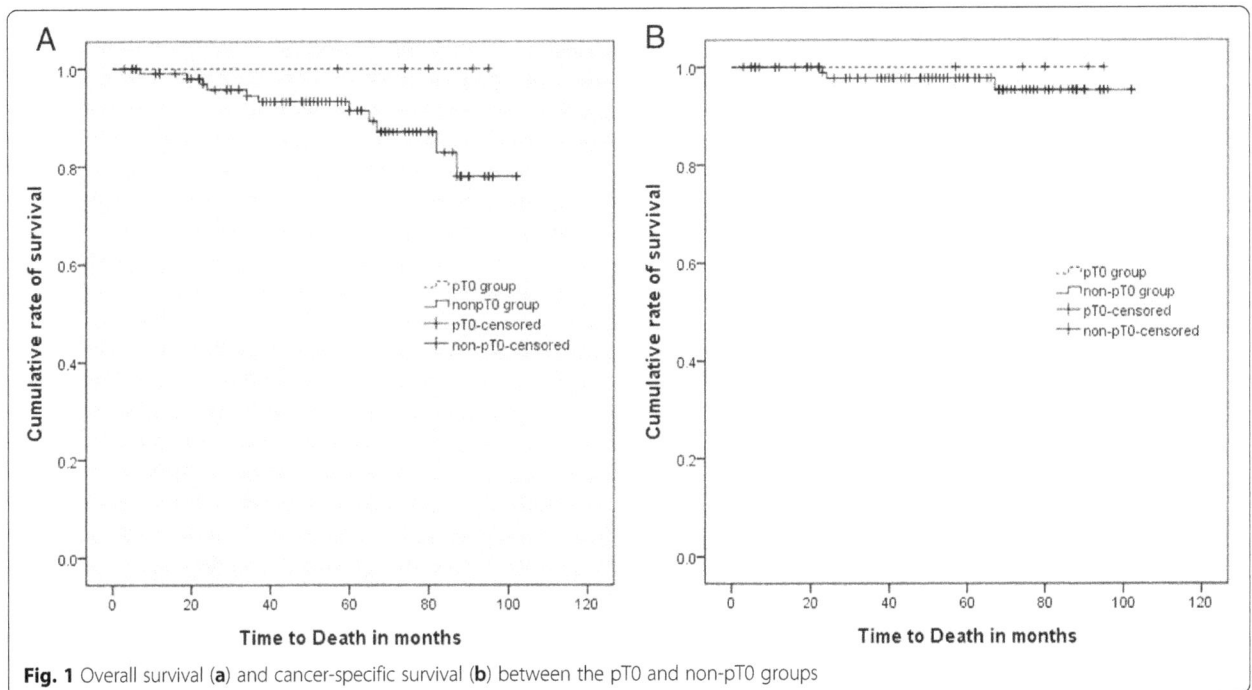

Fig. 1 Overall survival (a) and cancer-specific survival (b) between the pT0 and non-pT0 groups

high-risk or locally advanced prostate cancer, combined NHT and RP achieves a long-term PFS and OS comparable to the alternative strategy of combined RT and ADT [4, 5]. In the current study, we also achieved good results for the 5-year survival outcome, which was comparable to previous reports, despite a higher BCR rate.

With respect to the prevalence of pT0 disease after ADT, it is more common and has a wider prevalence compared with that in non-ADT cases. In one study, 36 (20.7 %) out of 174 patients who received NHT did not show any residual tumor in RP specimens [6]. In another study of high-risk disease, 2 (9.5 %) out of 21 patients did not show any residual tumor after 8 months of ADT before RP [7]. In the current study, pT0 disease was observed in 5.4 % of the patients with high-risk prostate cancer. This difference in the prevalence of pT0 after ADT may be related to the varying degree of diagnostic accuracy in detecting residual tumors that undergo histological changes following ADT, varying durations of ADT, and highly heterogeneous characteristics of tumors in each study.

In prostate cancer, diagnosis is generally made based on a routine pathological exam using standard processes such as H&E staining in a limited number of slides. In one study, after microscopic reassessment of the slides, very small tumor remnants with a mean volume of 0.2 ml were detected in 13 of the 20 prostatectomy specimens [16]. Considering our diagnostic procedure of using whole mounted sections and reexamination by pathologists who have excellent experience in the assessment of ADT-related cases, we are confident that the pT0 stage indicates a complete pathological response and eradication of the tumor following ADT.

The duration of ADT could also affect the incidence of pT0 disease. Prolonged NHT results in an additional decrease in tumor volume and positive surgical margin rates, and an increase in the rate of pathologically-confirmed organ-confined cancer and prevalence of pT0 disease [16, 17]. Based on the results of the current study, we found that ADT administered for only 3 months induced a complete pathological response in 2 patients.

The pathological response following ADT may be different depending on the tumor characteristics of each case. Among the prostatectomy cases that received NHT in a previous report, 43 % of patients still showed an unaltered area in tissues upon microscopic examination [11], indicating remarkable differences in the response of prostate cancer to ADT. In another previous study, after stratifying the rate of pT0 disease depending on the clinical stage (cT), pT0 was observed in 36.7 % of patients with cT1 prostate cancer, 33.9 % of patients with cT2 prostate cancer, and 5.9 % of patients with cT3 prostate cancer [6]. In a multi-institutional prospective trial including Japanese patients with high-risk disease, 8 months of ADT administration before RP resulted in no residual tumor (pT0) in 2 out of

21 patients (9.5 %) [7]. Despite being a retrospective study at a single institution, our present study included 111 patients with high-risk prostate cancer, of which 6 patients (5.4 %) were finally diagnosed as having pT0 disease, making this one of the largest data sets showing the rate of pT0 disease after NHT among patients in the high-risk group.

Theoretically, pT0 disease is assumed to have a good prognosis since relapse does not occur or occurs extremely rarely in pT0 patients. As expected, some studies have not shown biochemical or clinical progression of the disease [8, 18, 19]. However, Kollermann et al., showed that BCR was observed in 7 (18.4 %) of 38 patients with pT0 disease during a median follow-up of 47 months. Among these, 3 cases showed local or systemic tumor relapse [20]. Furthermore, PSA progression-free survival in the pT0 group was no different to that in the non-pT0 group in a matched pair analysis [6]. In a Japanese study of high-risk disease, BCR developed in half of the 21 patients with pT0 disease after 8 months of NHT [7]. These inconsistent results of clinical outcomes in pT0 disease are related to the diagnostic accuracy in detecting residual tumor and the length of follow-up. In fact, we cannot exclude the possibility that we may have experienced a relapse of the disease among patients with pT0 disease in the current study if the duration of the follow-up was longer. On the contrary, Bostwick et al., reported that none of the 34 pT0 patients had a relapse during a mean follow-up of 9.6 years, which is the longest follow-up data set to date [1].

Although we obtained encouraging results that showed no relapse of the disease, as well as the occurrence of pT0 disease in high-risk prostate cancer patients, there are some limitations to this study due to its retrospective nature.

Firstly, we only had 6 cases of pT0 disease. Although we analyzed some characteristics of the patients using a non-parametric method due to the very small number of pT0 patients, we could not compare the pT0 group with the non-pT0 group by performing a matched-pair analysis.

Secondly, the length of the follow-up period was limited. The median follow-up duration in the pT0 group was 59 months, which is not a sufficient time period to assess recurrence of the disease or the effect of pT0 disease on long-term survival in other localized prostate cancer with low or intermediate risk. Considering that BCR developed in more than 50 % of patients in the non-pT0 group of the current study, this follow-up duration may be sufficient to assess the clinical outcomes in high-risk prostate cancer.

Thirdly, there was no case of tumor relapse in the pT0 group. In some reports, pT0 patients have shown frequent recurrence of the tumor, which may be due to the probable over-diagnosis of pT0 disease due to insufficient partial sampling of prostatectomy specimens or missing small foci in the tumor. As already mentioned, we are confident that our pT0 stage indicates tumor eradication due to a complete pathological response to ADT, which led to good clinical outcomes of pT0 prostate cancer.

Although there was no statistically significant difference in the duration of ADT between the two groups, there was a wide variation in the duration of ADT due to the retrospective study design. It is assumed that the duration of NHT can affect the prevalence of pT0 disease and tumor relapse. Further prospectively-designed studies are required in order to refine and standardize the duration of therapy.

Conclusions

Among the 111 patients with high-risk prostate cancer who received NHT and RP, we found 6 cases (5.4 %) that had no apparent residual tumor, and they were diagnosed as having pT0 disease from the prostatectomy specimens. Of interest, we observed that none of the pT0 patients showed disease recurrence, indicating a potential benefit of NHT as a preoperative treatment in patients with high-risk prostate cancer. Furthermore, NHT may have the ability to eradicate prostate cancer. This is one of the largest studies showing the prevalence of pT0 disease after NHT among patients with high-risk prostate cancer.

Competing interests
The authors declare that they have no competing interests.

Authors' contributions
JYJ designed the study and wrote the manuscript. SHK participated in the study design. JEK helped to draft the manuscript. SHK did statistical analysis for the clinical factors of the patients. JEK managed and analyzed the raw data of the characteristics of the patients. WSP helped to design the study and draft the manuscript. JYJ and HKS analyzed the reference data. KHL and JC designed and supervised the study. JEK and EKH reviewed the previous data. All authors read and approved the final manuscript.

Acknowledgements
This study was supported by Korean National Cancer Center grants (nos. 1510170 and 1310330).

Author details
[1]Center for Prostate Cancer, National Cancer Center, Goyang, South Korea.
[2]Department of Pathology, National Cancer Center, Goyang, South Korea.

References
1. Bostwick DG, Bostwick KC. 'Vanishing' prostate cancer in radical prostatectomy specimens: incidence and long-term follow-up in 38 cases. BJU Int. 2004;94(1):57–8.
2. Cao D, Hafez M, Berg K, Murphy K, Epstein JI. Little or no residual prostate cancer at radical prostatectomy: vanishing cancer or switched specimen?: a microsatellite analysis of specimen identity. Am J Surg Pathol. 2005;29(4):467–73.
3. Hu J, Hsu J, Bergerot PG, Yuh BE, Stein CA, Pal SK. Preoperative therapy for localized prostate cancer: a comprehensive overview. Maturitas. 2013;74(1):3–9.
4. Berglund RK, Tangen CM, Powell IJ, Lowe BA, Haas GP, Carroll PR, et al. Ten-year follow-up of neoadjuvant therapy with goserelin acetate and flutamide before radical prostatectomy for clinical T3 and T4 prostate cancer: update on Southwest Oncology Group Study 9109. Urology. 2012;79(3):633–7.
5. Powell IJ, Tangen CM, Miller GJ, Lowe BA, Haas G, Carroll PR, et al. Neoadjuvant therapy before radical prostatectomy for clinical T3/T4 carcinoma of the prostate: 5-year followup, phase ii southwest oncology group study 9109. J Urol. 2002;168(5):2016–9.
6. Kollermann J, Hopfenmuller W, Caprano J, Budde A, Weidenfeld H, Weidenfeld M, et al. Prognosis of stage pT0 after prolonged neoadjuvant endocrine therapy of prostate cancer: a matched-pair analysis. Eur Urol. 2004;45(1):42–5.
7. Tabata K, Satoh T, Matsumoto K, Fujita T, Irie A, Iwamura M, et al. 8 months of neoadjuvant hormonal therapy prior to radical prostatectomy for high-risk prostate cancer. Nihon Hinyokika Gakkai Zasshi. 2006;97(5):712–8.
8. Trpkov K, Gao Y, Hay R, Yimaz A. No residual cancer on radical prostatectomy after positive 10-core biopsy: incidence, biopsy findings, and DNA specimen identity analysis. Arch Pathol Lab Med. 2006;130(6):811–6.
9. Mazzucchelli R, Barbisan F, Tagliabracci A, Lopez-Beltran A, Cheng L, Scarpelli M, et al. Search for residual prostate cancer on pT0 radical prostatectomy after positive biopsy. Virchows Arch. 2007;450(4):371–8.
10. Park J, Jeong IG, Bang JK, Cho YM, Ro JY, Hong JH, et al. Preoperative clinical and pathological characteristics of pt0 prostate cancer in radical prostatectomy. Korean J Urol. 2010;51(6):386–90.
11. Civantos F, Marcial MA, Banks ER, Ho CK, Speights VO, Drew PA, et al. Pathology of androgen deprivation therapy in prostate carcinoma. A comparative study of 173 patients. Cancer. 1995;75(7):1634–41.
12. van der Kwast TH, Tetu B, Candas B, Gomez JL, Cusan L, Labrie F. Prolonged neoadjuvant combined androgen blockade leads to a further reduction of prostatic tumor volume: three versus six months of endocrine therapy. Urology. 1999;53(3):523–9.
13. Gleave ME, La Bianca SE, Goldenberg SL, Jones EC, Bruchovsky N, Sullivan LD. Long-term neoadjuvant hormone therapy prior to radical prostatectomy: evaluation of risk for biochemical recurrence at 5-year follow-up. Urology. 2000;56(2):289–94.
14. Bolla M, de Reijke TM, Van Tienhoven G, Van den Bergh AC, Oddens J, Poortmans PM, et al. Duration of androgen suppression in the treatment of prostate cancer. N Engl J Med. 2009;360(24):2516–27.
15. Bolla M, Gonzalez D, Warde P, Dubois JB, Mirimanoff RO, Storme G, et al. Improved survival in patients with locally advanced prostate cancer treated with radiotherapy and goserelin. N Engl J Med. 1997;337(5):295–300.
16. Kollermann J, Feek U, Muller H, Kaulfuss U, Oehler U, Helpap B, et al. Nondetected tumor (pT0) after prolonged, neoadjuvant treatment of localized prostatic carcinoma. Eur Urol. 2000;38(6):714–20.
17. Kollermann MW, Pantel K, Enzmann T, Feek U, Kollermann J, Kossiwakis M, et al. Supersensitive PSA-monitored neoadjuvant hormone treatment of clinically localized prostate cancer: effects on positive margins, tumor detection and epithelial cells in bone marrow. Eur Urol. 1998;34(4):318–24.
18. Descazeaud A, Zerbib M, Flam T, Vieillefond A, Debre B, Peyromaure M. Can pT0 stage of prostate cancer be predicted before radical prostatectomy? Eur Urol. 2006;50(6):1248–52. discussion 1253.
19. Herkommer K, Kuefer R, Gschwend JE, Hautmann RE, Volkmer BG. Pathological T0 prostate cancer without neoadjuvant therapy: clinical presentation and follow-up. Eur Urol. 2004;45(1):36–41.
20. Kollermann J, Caprano J, Budde A, Weidenfeld H, Weidenfeld M, Hopfenmuller W, et al. Follow-up of nondetectable prostate carcinoma (pT0) after prolonged PSA-monitored neoadjuvant hormonal therapy followed by radical prostatectomy. Urology. 2003;62(3):476–80.

18

Genetic polymorphisms in key hypoxia-regulated downstream molecules and phenotypic correlation in prostate cancer

Avelino Fraga[1,2,3*], Ricardo Ribeiro[2,4,5], André Coelho[6], José Ramon Vizcaíno[6], Helena Coutinho[7], José Manuel Lopes[7,8], Paulo Príncipe[1,2], Carlos Lobato[9], Carlos Lopes[3] and Rui Medeiros[3,4]

Abstract

Background: In this study we sought if, in their quest to handle hypoxia, prostate tumors express target hypoxia-associated molecules and their correlation with putative functional genetic polymorphisms.

Methods: Representative areas of prostate carcinoma ($n = 51$) and of nodular prostate hyperplasia ($n = 20$) were analysed for hypoxia-inducible factor 1 alpha (HIF-1α), carbonic anhydrase IX (CAIX), lysyl oxidase (LOX) and vascular endothelial growth factor (VEGFR2) immunohistochemistry expression using a tissue microarray. DNA was isolated from peripheral blood and used to genotype functional polymorphisms at the corresponding genes (*HIF1A* +1772 C > T, rs11549465; *CA9* + 201 A > G; rs2071676; *LOX* +473 G > A, rs1800449; *KDR* – 604 T > C, rs2071559).

Results: Immunohistochemistry analyses disclosed predominance of positive CAIX and VEGFR2 expression in epithelial cells of prostate carcinomas compared to nodular prostate hyperplasia ($P = 0.043$ and $P = 0.035$, respectively). In addition, the VEGFR2 expression score in prostate epithelial cells was higher in organ-confined and extra prostatic carcinoma compared to nodular prostate hyperplasia ($P = 0.031$ and $P = 0.004$, respectively). Notably, for LOX protein the immunoreactivity score was significantly higher in organ-confined carcinomas compared to nodular prostate hyperplasia ($P = 0.015$). The genotype-phenotype analyses showed higher LOX staining intensity for carriers of the homozygous *LOX* +473 G-allele ($P = 0.011$). Still, carriers of the *KDR*–604 T-allele were more prone to have higher VEGFR2 expression in prostate epithelial cells ($P < 0.006$).

Conclusions: Protein expression of hypoxia markers (VEGFR2, CAIX and LOX) on prostate epithelial cells was different between malignant and benign prostate disease. Two genetic polymorphisms (*LOX* +473 G > A and *KDR*–604 T > C) were correlated with protein level, accounting for a potential gene-environment effect in the activation of hypoxia-driven pathways in prostate carcinoma. Further research in larger series is warranted to validate present findings.

Keywords: Genetic polymorphism, Hypoxia, Hypoxia-inducible factor 1, Prostate cancer

* Correspondence: avfraga@gmail.com
[1]Department of Urology, Porto Hospital Centre – St. António Hospital, Largo Prof. Abel Salazar, 4000-001 Porto, Portugal
[2]Center for Urological Research, Department of Urology, Porto Hospital Centre – St. António Hospital, Porto, Portugal
Full list of author information is available at the end of the article

Background

Prostate carcinoma is the most common cancer and the second cause of death due to malignancy in men [1]. It is clinically heterogeneous in aggressiveness, not with standing comparable clinicopathological features. Currently, only few biomarkers assist prostate carcinoma risk and aggressiveness prediction [2].

During tumor growth, malignant cells become progressively distant from the vasculature, oxygen supply and nutrients, urging tumor cells to signal to the microenvironment their needs. The hypoxia inducible factor 1 alpha (HIF-1α) is a key factor by which tumors regulate the response to hypoxia, triggering cascades with effects in angiogenesis, energy metabolism, vasomotor function and on apoptosis and proliferation activity [3–5]. In hypoxia, the HIF-1α/HIF-1β complex binds hypoxia response elements in promoters of many downstream target genes, notably vascular endothelial growth factor (VEGF), carbonic anhydrase IX (CAIX), and lysyl oxidase (LOX) promoters. They have been demonstrated to be up-regulated by hypoxia, ensuing aggressive and treatment-resistant tumor phenotypes [3, 5–9]. A large randomized study on radiotherapy and surgical cohorts described that markers of tumor hypoxia and angiogenesis were relevant for localized prostate carcinoma and outcome of radical treatment [10]. However, further studies at the genetic and protein levels are required to confirm molecules in hypoxia pathway as useful markers in prostate carcinoma.

Genetic variants may predispose to prostate carcinoma and influence the clinical outcome [2, 11, 12]. Single nucleotide polymorphisms (SNPs) in genes coding for molecules involved in the response to hypoxia, particularly a functional polymorphism in HIF1A gene at locus +1772 C > T [13–20], has been studied in association with prostate carcinoma with controversial results. Current knowledge suggests that we should consider a panel of genes in hypoxia pathway, in order to provide more accurate prediction of the response to tumor hypoxia [21, 22]. Therefore, despite functional SNPs in genes of pathways downstream of HIF-1α, such as KDR,

LOX and CAIX, have not been studied so far in prostate carcinoma patients, they merit further research as they represent key molecules in hypoxia-generated stimulus in cancer.

Based on the role of hypoxia-associated molecules in cancer cell biological behaviour and clinical outcome, we assumed there might be an association, at the genetic and protein level, between HIF1A, LOX, CA9 and KDR genetic variants, the protein expression and prostate carcinoma. Hence, if these polymorphisms modulate protein expression in response to tumor hypoxia, then the knowledge of the genotype could aid identify patients at higher risk for prostate carcinoma and eventually more aggressive disease, thereby making it possible to undertake chemoprevention strategies adjusted to the individual characteristics of the patient.

Methods

Patients

Sixty-seven patients with prostate pathology ($n = 49$ with carcinoma, and $n = 18$ with nodular hyperplasia) and elective for prostatic surgery [radical prostatectomy and simple (open) prostatectomy, respectively] at the Porto Hospital Centre - Sto. António Hospital and Porto Military Hospital were included in this study. Inclusion criteria were: 45–75 years of age and for prostate carcinoma absence of previous treatments. Clinicopathological data was collected from clinical files and pathological staging was determined according to European Association of Urology guidelines [23] as organ-confined (T1-T2) (OCPCa) or extra prostatic (T3-T4) (EPCa) disease. Descriptive data is depicted on Table 1. This study was conducted with informed written consent by participants and after approval by the Porto Hospital Centre Ethical Committee.

DNA extraction and genotyping

At the time of surgery, a venous blood sample was obtained by forearm venepuncture and the white cell fraction used to extract DNA (QIAmp DNA Blood Mini

Table 1 Descriptive clinicopathological data of participating patients

	BPH	OCPCa	EPCa
Age at diagnosis, yrs	67.8 ± 8.4	61.3 ± 6.4	63.3 ± 6.3
PSA at diagnosis, ng/mL	5.5 ± 5.1	6.6 ± 2.4	11.9 ± 5.6
Weight of the prostate, g	94.8 ± 32.1	45.9 ± 14.3	56.6 ± 22.7
Gleason Score			
<7	–	14 (43.8)	0 (0.0)
≥7	–	18 (56.3)	19 (100)
Percentage of tumor [a], %	–	15.0 (6.3–20.0)	57.0 (28.8–78.8)

Continuous variables were parametric (Shapiro-Wilk) (data presented as mean ± standard deviation) except for percentage of tumor [data shown as median (interquartile range)]. Categorical variable is depicted as number of observations and respective frequencies. BPH nodular prostate hyperplasia, EPCa extra prostatic cancer, OCPCa organ-confined prostate carcinoma, PSA prostate specific antigen
[a] on prostatectomy specimens

Kit, Qiagen). Candidate SNPs were selected from the best evidence from published studies that provide information on phenotypic risks. Candidate genes involved in key hypoxia pathways were selected. Four putative functional SNPs in 4 different genes were selected (*HIF1A* +1772 C > T, rs11549465; *CA9* + 201 A > G, rs2071676; *LOX* +473 G > A, rs1800449; *KDR*–604 T > C, rs2071559). These SNPs were genotyped by Real-Time PCR (TaqMan allelic discrimination) using pre-designed validated Taqman assays (Applied Biosystems). Quality control included non-template controls in all runs and blind replicate genotypes assessment in 5% of the samples.

Immunohistochemistry and scoring

Formalin–fixed paraffin embedded tissues were morphologically assessed on haematoxylin-eosin stained slides, before tissue microarray construction as previously described [24]. Representative areas of carcinoma and of nodular hyperplasia were selected and included into tissue arrays: prostate carcinoma (n = 51) and nodular hyperplasia (n = 20), to analyse HIF-1α, LOX, CAIX and VEGFR2 immunohistochemistry expression. Slides were stained with mouse monoclonal antibody to HIF-1α (dilution 1:100, NB100-105, Novus Biologicals), and rabbit polyclonal antibodies to LOX, (dilution 1:100, ab 31238, Abcam), VEGFR2 (dilution 1:200, ab 2349, Abcam) and CAIX, (dilution 1:1000, NB100-417, Novus Biologicals) using the VENTANA BenchMark XT series slide-staining instrument (with the VENTANA ultraView DAB IHC detection kit) (VENTANA, Tucson, AZ, United States). Negative controls omitting the primary antibody confirmed specificity. Immunohistochemistry evaluation was independently reviewed by two pathologists (JRV and AC) to assess VEGFR2 expression in carcinoma vasculature and prostate epithelial cells (carcinoma and nodular hyperplasia), and HIF-1α, LOX and CAIX in prostate epithelial cells (carcinoma and nodular hyperplasia). Discordant cases were discussed in order to attain a final consensus. For VEGFR2 different scoring approaches were evaluated for vessels and epithelial cells as described by Holzer et al. [25], whereas analysis of CAIX, HIF-1α and LOX expression in prostatic epithelial cells (both in carcinoma and nodular hyperplasia) were performed according to Smyth et al. [26], Vergis et al. [10] and Albinger-Hegyi [27], respectively. Briefly, for VEGFR the level of intensity of tumor cell staining (0, no staining; 1+, weak staining; 2+, moderate staining; 3+, intense staining) was made in the cytoplasmic and nuclear compartments simultaneously. The value of each staining level (0, 1, 2 or 3) was multiplied by the respective percentage of tumor cells at that intensity level. A total VEGFR2 H-score represents the sum of the three scores. Regarding LOX, only cytoplasmic immunoreactivity of epithelial cells was considered positive expression,

whereas staining in the stromal component was not used. The LOX immunoreactivity score (IRS), was calculated multiplicating the percentage of positive cells (scored 0 if 0% cells; 1 if 1–20% cells; 2 if 21–40% cells; 3 if 41–60% cells; 4 if 61–80%; 5 if 81–100% cells) with staining intensity (with 0 if negative; 1 if weak; 2 if moderate; 3 if strong staining intensity). A representative image of the expression of each aforementioned protein is shown in Fig. 1.

Statistical analysis

We used means as descriptive statistics for continuous variables and the Shapiro-Wilk test to assess their departure from normality. As appropriate, the Mann–Whitney test and Student t-test were used to compare means between prostatic disease groups. The Kruskal Wallis followed by Mann–Whitney two samples tests were used for analyses of non-parametric variables. The Pearson chi-square was used to test for association between categorical variables based on the distribution among diseases, protein expression or genotype groups. Odds ratios (ORs) and 95% confidence intervals (95%CIs) were calculated to evaluate the associations between CAIX expression with risk for developing organ-confined and extra prostatic carcinoma. When appropriate, non-parametric Spearman's correlation was computed to assess the statistical dependence between variables. Analyses were performed using SPSS 17.0. The datasets analysed during the current study are available from the corresponding author on reasonable request.

Results

Association of hypoxia proteins with prostate cancer and extra-prostatic disease

To assess the prevalence of the key hypoxia-associated proteins in prostate carcinomas and nodular prostate hyperplasia, a tissue microarray was constructed for immunohistochemistry analyses. Immunohistochemistry for cytoplasmic HIF-1α demonstrated a non-significant trend (P = 0.111) for increased proportion of localized prostate carcinoma patients with positive malignant prostatic epithelial cells (Fig. 2). CAIX immunoreactivity was observed in the cytoplasm of epithelial cells and significant differences were found among disease groups: CAIX expression was predominantly positive in epithelial cells of carcinomas (P = 0.043) (Fig. 2).

Lysyl oxidase protein expression was found in prostate epithelial cells of a high percentage of cases, notably in carcinomas of patients with organ-confined malignancy (92.0%), but no significant differences were found among pathologic groups (P = 0.266) (Fig. 2). Nevertheless, the immunoreactivity score (IRS), which combines intensity with amount of cells positive for LOX in prostate epithelial cells, was significantly higher in organ-confined carcinomas compared to nodular prostate hyperplasia (P = 0.015)

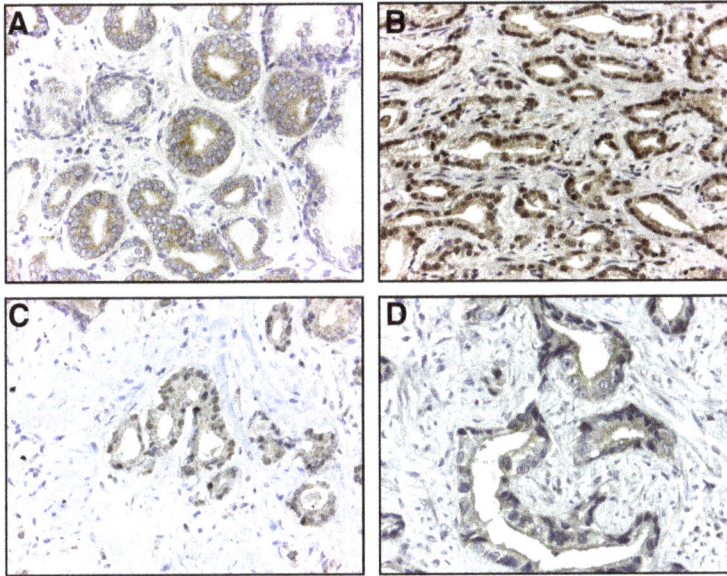

Fig. 1 Representative microscopy images of staining for hypoxia markers in prostate tissues (MO, 400×). A) HIF-1α - notice the granular cytoplasmic immunoreactivity of the malignant epithelial cells. In this case, more than 50% of the glands stained. B) LOX - strong and diffuse nuclear immunoreactivity of the epithelial cells. C) CAIX - note a focal apical cytoplasmic immunoreactivity in epithelial cells. D) VEGFR2 - moderate nuclear and weak cytoplasmic expression of the epithelial cells

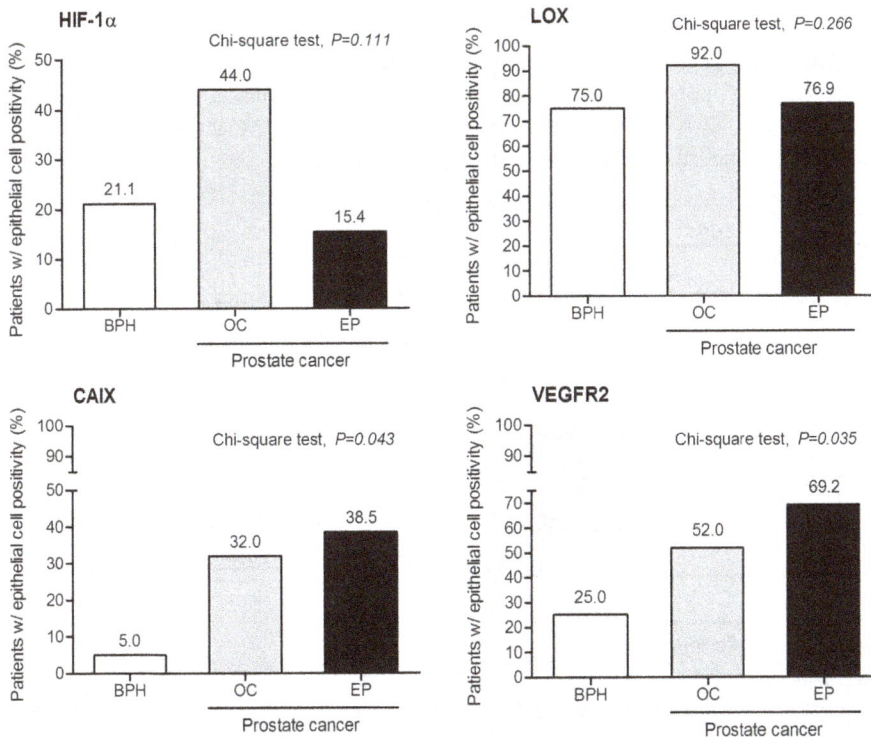

Fig. 2 Frequency of patients with positive staining in benign (BPH) and malignant (organ-confined and extra prostatic disease) epithelial cells. CAIX, carbonic anhydrase IX; HIF-1α, hypoxia inducible factor - 1 alpha; LOX, lysyl oxidase; VEGFR2, vascular endothelial growth factor receptor 2. BPH, nodular prostate hyperplasia; EP, extra prostatic disease; OC, organ-confined disease

(Fig. 3). Noteworthy, patients with positive HIF-1α expression were more prone to have higher immunoreactivity score for LOX (*P* = 0.053) (Fig. 4). In addition, a trend exists for HIF-1α immunostaining grade to be correlated with LOX IRS expression (Spearman correlation coefficient, *r²* = 0.255, *P* = 0.055).

Cytoplasmic and nuclear VEGFR2 immunoreactivity was observed in vascular endothelial cells of approximately 20% of all samples. The difference between vascular positivity for VEGFR2 in nodular prostate hyperplasia and both organ-confined and extra prostatic carcinomas was not statistically significant (*P* = 0.971). As for VEGFR2 staining in epithelial prostate cells, almost 70% of patients with extra prostatic carcinomas and approximately half of organ-confined carcinomas showed tumor cell immunoreactivity for VEGFR2, whereas only 25% of nodular prostate hyperplasia were positive (*P* = 0.035) (Fig. 2). The VEGFR2 expression scores in the prostate epithelial cells in nodular prostate hyperplasia (5.6 ± 3.9) compare to either organ-confined (41.6 ± 16.5) or extra prostatic carcinomas (68.7 ± 28.4) were statistically different (*P* = 0.031 and *P* = 0.004, respectively) (Fig. 5). The VEGFR2 epithelial cell H-score for samples that were positive for VEGFR2 in the vasculature showed a trend for being higher than those with negative immunoreactivity status (*P* = 0.062), indicating a positive association between the expression of VEGFR2 in the prostatic epithelial cells and the vasculature.

Genotype-phenotype correlation

The genotypic distribution in polymorphisms *HIF1A* +1772 C > T, *LOX* +473 G > A, *CA9* + 201 A > G and *KDR* −604 T > C is shown in Additional file 1: Table S1. There

was no over-represented genotype in disease groups using either the additive or recessive models.

There was lack of association between both *HIF1A* +1772 C > T and *CA9* + 201 A > G genotypes and positivity or intensity for HIF-1α and CAIX protein expression (Table 2). Conversely, the LOX immunoreactivity intensity was significantly higher in individuals carrying the *LOX* +473 homozygous G allele (GG, 2.0 ± 0.2) compare to A carriers (1.1 ± 0.2) (*P* = 0.011) (Fig. 6), despite no significance was achieved for IRS (but with similar trend) according to *LOX* genotypes in recessive model. Patients

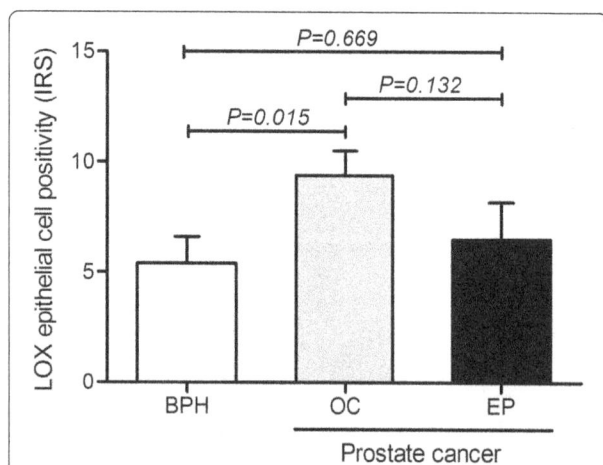

Fig. 4 LOX immunoreactivity score by HIF-1α positivity in epithelial cells. Patients with positive HIF-1α expression are prone to higher LOX IRS. HIF-1α, hypoxia inducible factor – 1 alpha; LOX, lysyl oxidase. IRS, immunoreactivity score. Mann–Whitney non-parametric test was used to calculate differences between positive and negative HIF-1α expression

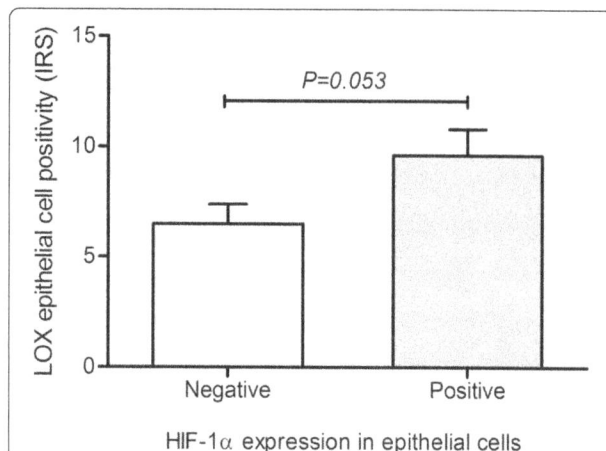

Fig. 3 Comparison of LOX immunoreactivity score in prostate epithelial cells of benign and malignant patients. BPH, nodular prostate hyperplasia; EP, extra prostatic disease; OC, organ-confined disease. LOX, lysyl oxidase; IRS, immunoreactivity score. Kruskall-Wallis followed by Mann–Whitney non-parametric tests were used to calculate differences between prostatic pathologies

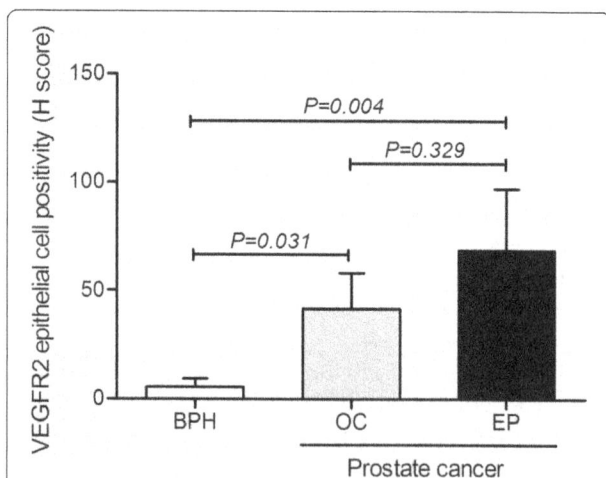

Fig. 5 Expression of VEGFR2 (H score) in prostate epithelial cells according to prostatic diseases. BPH, nodular prostate hyperplasia; EP, extra prostatic disease; OC, organ-confined disease. VEGFR2, vascular endothelial growth factor receptor 2. Kruskall-Wallis followed by Mann–Whitney non-parametric tests were used to calculate differences between prostatic pathologies

Table 2 Association of the genetic polymorphisms in *HIF1A* +1772 C > T and *CA9*+ 201 A > G with HIF-1α and CAIX immunoreactivity in prostatic epithelial cells

HIF-1α expression	Recessive model (*HIF1A* and *CA9*)		
	CC	TT/CT	P [a]
Negative	28 (0.76)	9 (0.24)	
Positive	10 (0.77)	3 (0.23)	0.928
<50%	32 (0.74)	11 (0.26)	
≥50%	6 (0.86)	1 (0.14)	0.516
CAIX expression	GG	GA/AA	
Negative	9 (0.75)	20 (0.69)	
Positive	3 (0.25)	9 (0.31)	0.699

[a] Fisher exact test

with at least one *KDR*–604 T-allele were more prone to have VEGFR2 expression in prostate epithelial cells but not in vessels (Table 3). Since the presence of VEGFR2 immunoreactivity in epithelial cells, but not in vessels, was associated with the *KDR* genetic polymorphism, we looked for its association with VEGFR2 H-score only in prostate epithelial cells. The H-score was significantly higher in cases carrying the T allele (CT, 38.9 ± 13.0 and TT, 74.7 ± 33.0) compare to homozygous C (1.64 ± 1.0) (Fig. 7). Both additive and recessive models show that the allele T was related with increased VEGFR2 epithelial cell positivity ($P = 0.017$ and $P = 0.006$, respectively).

Only data from prostate carcinomas was used to evaluate if hypoxia proteins associated with Gleason score or prostate specific antigen (PSA) > 10 ng/mL (Table 4). Trends were observed for higher VEGFR2 H-score expression in more undifferentiated carcinomas (Gleason ≥7) ($P = 0.099$) and in patients with PSA ≥ 10 ng/mL ($P = 0.085$), and for positive CAIX expression in prostate carcinomas from patients with PSA above 10 ng/mL ($P = 0.078$).

Discussion

Tumor-associated hypoxia was found in over 70% of solid malignancies, including prostate carcinoma [3]. It promotes tumor progression and resistance to therapies through an effect in reducing apoptosis, and increasing tumor cell proliferation and neoangiogenesis [5]. However, the hypoxia-driven HIF-1α upregulation also activates downstream pathways involved in metabolism (e.g. CAIX), angiogenesis (e.g. VEGF/VEGFR2 pathway) and extracellular matrix activity (e.g. LOX), which can modulate cancer behavior [28].

Experimental studies with prostate cancer cells demonstrated that HIF-1α overexpression was associated with higher proliferation and metastatic potential [29]. Likewise, a greater expression of HIF-1α has been found in human prostate carcinomas compared to nodular prostate hyperplasia [30, 31]. For prostate carcinoma and other oncologic models, besides the observed higher amount of HIF-1α in tumors, increased HIF-1α expression was also associated with prognosis [10, 32–35]. In the current study, we found a trend for higher HIF-1α protein expression in prostate carcinomas compared to nodular prostate hyperplasia, which may be explained by the limited samples analysed. The use of cytoplasmic rather than nuclear staining, is unlikely to have influenced our results, since this method has been published before, reporting positive associations of HIF-1α with prostate carcinoma and prognosis [10, 30].

Albeit mainly distributed in vascular endothelial cells, also epithelial cells express VEGFR2 that signals through signal transducer and activator of transcription 3 (STAT3), mitogen-activated protein kinase (MAPK) or phosphoinositide-3-kinase (PI3K) intracellular signalling cascades [36–38]. Unambiguously, the VEGFR2 was shown to regulate protein kinase B (Akt)/mammalian target of rapamycin (mTOR)/ribosomal protein S6 kinase beta-1 (P70S6K) signalling pathway in PC-3 prostate cancer cell line [39]. In the present study, VEGFR2 was more frequently expressed in epithelial tumor cells of organ confined or extra prostatic carcinomas than in nodular prostate hyperplasia, and to lower extent in endothelial cells. Hence, at least in prostate tissue,

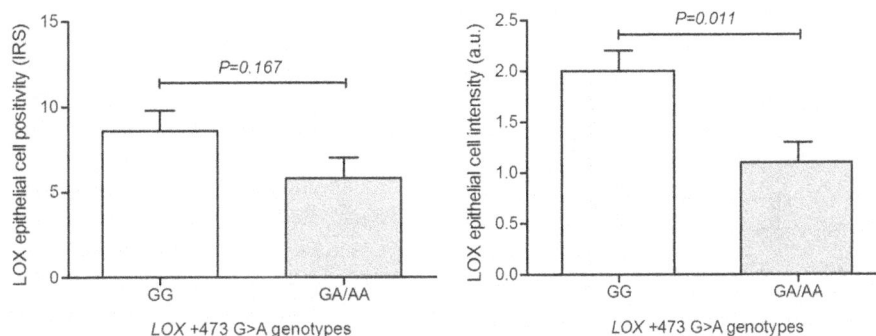

Fig. 6 LOX protein expression (both for immunoreactivity score and staining intensity) according to *LOX* +473 G > A polymorphism. IRS, immunoreactivity score; *LOX*, lysy oxidase; a.u., arbitrary units

Table 3 Association of the *KDR-604 T > C* genetic polymorphism with VEGFR2 immunoreactivity in vessels and in prostatic epithelial cells

	Additive model				Recessive model		
	CC	CT	TT	P [a]	CC	TT/CT	P [a]
Vessels VEGFR+							
Negative	11 (0.26)	22 (0.53)	9 (0.21)		11 (0.26)	31 (0.78)	
Positive	3 (0.25)	5 (0.42)	4 (0.33)	0.681	3 (0.25)	9 (0.22)	0.626
Epithelial cells VEGFR+							
Negative	11 (0.39)	13 (0.47)	4 (0.14)		11 (0.39)	17 (0.42)	
Positive	3 (0.11)	14 (0.54)	9 (0.35)	0.039	3 (0.11)	23 (0.58)	0.030

[a] Fisher exact test

VEGFR2 expression is not specific of endothelial cells; it is mainly expressed in malignant epithelium where VEGF can act as a promoter of tumor cell proliferation. The expression of VEGFR2 in epithelial prostate carcinoma cells has been rarely reported, and its role in the occurrence and development of prostate cancer remains unclear. Previous immunohistochemistry studies reported VEGFR2 expression in high-grade prostate intra-epithelial neoplasia and carcinomas of the prostate [40–42], whereas gene expression findings evidenced expression of *KDR* mRNA in prostate cancer cell lines and a functional impact of using a *KDR* antisense oligonucleotide in suppressing cell proliferation and promoting apoptosis [43, 44].

The body of past evidences, taken together with present findings indicates that the distribution of VEGFR2 expression towards epithelial prostate carcinoma cells supports a function for VEGF that is not limited to angiogenesis. Thus, abrogation of VEGFR2 signalling in malignant epithelial cells may prove an effective therapeutic modality for the treatment of prostate cancer. At present, two anti-angiogenic drugs are being tested in the phase III setting for men with prostate cancer, carbozantinib (a dual VEGFR2/MET inhibitor) and tasquinimod (down-regulator of HIF-1α), which previously showed beneficial and encouraging results on phase II trials [45].

Cancer-associated hypoxia switches cell metabolism towards increased production of acidic metabolites. However, tumor cells have to adapt to hypoxia and acidosis in order to survive. CAIX is a membrane-bound protein crucial to a wide variety of processes, including pH regulation in the highly metabolically active malignant cells. Expression of CAIX is associated with tumor cell hypoxia in a variety of human tumors, including urologic cancers [46–49]. Carbonic anhydrase IX gene (*CA9*) is a target of HIF-1α that is up-regulated in response to hypoxia [50]. The expression of CAIX in prostate carcinoma has been rarely reported. *CA9* mRNA expression increases reliably following hypoxia incubation of PC-3 cells [51], although no significant differences in *CA9* mRNA expression were found when comparing nodular prostate hyperplasia with prostate carcinomas [7]. However, other studies reported lack of CAIX expression in primary prostate carcinoma and hypothesized that alternative pathway for maintaining pH balance (e.g. monocarboxylate transporters 2 and 4) [26, 52, 53] may be more relevant than CAIX.

Our results disclosed increased frequency of cases with epithelial cell positivity for CAIX expressing in organ confined and extra prostatic carcinomas compared to BPH. Despite recent concern arisen for the specificity of the CAIX polyclonal antibody generated against a C-terminal peptide in detecting CAIX (except when used at high dilution, in prostate tissues) [54], in this study we used the antibody at a dilution of 1:1000 and found membrane-bound staining for CAIX. Therefore, our findings are likely to reflect reliable expression of CAIX in epithelial prostate cells. Our findings taken together with reports of CAIX expression in malignant prostate epithelial cells [7, 51, 55] sustains the need for reconsidering CAIX role in prostate carcinoma. CAIX may serve as one of the mechanisms by which prostate carcinoma cells regulate extracellular pH and induce cytoplasmic alkalization.

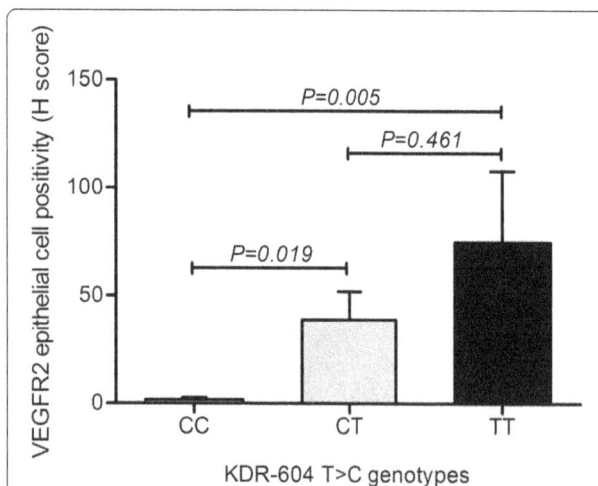

Fig. 7 VEGFR2 protein expression (H score) according to *KDR* −604 T > C polymorphism. *KDR*, gene coding for VEGFR2 protein; VEGFR2, vascular endothelial growth factor receptor 2

Table 4 Expression of proteins from hypoxia pathways in prostate cancer patients, by Gleason grade and PSA value

	Gleason grade (n = 38)			PSA at diagnosis (n = 36)		
	<7	≥7	P	<10	≥10	P
VEGFR2 H-score[a]	30.9 ± 24.7	60.1 ± 17.9	0.099	30.2 ± 1.2	80.0 ± 33.5	0.085
LOX immunoreactivity score[a]	10.2 ± 1.6	7.6 ± 1.1	0.184	9.2 ± 1.1	6.6 ± 1.8	0.242
HIF-1α expression[b]						
Negative	6 (0.50)	19 (0.73)		17 (0.65)	8 (0.80)	0.335[c]
Positive	6 (0.50)	7 (0.27)	0.163	9 (0.35)	2 (0.20)	
CAIX expression[b]						
Negative	10 (0.83)	15 (0.58)		19 (0.73)	5 (0.50)	
Positive	2 (0.17)	11 (0.42)	0.117[c]	7 (0.27)	5 (0.50)	0.078

PSA prostate specific antigen, *VEGFR2* vascular endothelial growth factor receptor 2, *LOX* lysyl oxidase, *HIF1a* hypoxia inducible factor 1 alpha, *CAIX* carbonic anhydrase IX

[a] Kruskal Wallis and Mann–Whitney U tests for VEGFR2 H-score in epithelial cells; [b] Chi-square test. [c] Fisher exact test

The lysyl oxidase gene (*LOX*), one of the overexpressed genes among a tumor hypoxia signature [56, 57], was shown to be directly regulated by HIF-1α transcription factor and is essential for hypoxia-induced metastasis and cancer cell proliferation [58]. Hypoxia-driven cancer cell invasion is severely impaired when LOX expression or oxidase activity were inhibited [59]. In prostate tissue we found that the LOX immunoreactivity score correlated with HIF-1α expression, thus supporting the regulatory nature of HIF-1α in LOX expression. Furthermore, although we have not observed an overrepresentation of cases with positive LOX expression in carcinomas compared to nodular prostate hyperplasia, the LOX immunoreactivity score was significantly higher in organ confined prostate carcinomas compared to nodular prostate hyperplasia. Interestingly, previous reports showed significantly increased expression of *LOX* mRNA in prostate carcinomas compared to nodular prostate hyperplasia [7], whereas stronger LOX expression was also observed in other solid malignancies [27, 60, 61]. LOX is known to participate in critical biological functions that include cell migration, cell polarity, epithelial-to-mesenchymal transition (EMT) and angiogenesis [58] (reviewed in Fraga et al., 2015) [62], which fits with the increased LOX expression found in our carcinomas. Altogether, we suggest the possibility that a HIF-1α/LOX regulatory mechanism may act in synergy to foster tumor formation along with the adaptation of tumor cells to hypoxia.

The analysis of protein expression in distinct pathological groups (by stage, differentiation score and PSA serum levels at diagnosis), which are predictive of prostate cancer aggressiveness, showed at most only trends for increased expression of VEGFR2 in carcinomas with Gleason >7 or patients with PSA > 10 ng/mL, and of CAIX in patients with PSA > 10 ng/mL. These findings indicate relevant clues but require further studies.

The genotypic distributions for the putative functional target SNPs in *HIF1A*, *LOX*, *CA9* and *KDR* were similar between nodular prostate hyperplasia and prostate carcinomas. We might have hypothesized that carriers of variant alleles are prone to be more susceptible to have cancer, but the underpowered sample size limits conclusions regarding genetic association for these SNPs. Nevertheless, it is expected that only the combination of several SNPs within pathways or mechanisms may have significant impact in the association with complex diseases as prostate carcinoma. Further studies are warranted to evaluate the predictive/prognostic value of these genetic polymorphisms in prostate cancer.

In this study, evaluation of protein expression according to SNPs in the respective coding genes disclosed a genotype-phenotype effect for the *LOX* and *KDR* SNPs, but no functional validation at the protein level was observed for the studied *HIF1A* and *CA9* SNPs. In the *HIF1A* gene, a C-to-T substitution at locus +1772 (rs11549465) results in non-synonymous proline-by-serine aminoacid substitution at codon 582. Association studies of this SNP with prostate carcinoma risk and with microvessel density, yielded conflicting results [13, 16, 19, 20, 63–65]. This SNP localizes in the oxygen-dependent domain of the gene where the variant allele was shown to stabilize *HIF1A* mRNA and enhance *HIF1A* transcriptional activity [64]. In our study there were no differences in HIF-1α protein expression according to the *HIF1A* +1772 C > T genotypes as reported previously in localised prostatic carcinomas [16]. As we measured HIF-1α protein levels and it is known that *HIF1A* is subjected to post-transcriptional and post-translational regulation [66], this SNP may indeed influence mRNA transcription that is not reflected in protein expression. The low frequency of T homozygous genotype in our sample (only 2 cases carried TT genotype) may have influenced statistical power, since the HIF-1α protein and mRNA overexpression have been associated with the *HIF1A* +1772 TT [14, 67, 68].

A functional genetic variant on *KDR* gene that codifies for VEGFR2 is located in the promoter region (−604, rs2071559), where a T-to-C substitution occurs. Preceding in vitro luciferase assays showed that the C-allele was associated with lower transcription activity than T-allele, whereas serum VEGFR2 levels were significantly lower in CC versus TT carriers [69]. Interestingly, we found that CT and TT carriers had significantly increased VEGFR2 expression in prostate epithelial cells. We postulate that this SNP might prove useful for predictive and/or prognostic evaluations in prostate carcinoma. Studies in colorectal cancer reported association of this SNP in *KDR* with susceptibility and recurrence [70, 71], whereas, to the best of our knowledge, no studies using this SNP were conducted in prostate carcinoma patients. Likewise, it is expected that this SNP might increase susceptibility to prostate cancer by upregulating the number of available VEGFR2 proteins in malignant cells.

A SNP in exon 1 of *CA9* gene is located at locus +201 (rs2071676), where an A-to-G substitution leads to a change of valine-by-methionine in codon 33. Although we observed an overrepresentation of CAIX positive immunoreactivity in prostate carcinoma compared to BPH, the nonsynonymous SNP in *CA9* + 201 were unable to explain variations in the levels of CAIX protein expression in the prostatic tissue. Likewise, a recent report described lack of association between the *CA9* + 201 SNP with CAIX protein expression in renal cell carcinoma [72]. These findings may suggest that lack of influence of this SNP in protein expression, even though the potential molecular structure modifications of this nonsynonymous substitution (valine to methionine) in CAIX protein activity remains to be confirmed. In fact, genetic association studies that included the *CA9* + 201 A > G polymorphism showed neither risk for renal cell carcinoma [72] nor for oral squamous cell carcinoma [73]. Noteworthy, the G-allele was associated with lymph node metastasis in oral cancer and represented increased risk for cancer when combined into a haplotype with other two SNPs in this gene [73]. Furthermore, another SNP in *CA9* (rs12553173) was independently associated with improved overall survival and greater likelihood of response to therapy in renal cell carcinoma [72], thus warranting further functional analysis. In our study, although we are aware that haplotype analyses can be expedite over analysis of individual SNPs for detecting an association between alleles and a disease phenotype, the small size sample prevented the consideration of such evaluation.

The *LOX* gene is translated and secreted as a pro-enzyme (Pro-LOX), and then processed to a functional enzyme (LOX) and a propeptide (LOX-PP) [74, 75]. While LOX-PP was described as a Ras tumor suppressor, reversing mesenchymal tumor cells to a more epithelial phenotype [76–78], the LOX enzyme was found to facilitate a more migratory and invasive phenotype during breast cancer progression [58, 79]. We studied a SNP in *LOX* gene that has been identified at locus +473 (rs1800449), presenting a G-to-A substitution that cause an aminoacid substitution arginine-by-glutamine in codon 158. This SNP located in a highly conserved region within LOX-PP has been associated with attenuated ability of LOX-PP to oppose the effects of LOX, resulting in tumor cell invasive phenotype. Functional studies revealed that the A-allele decreases the protective capacity of LOX-PP, while increasing the Pro-LOX-associated invasive ability of tumor cells [78]. When evaluating LOX immunoreactivity and expression intensity by immunohistochemistry in prostate tissues, we found it significantly lower in carriers of the *LOX* +473 A-allele. Indeed, *LOX* A-carriers disclosed decreased LOX protein expression in the nucleus of prostate epithelial cells.

The complex nature of LOX protein domain structure and biological functions makes noticeable that it can act as both a tumor suppressor and a metastasis promoter gene in cancer [80]. Under hypoxic conditions, the increased expression of LOX enzyme correlates with tumor invasiveness [81, 82]. In the present study, we found that lysyl oxidase was present primarily intracellular in the nucleus of epithelial cells, which fits with other reports asserting that this enzyme may have important functions in secretory cells, either as catalyser of histones in the nucleus or in association with cytoskeletal proteins at the cytoplasm [83, 84]. Thus, our findings seem to suggest a wider variety of functions for LOX in prostate epithelial cells, beyond those related to cross-link formation in collagen and elastin, which merit further research. We hypothesize that the trafficking of LOX towards inside the cell or a specific cell compartment may be subordinated to the structural molecular characteristics and folding of the protein, which could be determined by *LOX* +473 G > A polymorphism. Further studies should clarify the meaning of increased nuclear LOX intensity for PCa development.

Our endeavour to study the genotype-phenotype correlation in key hypoxia markers and its association with prostate cancer yielded novel and interesting findings, nevertheless our results should be interpreted in the context of several potential limitations. Sample size was a major issue as conclusions were impracticable for genetic association analysis and limited for genotype-phenotype inferences. Nevertheless, considering the hypothesis-generating nature of this study, we report findings that provide important clues to further work in larger samples. The use of tissue microarrays for immunohistochemical evaluation has been subject of concern mainly due to limited sample of diagnostic tissue, although in our series the representative tumor sections were adequately selected by an experienced pathologist. The comparison of hypoxia markers between patients with benign and malignant prostate disease might attenuate differences since it is known that hypoxia is altered in cancer but also in benign hyperproliferative diseases. The group of benign prostate disease seemed adequate for several order of reasons: 1) the diagnosis was contemporary with that of cancers; 2) their advanced age at diagnosis allowed matching with elderly prostate cancer patients; 3) all patients underwent digital rectal examination, PSA testing and prostate needle biopsy, making the possibility of crossover remote, and 4) most men develop nodular prostate hyperplasia or chronic prostatitis by the 7th–8th decades of life, making it normal in men of that age to carry benign prostatic disease.

Conclusions

Prostate carcinoma triggers an increase in hypoxia, which regulates *HIF1A* that in turn impacts downstream the expression of LOX, CAIX and VEGFR2 in tumor cells. In this study we observed that the inherited genetic variants in *LOX* and *KDR* seem to modulate the expression of LOX and VEGFR2 in carcinoma cells, supporting a gene-tumor microenvironment interaction in the activation of hypoxia-driven pathways in prostate carcinoma. Results presented here warrant further research in larger samples in order to evaluate the predictive and prognostic value of *KDR* and *LOX* SNPs in prostate carcinoma.

Additional file

Additional file 1: Table S1. Genotypic distribution of functional SNPs in genes of hypoxia pathways by disease status using additive and recessive models analyses. The genotypic distribution of studied SNPs in genes of hypoxia pathways, using additive and recessive models, are shown according to disease status.

Abbreviations

95%CI: 95% confidence interval; Akt: Protein kinase B; BPH: Nodular prostate hyperplasia; CA9: Carbonic anhydrase IX gene; CAIX: Carbonic anhydrase IX; EMT: Epithelial-to-mesenchymal transition; EPCa: Extra prostatic (T3–T4) Prostate Cancer; HIF-1α: Hypoxia-inducible factor 1 alpha; HIF-1β: Hypoxia-inducible factor 1 beta; HIF1A: HIF-1α gene; IRS: Immunoreactivity score; KDR: VEGFR2 gene; LOX: Lysyl oxidase; LOX-PP: Lysyl oxidase propeptide; MAPK: Mitogen-activated protein kinase; mTOR: Mammalian target of rapamycin; OCPCa: Organ-confined (T1–T2) Prostate Cancer; OR: Odds ratio; P70S6K: Ribosomal protein S6 kinase beta-1; PCR: Polymerase chain reaction; PI3K: Phosphoinositide-3-kinase; PSA: Prostate specific antigen; SNP: Single nucleotide polymorphisms; STAT3: Signal transducer and activator of transcription 3; VEGF: Vascular endothelial growth factor; VEGFR2: Vascular endothelial growth factor receptor 2

Acknowledgements

Authors acknowledge the support of the Portuguese League Against Cancer – North Centre.

Funding

RR was supported by the Portuguese League Against Cancer – North Centre. We declare no role of the funding body in the design of the study and collection, analysis, and interpretation of data and in writing the manuscript.

Authors' contributions

AF: Conception and design, Acquisition of data, Drafting the manuscript; RR: Conception and design, Analysis and interpretation of data, Drafting the manuscript; AC: Acquisition of data, Drafting the manuscript; JRV: Acquisition of data, Revising the manuscript critically for important intellectual content; HC: Acquisition of data, Drafting the manuscript; JML: Analysis and interpretation of data, Revising the manuscript critically for important intellectual content; PP: Acquisition of data, Drafting the manuscript; CLobato: Acquisition of data, Revising the manuscript critically for important intellectual content; CLopes: Conception and design, Revising the manuscript critically for important intellectual content; RM: Analysis and interpretation of data, Revising the manuscript critically for important intellectual content. All authors provided final approval of the version to be published and agreed to be accountable for all aspects of the work.

Competing interests

The authors declare that they have no competing interests.

Author details

[1]Department of Urology, Porto Hospital Centre – St. António Hospital, Largo Prof. Abel Salazar, 4000-001 Porto, Portugal. [2]Center for Urological Research, Department of Urology, Porto Hospital Centre – St. António Hospital, Porto, Portugal. [3]ICBAS, Abel Salazar Biomedical Sciences Institute, University of Porto, Porto, Portugal. [4]Molecular Oncology Group - CI, Portuguese Institute of Oncology, Porto, Portugal. [5]Genetics Laboratory, Faculty of Medicine, University of Lisbon, Lisbon, Portugal. [6]Department of Pathology, Porto Hospital Centre – St. António Hospital, Porto, Portugal. [7]Department of Pathology and Oncology, Faculty of Medicine, University of Porto, Porto, Portugal. [8]Institute of Pathology and Molecular Immunology of University of Porto (IPATIMUP), Porto, Portugal. [9]Department of Urology, Porto Military Hospital, Porto, Portugal.

References

1. Jemal A, Bray F, Center MM, Ferlay J, Ward E, Forman D. Global cancer statistics. CA Cancer J Clin. 2011;61(2):69–90.
2. Wiklund F. Prostate cancer genomics: can we distinguish between indolent and fatal disease using genetic markers? Genome Med. 2010;2(7):45.
3. Fraga A, Ribeiro R, Medeiros R. Tumor hypoxia: the role of HIF. Actas Urol Esp. 2009;33(9):941–51.
4. Pouysségur J, Dayan F, Mazure NM. Hypoxia signalling in cancer and approaches to enforce tumour regression. Nature. 2006;441(7092):437–43.
5. Harris AL. Hypoxia–a key regulatory factor in tumour growth. Nat Rev Cancer. 2002;2(1):38–47.
6. Brahimi-Horn MC, Pouysségur J. The hypoxia-inducible factor and tumor progression along the angiogenic pathway. Int Rev Cytol. 2005;242:157–213.
7. Stewart GD, Gray K, Pennington CJ, Edwards DR, Riddick AC, Ross JA, Habib FK. Analysis of hypoxia-associated gene expression in prostate cancer: lysyl oxidase and glucose transporter-1 expression correlate with Gleason score. Oncol Rep. 2008;20(6):1561–7.

8. Gupta S, Srivastava M, Ahmad N, Bostwick DG, Mukhtar H. Over-expression of cyclooxygenase-2 in human prostate adenocarcinoma. Prostate. 2000; 42(1):73–8.

9. Baltaci S, Orhan D, Gogus C, Turkolmez K, Tulunay O, Gogus O. Inducible nitric oxide synthase expression in benign prostatic hyperplasia, low- and high-grade prostatic intraepithelial neoplasia and prostatic carcinoma. BJU Int. 2001;88(1):100–3.

10. Vergis R, Corbishley CM, Norman AR, Bartlett J, Jhavar S, Borre M, Heeboll S, Horwich A, Huddart R, Khoo V, et al. Intrinsic markers of tumour hypoxia and angiogenesis in localised prostate cancer and outcome of radical treatment: a retrospective analysis of two randomised radiotherapy trials and one surgical cohort study. Lancet Oncol. 2008;9(4):342–51.

11. Teixeira AL, Ribeiro R, Morais A, Lobo F, Fraga A, Pina F, Calais-da-Silva FM, Calais-da-Silva FE, Medeiros R. Combined analysis of EGF + 61G > A and TGFB1 + 869T > C functional polymorphisms in the time to androgen independence and prostate cancer susceptibility. Pharmacogenomics J. 2009;9(5):341–6.

12. Ribeiro RJ, Monteiro CP, Azevedo AS, Cunha VF, Ramanakumar AV, Fraga AM, Pina FM, Lopes CM, Medeiros RM, Franco EL. Performance of an adipokine pathway-based multilocus genetic risk score for prostate cancer risk prediction. PLoS ONE. 2012;7(6), e39236.

13. Fraga A, Ribeiro R, Principe P, Lobato C, Pina F, Mauricio J, Monteiro C, Sousa H, CalaisdaSilva F, Lopes C, et al. The HIF1A functional genetic polymorphism at locus +1772 associates with progression to metastatic prostate cancer and refractoriness to hormonal castration. Eur J Cancer. 2014;50(2):359–65.

14. Vainrib M, Golan M, Amir S, Dang DT, Dang LH, Bar-Shira A, Orr-Urtreger A, Matzkin H, Mabjeesh NJ. HIF1A C1772T polymorphism leads to HIF-1alpha mRNA overexpression in prostate cancer patients. Cancer Biol Ther. 2012; 13(9):720–6.

15. Ye Y, Wang M, Hu S, Shi Y, Zhang X, Zhou Y, Zhao C, Wang G, Wen J, Zong H. Hypoxia-inducible factor-1alpha C1772T polymorphism and cancer risk: a meta-analysis including 18,334 subjects. Cancer Investig. 2014;32(4):126–35.

16. Foley R, Marignol L, Thomas AZ, Cullen IM, Perry AS, Tewari P, O'Grady A, Kay E, Dunne B, Loftus B, et al. The HIF-1alpha C1772T polymorphism may be associated with susceptibility to clinically localised prostate cancer but not with elevated expression of hypoxic biomarkers. Cancer Biol Ther. 2009;8(2):118–24.

17. Chau CH, Permenter MG, Steinberg SM, Retter AS, Dahut WL, Price DK, Figg WD. Polymorphism in the hypoxia-inducible factor 1alpha gene may confer susceptibility to androgen-independent prostate cancer. Cancer Biol Ther. 2005;4(11):1222–5.

18. Fu XS, Choi E, Bubley GJ, Balk SP. Identification of hypoxia-inducible factor-1alpha (HIF-1alpha) polymorphism as a mutation in prostate cancer that prevents normoxia-induced degradation. Prostate. 2005; 63(3):215–21.

19. Li P, Cao Q, Shao PF, Cai HZ, Zhou H, Chen JW, Qin C, Zhang ZD, Ju XB, Yin CJ. Genetic polymorphisms in HIF1A are associated with prostate cancer risk in a Chinese population. Asian J Androl. 2012;14(6):864–9.

20. Li H, Bubley GJ, Balk SP, Gaziano JM, Pollak M, Stampfer MJ, Ma J. Hypoxia-inducible factor-1alpha (HIF-1alpha) gene polymorphisms, circulating insulin-like growth factor binding protein (IGFBP)-3 levels and prostate cancer. Prostate. 2007;67(12):1354–61.

21. Ranasinghe WK, Baldwin GS, Bolton D, Shulkes A, Ischia J, Patel O. HIF1alpha expression under normoxia in prostate cancer: which pathways to target? J Urol. 2014;193:763–70.

22. Zhao T, Lv J, Zhao J, Nzekebaloudou M. Hypoxia-inducible factor-1alpha gene polymorphisms and cancer risk: a meta-analysis. J Exp Clin Cancer Res. 2009;28:159.

23. Heidenreich A, Bastian PJ, Bellmunt J, Bolla M, Joniau S, van der Kwast T, Mason M, Matveev V, Wiegel T, Zattoni F, et al. EAU guidelines on prostate cancer. part 1: screening, diagnosis, and local treatment with curative intent-update 2013. Eur Urol. 2014;65(1):124–37.

24. Pertega-Gomes N, Vizcaino JR, Miranda-Goncalves V, Pinheiro C, Silva J, Pereira H, Monteiro P, Henrique RM, Reis RM, Lopes C, et al. Monocarboxylate transporter 4 (MCT4) and CD147 overexpression is associated with poor prognosis in prostate cancer. BMC Cancer. 2011;11:312.

25. Holzer TR, Fulford AD, Nedderman DM, Umberger TS, Hozak RR, Joshi A, Melemed SA, Benjamin LE, Plowman GD, Schade AE, et al. Tumor cell expression of vascular endothelial growth factor receptor 2 is an adverse prognostic factor in patients with squamous cell carcinoma of the lung. PLoS ONE. 2013;8(11), e80292.

26. Smyth LG, O'Hurley G, O'Grady A, Fitzpatrick JM, Kay E, Watson RW. Carbonic anhydrase IX expression in prostate cancer. Prostate Cancer Prostatic Dis. 2010;13(2):178–81.

27. Albinger-Hegyi A, Stoeckli SJ, Schmid S, Storz M, Iotzova G, Probst-Hensch NM, Rehrauer H, Tinguely M, Moch H, Hegyi I. Lysyl oxidase expression is an independent marker of prognosis and a predictor of lymph node metastasis in oral and oropharyngeal squamous cell carcinoma (OSCC). Int J Cancer J International du cancer. 2010;126(11):2653–62.

28. Semenza GL. Hypoxia-inducible factors in physiology and medicine. Cell. 2012;148(3):399–408.

29. Zhong H, Agani F, Baccala AA, Laughner E, Rioseco-Camacho N, Isaacs WB, Simons JW, Semenza GL. Increased expression of hypoxia inducible factor-1alpha in rat and human prostate cancer. Cancer Res. 1998; 58(23):5280–4.

30. Zhong H, De Marzo AM, Laughner E, Lim M, Hilton DA, Zagzag D, Buechler P, Isaacs WB, Semenza GL, Simons JW. Overexpression of hypoxia-inducible factor 1alpha in common human cancers and their metastases. Cancer Res. 1999; 59(22):5830–5.

31. Saramaki OR, Savinainen KJ, Nupponen NN, Bratt O, Visakorpi T. Amplification of hypoxia-inducible factor 1alpha gene in prostate cancer. Cancer Genet Cytogenet. 2001;128(1):31–4.

32. Ranasinghe WK, Xiao L, Kovac S, Chang M, Michiels C, Bolton D, Shulkes A, Baldwin GS, Patel O. The role of hypoxia-inducible factor 1alpha in determining the properties of castrate-resistant prostate cancers. PLoS ONE. 2013;8(1), e54251.

33. Bos R, Zhong H, Hanrahan CF, Mommers EC, Semenza GL, Pinedo HM, Abeloff MD, Simons JW, Van Diest PJ, van der Wall E. Levels of hypoxia-inducible factor-1 alpha during breast carcinogenesis. J Natl Cancer Inst. 2001;93(4):309–14.

34. Birner P, Schindl M, Obermair A, Breitenecker G, Oberhuber G. Expression of hypoxia-inducible factor 1alpha in epithelial ovarian tumors: its impact on prognosis and on response to chemotherapy. Clin Cancer Res. 2001;7(6):1661–8.

35. Aebersold DM, Burri P, Beer KT, Laissue J, Djonov V, Greiner RH, Semenza GL. Expression of hypoxia-inducible factor-1alpha: a novel predictive and prognostic parameter in the radiotherapy of oropharyngeal cancer. Cancer Res. 2001;61(7):2911–6.

36. Waldner MJ, Wirtz S, Jefremow A, Warntjen M, Neufert C, Atreya R, Becker C, Weigmann B, Vieth M, Rose-John S, et al. VEGF receptor signaling links inflammation and tumorigenesis in colitis-associated cancer. J Exp Med. 2010;207(13):2855–68.

37. Kroll J, Waltenberger J. The vascular endothelial growth factor receptor KDR activates multiple signal transduction pathways in porcine aortic endothelial cells. J Biol Chem. 1997;272(51):32521–7.

38. Gerber HP, McMurtrey A, Kowalski J, Yan M, Keyt BA, Dixit V, Ferrara N. Vascular endothelial growth factor regulates endothelial cell survival through the phosphatidylinositol 3'-kinase/Akt signal transduction pathway. Requirement for Flk-1/KDR activation. J Biol Chem. 1998;273(46):30336–43.

39. Saraswati S, Kumar S, Alhaider AA. alpha-santalol inhibits the angiogenesis and growth of human prostate tumor growth by targeting vascular endothelial growth factor receptor 2-mediated AKT/mTOR/P70S6K signaling pathway. Mol Cancer. 2013;12:147.

40. Hahn D, Simak R, Steiner GE, Handisurya A, Susani M, Marberger M. Expression of the VEGF-receptor Flt-1 in benign, premalignant and malignant prostate tissues. J Urol. 2000;164(2):506–10.

41. Ferrer FA, Miller LJ, Lindquist R, Kowalczyk P, Laudone VP, Albertsen PC, Kreutzer DL. Expression of vascular endothelial growth factor receptors in human prostate cancer. Urology. 1999;54(3):567–72.

42. Pallares J, Rojo F, Iriarte J, Morote J, Armadans LI, De Torres I. Study of microvessel density and the expression of the angiogenic factors VEGF, bFGF and the receptors Flt-1 and FLK-1 in benign, premalignant and malignant prostate tissues. Histol Histopathol. 2006;21(8):857–65.

43. Bai AS, Zeng H, Li X, Wei Q, Li H, Yang YR. Expression of kinase insert domain-containing receptor in prostate adenocarcinoma. Zhonghua nan ke xue = National journal of andrology. 2007;13(4):324–6.

44. Song J, Song Y, Guo W, Jia J, Jin Y, Bai A. Regulatory roles of KDR antisense oligonucleotide on the proliferation of human prostate cancer cell line PC-3. J BUON. 2014;19(3):770–4.

45. Schweizer MT, Carducci MA. From bevacizumab to tasquinimod: angiogenesis as a therapeutic target in prostate cancer. Cancer J. 2013; 19(1):99–106.

46. Sherwood BT, Colquhoun AJ, Richardson D, Bowman KJ, O'Byrne KJ, Kockelbergh RC, Symonds RP, Mellon JK, Jones GD. Carbonic anhydrase IX expression and outcome after radiotherapy for muscle-invasive bladder cancer. Clin Oncol. 2007;19(10):777–83.

47. Swinson DE, Jones JL, Richardson D, Wykoff C, Turley H, Pastorek J, Taub N, Harris AL, O'Byrne KJ. Carbonic anhydrase IX expression, a novel surrogate marker of tumor hypoxia, is associated with a poor prognosis in non-small-cell lung cancer. J Clin Oncol. 2003;21(3):473–82.

48. Bui MH, Seligson D, Han KR, Pantuck AJ, Dorey FJ, Huang Y, Horvath S, Leibovich BC, Chopra S, Liao SY, et al. Carbonic anhydrase IX is an independent predictor of survival in advanced renal clear cell carcinoma: implications for prognosis and therapy. Clin Cancer Res. 2003;9(2):802–11.

49. Ord JJ, Agrawal S, Thamboo TP, Roberts I, Campo L, Turley H, Han C, Fawcett DW, Kulkarni RP, Cranston D, et al. An investigation into the prognostic significance of necrosis and hypoxia in high grade and invasive bladder cancer. J Urol. 2007;178(2):677–82.

50. Wykoff CC, Beasley NJ, Watson PH, Turner KJ, Pastorek J, Sibtain A, Wilson GD, Turley H, Talks KL, Maxwell PH, et al. Hypoxia-inducible expression of tumor-associated carbonic anhydrases. Cancer Res. 2000;60(24):7075–83.

51. Stewart GD, Nanda J, Brown DJ, Riddick AC, Ross JA, Habib FK. NO-sulindac inhibits the hypoxia response of PC-3 prostate cancer cells via the Akt signalling pathway. Int J Cancer J International du cancer. 2009;124(1):223–32.

52. Pertega-Gomes N, Vizcaino JR, Attig J, Jurmeister S, Lopes C, Baltazar F. A lactate shuttle system between tumour and stromal cells is associated with poor prognosis in prostate cancer. BMC Cancer. 2014;14:352.

53. Pertega-Gomes N, Vizcaino JR, Gouveia C, Jeronimo C, Henrique RM, Lopes C, Baltazar F. Monocarboxylate transporter 2 (MCT2) as putative biomarker in prostate cancer. Prostate. 2013;73(7):763–9.

54. Li Y, Wang H, Oosterwijk E, Selman Y, Mira JC, Medrano T, Shiverick KT, Frost SC. Antibody-specific detection of CAIX in breast and prostate cancers. Biochem Biophys Res Commun. 2009;386(3):488–92.

55. Weber DC, Tille JC, Combescure C, Egger JF, Laouiti M, Hammad K, Granger P, Rubbia-Brandt L, Miralbell R. The prognostic value of expression of HIF1alpha, EGFR and VEGF-A, in localized prostate cancer for intermediate- and high-risk patients treated with radiation therapy with or without androgen deprivation therapy. Radiat Oncol. 2012;7:66.

56. Denko NC, Fontana LA, Hudson KM, Sutphin PD, Raychaudhuri S, Altman R, Giaccia AJ. Investigating hypoxic tumor physiology through gene expression patterns. Oncogene. 2003;22(37):5907–14.

57. Chi JT, Wang Z, Nuyten DS, Rodriguez EH, Schaner ME, Salim A, Wang Y, Kristensen GB, Helland A, Borresen-Dale AL, et al. Gene expression programs in response to hypoxia: cell type specificity and prognostic significance in human cancers. PLoS Med. 2006;3(3), e47.

58. Erler JT, Bennewith KL, Nicolau M, Dornhofer N, Kong C, Le QT, Chi JT, Jeffrey SS, Giaccia AJ. Lysyl oxidase is essential for hypoxia-induced metastasis. Nature. 2006;440(7088):1222–6.

59. Kirschmann DA, Seftor EA, Fong SF, Nieva DR, Sullivan CM, Edwards EM, Sommer P, Csiszar K, Hendrix MJ. A molecular role for lysyl oxidase in breast cancer invasion. Cancer Res. 2002;62(15):4478–83.

60. Peyrol S, Raccurt M, Gerard F, Gleyzal C, Grimaud JA, Sommer P. Lysyl oxidase gene expression in the stromal reaction to in situ and invasive ductal breast carcinoma. Am J Pathol. 1997;150(2):497–507.

61. Trivedy C, Warnakulasuriya KA, Hazarey VK, Tavassoli M, Sommer P, Johnson NW. The upregulation of lysyl oxidase in oral submucous fibrosis and squamous cell carcinoma. J Oral Pathol Med. 1999;28(6):246–51.

62. Ribeiro R, Monteiro C, Cunha V, Oliveira MJ, Freitas M, Fraga A, Principe P, Lobato C, Lobo F, Morais A, et al. Human periprostatic adipose tissue promotes prostate cancer aggressiveness in vitro. J Exp Clin Cancer Res. 2012;31:32.

63. Orr-Urtreger A, Bar-Shira A, Matzkin H, Mabjeesh NJ. The homozygous P582S mutation in the oxygen-dependent degradation domain of HIF-1 alpha is associated with increased risk for prostate cancer. Prostate. 2007;67(1):8–13.

64. Tanimoto K, Yoshiga K, Eguchi H, Kaneyasu M, Ukon K, Kumazaki T, Oue N, Yasui W, Imai K, Nakachi K, et al. Hypoxia-inducible factor-1alpha polymorphisms associated with enhanced transactivation capacity, implying clinical significance. Carcinogenesis. 2003;24(11):1779–83.

65. Fransen K, Fenech M, Fredrikson M, Dabrosin C, Soderkvist P. Association between ulcerative growth and hypoxia inducible factor-1alpha polymorphisms in colorectal cancer patients. Mol Carcinog. 2006;45(11):833–40.

66. Kallio PJ, Pongratz I, Gradin K, McGuire J, Poellinger L. Activation of hypoxia-inducible factor 1alpha: posttranscriptional regulation and conformational change by recruitment of the Arnt transcription factor. Proc Natl Acad Sci U S A. 1997;94(11):5667–72.

67. Wu F, Zhang J, Liu Y, Zheng Y, Hu N. HIF1alpha genetic variants and protein expressions determine the response to platinum based chemotherapy and clinical outcome in patients with advanced NSCLC. Cell Physiol Biochem. 2013;32(6):1566–76.

68. Kim HO, Jo YH, Lee J, Lee SS, Yoon KS. The C1772T genetic polymorphism in human HIF-1alpha gene associates with expression of HIF-1alpha protein in breast cancer. Oncol Rep. 2008;20(5):1181–7.

69. Wang Y, Zheng Y, Zhang W, Yu H, Lou K, Zhang Y, Qin Q, Zhao B, Yang Y, Hui R. Polymorphisms of KDR gene are associated with coronary heart disease. J Am Coll Cardiol. 2007;50(8):760–7.

70. Jang MJ, Jeon YJ, Kim JW, Cho YK, Lee SK, Hwang SG, Oh D, Kim NK. Association of VEGF and KDR single nucleotide polymorphisms with colorectal cancer susceptibility in Koreans. Mol Carcinog. 2013;52 Suppl 1:E60–69.

71. Dong G, Guo X, Fu X, Wan S, Zhou F, Myers RE, Bao G, Burkart A, Yang H, Xing J. Potentially functional genetic variants in KDR gene as prognostic markers in patients with resected colorectal cancer. Cancer Sci. 2012;103(3):561–8.

72. De Martino M, Klatte T, Seligson DB, LaRochelle J, Shuch B, Caliliw R, Li Z, Kabbinavar FF, Pantuck AJ, Belldegrun AS. CA9 gene: single nucleotide polymorphism predicts metastatic renal cell carcinoma prognosis. J Urol. 2009;182(2):728–34.

73. Chien MH, Yang JS, Chu YH, Lin CH, Wei LH, Yang SF, Lin CW. Impacts of CA9 gene polymorphisms and environmental factors on oral-cancer susceptibility and clinicopathologic characteristics in Taiwan. PLoS ONE. 2012;7(12), e51051.

74. Trackman PC, Bedell-Hogan D, Tang J, Kagan HM. Post-translational glycosylation and proteolytic processing of a lysyl oxidase precursor. J Biol Chem. 1992;267(12):8666–71.

75. Uzel MI, Scott IC, Babakhanlou-Chase H, Palamakumbura AH, Pappano WN, Hong HH, Greenspan DS, Trackman PC. Multiple bone morphogenetic protein 1-related mammalian metalloproteinases process pro-lysyl oxidase at the correct physiological site and control lysyl oxidase activation in mouse embryo fibroblast cultures. J Biol Chem. 2001;276(25):22537–43.

76. Min C, Kirsch KH, Zhao Y, Jeay S, Palamakumbura AH, Trackman PC, Sonenshein GE. The tumor suppressor activity of the lysyl oxidase propeptide reverses the invasive phenotype of Her-2/neu-driven breast cancer. Cancer Res. 2007;67(3):1105–12.

77. Jeay S, Pianetti S, Kagan HM, Sonenshein GE. Lysyl oxidase inhibits ras-mediated transformation by preventing activation of NF-kappa B. Mol Cell Biol. 2003;23(7):2251–63.

78. Min C, Yu Z, Kirsch KH, Zhao Y, Vora SR, Trackman PC, Spicer DB, Rosenberg L, Palmer JR, Sonenshein GE. A loss-of-function polymorphism in the propeptide domain of the LOX gene and breast cancer. Cancer Res. 2009;69(16):6685–93.

79. Payne SL, Fogelgren B, Hess AR, Seftor EA, Wiley EL, Fong SF, Csiszar K, Hendrix MJ, Kirschmann DA. Lysyl oxidase regulates breast cancer cell migration and adhesion through a hydrogen peroxide-mediated mechanism. Cancer Res. 2005;65(24):11429–36.

80. Payne SL, Hendrix MJ, Kirschmann DA. Paradoxical roles for lysyl oxidases in cancer–a prospect. J Cell Biochem. 2007;101(6):1338–54.

81. Erler JT, Bennewith KL, Cox TR, Lang G, Bird D, Koong A, Le QT, Giaccia AJ. Hypoxia-induced lysyl oxidase is a critical mediator of bone marrow cell recruitment to form the premetastatic niche. Cancer Cell. 2009;15(1):35–44.

82. Erler JT, Weaver VM. Three-dimensional context regulation of metastasis. Clin Exp Metastasis. 2009;26(1):35–49.

83. Kobayashi H, Ishii M, Chanoki M, Yashiro N, Fushida H, Fukai K, Kono T, Hamada T, Wakasaki H, Ooshima A. Immunohistochemical localization of lysyl oxidase in normal human skin. Br J Dermatol. 1994;131(3):325–30.

84. Wakasaki H, Ooshima A. Immunohistochemical localization of lysyl oxidase with monoclonal antibodies. Lab Investig. 1990;63(3):377–84.

19

Assessment of a new point-of-care system for detection of prostate specific antigen

Steffen Rausch[1], Joerg Hennenlotter[1], Josef Wiesenreiter[1], Andrea Hohneder[1], Julian Heinkele[1], Christian Schwentner[1], Arnulf Stenzl[1] and Tilman Todenhöfer[1,2]*

Abstract

Background: Measurement of the prostate specific antigen (PSA) remains an important tool in prostate cancer (PC) diagnosis. Due to limited availability of laboratory devices in an outpatient setting, compact and easy-to-handle point-of-care (POC) systems are desirable. Recently, a chip for PSA measurement on the concile® Ω100 POC reader platform was introduced. To investigate the clinical applicability, we evaluated the system in a consecutive cohort of patients undergoing PSA measurement in our outpatient clinic.

Methods: Between 07/2014 and 01/2015, PSA was analyzed in a total of 198 patients by the POC reader system and in parallel by an Immulite 2000® and Centaur® standard laboratory system, respectively. By standard (Immulite®) measurement, 67 (34,2 %) had PSA > 4 ng/ml and 131 (65,8 %) had PSA ≤ 4 ng/ml. Results were correlated by linear regression analyses for all patients and within PSA subgroups. For patients with available prostate histology after PSA measurement ($n = 68$), receiver-operating characteristic curves were created and area under the curve (AUC), sensitivity and specificity for the prediction of PC at best cut-off value were calculated.

Results: The coefficients of determination (r^2) for the POC device compared to laboratory testing were 0.72 (Immulite®) and 0.63 (Centaur®), respectively (both $p < 0.0001$). In the PSA range of ≤4 ng/ml, the observed correlations were 0.75 and 0.70, respectively. For the POC test system, AUC for detection of PC was calculated with 0.745 while the standard laboratory tests showed 0.778 (Immulite®) and 0.771 (Centaur®). At best cut-off of 3.64 ng/ml, PSA analysis by the POC system showed a sensitivity of 85.7 % and a specificity of 66.7 %.

Conclusions: The POC system obtained good concordance to elaborate laboratory measurement. In a screening scenario, the system provides quick and reliable PSA measurement, especially in the PSA range up to 4 ng/ml.

Keywords: Point-of-care, Prostate cancer, Prostate specific antigen

Background

Since its discovery in 1979 by Wang et al. [1] prostate specific antigen (PSA) has become the gold standard biomarker for screening, diagnosis, and therapeutic monitoring of prostate cancer (PC), and a routine clinical parameter for the management of benign hyperplasia and inflammatory disorders of the prostate [2–7].

Despite country and health-system dependent approaches to prostate cancer screening and PSA testing, patients with clinical symptoms of urinary and prostatic disorders or the intention to undergo screening for prostate cancer are often primarily seen and tested for PSA in an outpatient setting. However, laboratory tests for PSA are usually performed in centralized institutions and therefore most often not available in proximity to the urologists' or general practitioners' office, resulting in a delayed information and putative psychological discomfort for patients [8].

Point-of-care (POC) test systems for a rapid and reliable testing at the practitioners' office have been already introduced for several medical conditions. For the evaluation of diabetes or acute inflammation, POC systems measuring blood count, CRP or HbA1c have shown to provide reliable test results [9–12].

The present prospective study was performed in order to evaluate the reproducibility and clinical applicability

* Correspondence: Tilman.todenhoefer@med.uni-tuebingen.de
[1]Department of Urology, Eberhard-Karls-University Tuebingen, Hoppe-Seyler-Str. 3, 72076 Tuebingen, Germany
[2]Vancouver Prostate Centre, University of British Columbia, 2660 Oak Street, Vancouver V6H 3Z6, Canada

of a novel quantitative POC PSA assay (CancerCheck® PSA, concile GmbH, Freiburg, Germany) using a portable device (concile® Ω100) in comparison to established standard routine laboratory PSA test systems.

Methods

Patient cohort

We prospectively included 200 patients, who underwent routine PSA measurement at the University hospital of Tuebingen. To cover a broad range of PSA values, patients were recruited based on PSA analysis using the Immulite® system, which was set as reference method. We evaluated 150, 25 and 25 patients with PSA values in the range of ≤4 ng/ml, 4–10 ng/ml and >10 ng/ml. Patients referred for PC screening, and patients designated to undergo surgery for PC or lower urinary tract symptoms due to benign prostatic hyperplasia were included. Patients with a history of other urogenital malignancy were excluded from the study.

Patient samples were prospectively analyzed with two elaborated test systems, Immulite 2000® (Siemens Healthcare Diagnostics, Deerfield, USA) and Centaur® (Siemens Healthcare Diagnostics), and the POC test system (CancerCheck® PSA, on the concile® Ω100 reader, concile GmbH, Freiburg, Germany) in parallel. Blood samples were collected one day prior to the analyses and stored at 2–8 °C to provide simultaneous application of the tests. All three tests were performed within a time-span of one hour.

Baseline patients' characteristics (age, history of prior prostatic disease), subsequent interventions and clinical parameters after PSA-measurement (biopsy, surgery, histology) were recorded.

Written informed consent was obtained by all participants, and the study was approved by the local ethics committee of the University hospital Tübingen (No. 122/2012BO2).

POC-Test system principle

The POC system consists of a portable device (concile® Ω100 reader, and a test cassette containing a one-step chromatographic sandwich immunoassay, which is analyzed by a charged-couple device (CCD).

After addition of sample, PSA binds to a colloidal gold-labeled antibody. The resulting complex is captured by a specific antibody pre-coated at the test zone and forming a red test line. The concentration of PSA is measured using complimentary light and the intensity of the test line is measured by the CCD sensor. The volume of the signal is directly proportional to the concentration of PSA in the sample and can be measured by the concile® Ω100 reader with a pre-set calibration curve. The concentration of PSA is displayed as numeric result with one decimal place.

Statistics

For data analyses, patients were classified into different categories of total PSA (tPSA) range ≤4, ≤10 ng/ml and >10 ng/ml according to the Immulite® measurement.

Linear regression analyses were performed to correlate individual test results given by the POC reader and Immulite® and Centaur® measurement in the whole group and in the three subgroups, respectively. In the subgroup of patients with available histology, receiver-operator-characteristics (ROC) analyses were performed to evaluate the diagnostic performance of the tests with respect to the correct identification of PC and the area-under-the-curve (AUC) was calculated. Youden's index was used to identify the optimum cut-off for each test system. Comparison of ROC curves was performed according to the method of DeLong. Analyses were performed using commercial software (MedCalc, version 12.5, Ostend, Belgium). Statistical significance was defined as $p < 0.05$.

Results

Samples of a total of 198 (99 %) patients were available for the analyses. Two patients were excluded from the collective due to insufficient sample preparation or extreme PSA values (>800 ng/ml). Median patient age was 66.15 years. Histological workup was performed in 68 patients (34.7 %). Of those, $n = 36$ (52.2 %) were diagnosed with PC. Patients' characteristics are summarized in Table 1.

Figure 1 illustrates PSA values determined by POC concile® measurement compared to the Immulite® (A) and Centaur® test results (B). The correlation of the three systems in different PSA ranges is illustrated in Fig. 2. The coefficient of determination (r^2) for the POC measurement compared to routine lab testing was 0.72 (Immulite®) and 0.63 (Centaur®), respectively. In the PSA ≤4 ng/ml subgroup, r^2 were 0.75 (Immulite®) and 0.70 (Centaur®) (both $p < 0.0001$). For patients with PSA ≤10 ng/ml the coefficients of determination observed were both 0.88 (Immulite® and Centaur®), respectively. In the high PSA group of >10 ng/ml, r^2 was 0.72 (Immulite®) and 0.70 (Centaur®) (Table 2). With regard to the correct prediction of prostate cancer, ROC analysis (Fig. 3) revealed an AUC of 0.745 (95 % CI: 0.625 to 0.843) for the POC test system, while the AUCs for the standard laboratory tests were calculated with 0.778 (95 % CI: 0.661 to 0.870) (Immulite®) and 0.771 (95 % CI: 0.653 to 0.864) (Centaur®). The comparison of ROC curves revealed no significant difference between POC and Centaur® measurement, while a significant difference of AUCs from POC and Immulite® analyses was noted ($P = 0.03$) (Table 3). From ROC analysis, optimal PSA cut-off values for the individual PSA test systems were determined. Sensitivity and specificity for the detection of prostate cancer and

Table 1 Patients' characteristics

Median patient age, years (Range)	66.15	(42.06–90.09)	
Patient groups according to Immulite® measurement		n=	%
	≤4 ng/ml	131	65.8 %
	>4 ng/ml	67	34.2 %
	≤10 ng/ml	168	84.8 %
	>10 ng/ml	30	15.2 %
Further diagnostic workup			
Histology available[a]	Yes	69	34.7 %
	No	130	65.3 %
Histologic evidence of prostate cancer	Yes	36	52.2 %
	No	30	43.5 %
		Median	95 % CI
PSA values	Immulite®	2.34	2.07 to 3.10
	Centaur®	1.90	1.70 to 2.33
	concile®	2.53	2.10 to 3.15

[a]from radical prostatectomy, TUR-P, or prostate biopsy

optimal PSA cut-off values for the respective test systems are shown in Table 4. At best cut-off (3.64 ng/ml), the POC system showed a sensitivity of 85.7 and a specificity of 66.7, respectively. Table 5 illustrates the association between PSA at cut-off 4 ng/ml and the presence of PC in the sub-cohort of patients with available histology. POC measurement showed the highest negative predictive value (81.5 %). No further false negative result was observed compared to Immulite®, however two patients (2.9 %) that were

negatively tested in the Centaur® assay were correctly classified as PC patients by POC measurement.

Within POC measurement, the rate of false positive subjects at cut-off PSA 4 ng/ml was 16.2 % ($n = 11$), while the rates of Centaur® and Immulite® were 11.8 ($n = 8$) and 19.1 % ($n = 13$). On the other hand, rates of patients with a PSA value >4 ng/ml in the Immulite® or Centaur® but <4 ng/ml in POC analysis were 1.0 % ($n = 2$, Immulite®) and 0 % ($n = 0$, Centaur®), respectively (Table 6).

Discussion

In the present study, we detected a close correlation between a new POC test system and standard laboratory tests, as documented by a coefficient of determination of 0.72 for the overall patient population comparing concile® Ω100 reader and Immulite® measurement. In the clinically relevant PSA range of ≤4 ng/ml with regard to the prediction of a negative result in a PC screen scenario, the observed correlation was even higher, with r^2 of 0.75.

Nevertheless, AUC analysis revealed a higher accuracy for the established standard assays, which has also been reported in earlier publications on POC PSA test systems [13].

However, in urologist's daily practice it is well known, that even the established laboratory systems differ in their results. Therefore, the decision of clinicians whether a biopsy should be recommended or not is dependent on the PSA system used. Slev et al. analyzed the intermethod differences for six different laboratory PSA assays, including Immulite® and Centaur® and reported relative differences of more than 10 % at PSA of 4.0 ng/ml [14].

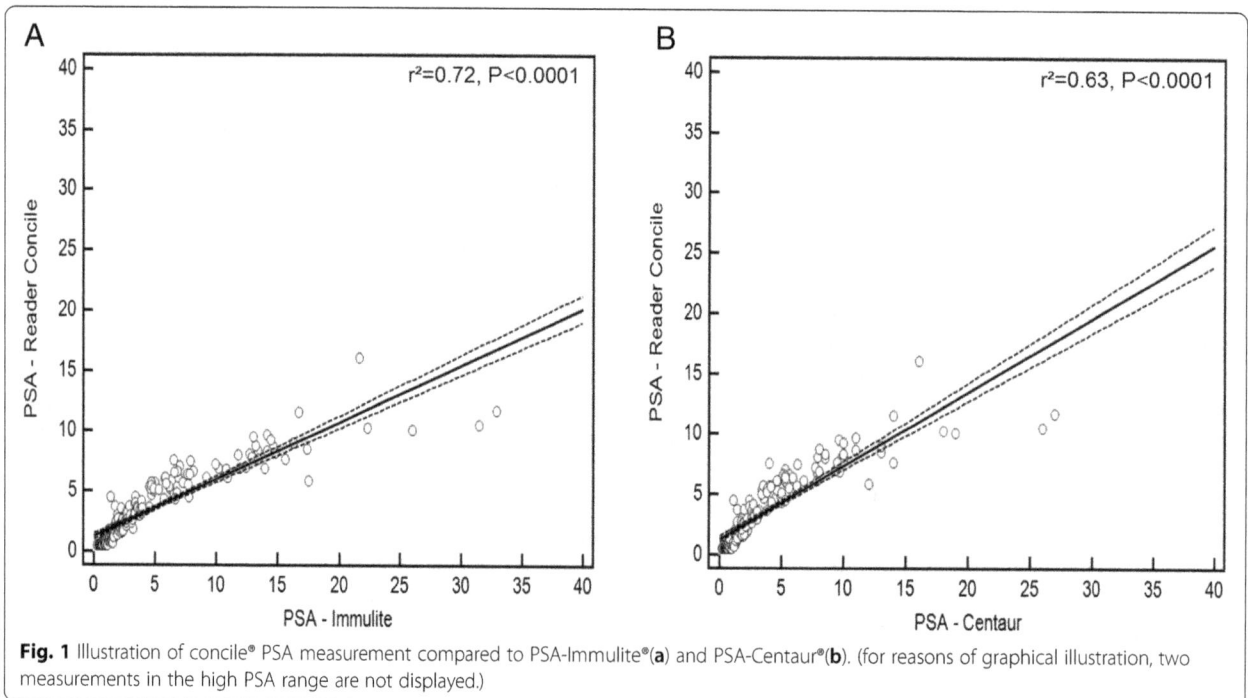

Fig. 1 Illustration of concile® PSA measurement compared to PSA-Immulite®(**a**) and PSA-Centaur®(**b**). (for reasons of graphical illustration, two measurements in the high PSA range are not displayed.)

Assessment of a new point-of-care system for detection of prostate specific antigen

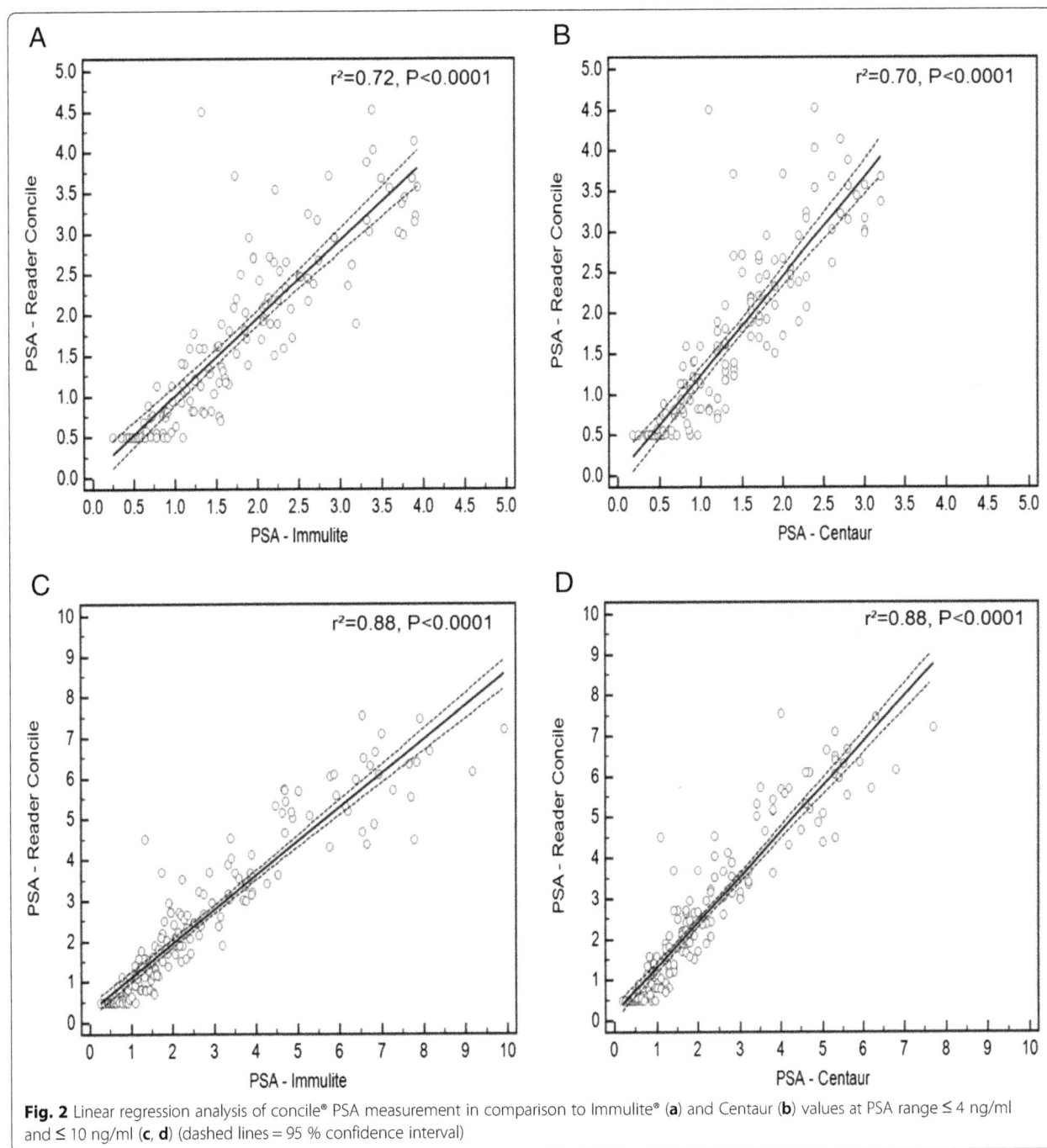

Fig. 2 Linear regression analysis of concile® PSA measurement in comparison to Immulite® (**a**) and Centaur (**b**) values at PSA range ≤ 4 ng/ml and ≤ 10 ng/ml (**c, d**) (dashed lines = 95 % confidence interval)

Table 2 Results from linear regression analysis

	Collective (n = 198)		PSA ≤ 4 ng/ml (n = 131)		PSA ≤ 10 ng/ml (n = 161)		PSA > 10 ng/ml (n = 37)	
	r^2	P=	r^2	P=	r^2	P=	r^2	P=
Concile® vs. Immulite®	0.7181	<0.0001	0.7518	<0.0001	0.8775	<0.0001	0.7155	<0.0001
Concile® vs. Centaur®	0.6346	<0.0001	0.7037	<0.0001	0.8782	<0.0001	0.7031	<0.0001

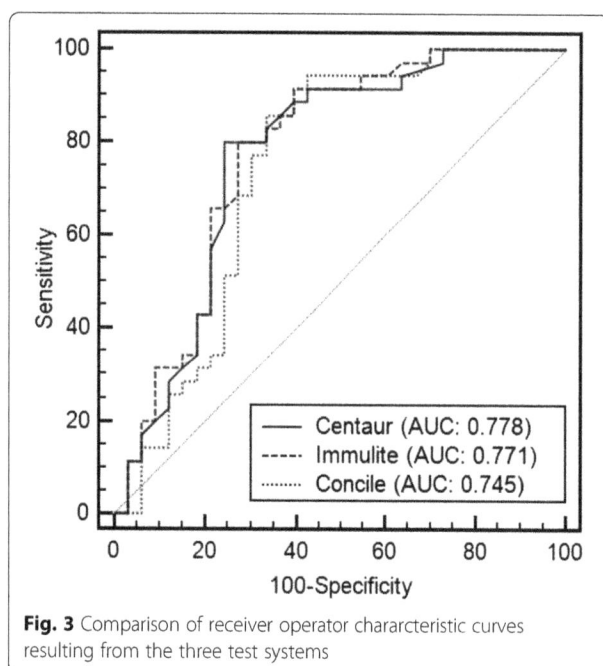

Fig. 3 Comparison of receiver operator chararcteristic curves resulting from the three test systems

Table 4 Prostate specific antigen best cut-off, sensitivity and specificity from receiver operator characteristic analysis

	Best cut off	Sensitivity	95 % CI	Specificity	95 % CI
Immulite®	5.02	80.0	63.1–91.6	72.7	54.5–86.7
Centaur®	4.00	80.0	63.1–91.6	75.8	57.7–88.9
Concile®	3.64	85.7	69.7–95.2	66.7	48.2–82.0

In this context it is noteworthy that a PSA-POC system may not provide meticulous correlation to all of the standard laboratory tests, it should however try to give the PSA value on a level that is located in an appropriate range compared to standard assays. A valid variable for determining this level is the comparison of individual system's best cut- offs. With 3.64 ng/ml the POC system ranged in its level at an adequate best cut-off value.

A PSA value of 4 ng/ml is considered a common threshold for a biopsy decision. At a cut-off PSA value of 4 ng/ml, POC measurement outperformed Immulite® and Centaur® with regard to the negative predictive value, which underlines the effectiveness of POC measurement as a screening tool. POC test systems used at a general practitioners office could be used as pre-screening tests and avoid unnecessary referrals to urologists in cases of inconspicuous digital rectal examination and low POC PSA values. Despite the fact, that PSA standard lab test results may in some cases be available within a few hours according to specific health system dependent or institutional conditions, the main rationale for the use of POC tests is the option to receive a test result within 20 min, which makes a discussion of the test result with the patient possible in the same session.

As a general rule, POC tests should not be applied as a diagnostic following radical prostatectomy, where ultrasensitive monitoring of PSA is recommended [15, 16]. In patients with POC PSA values in the range of 2.5 to 4.0 ng/ml [17] and beyond, POC measurement should be regarded as a pre-screening test and an immediate routine lab testing should follow. In addition, the confirmation of an elevated PSA after three weeks, as recommended by current PC treatment guidelines in cases of cancer suspicion, should not exclusively been performed by concile® Ω100 measurement [15]. Hence, POC measurement is subject to the same restrictions in men undergoing active surveillance for PC. However, the POC assay appears appropriate for the identification of patients with a low risk of prostate cancer in the PSA range of <2.5 ng/ml. The evaluation of other frequent prostatic diseases like benign hyperplasia, prostatitis, and follow-up studies for prostate cancer after radiotherapy or hormonal treatment may also be performed based on concile® PSA analysis. In PSA ranges >10 ng/ml, up to extreme PSA values, the diagnostic precision of POC measurement is impaired. Follow up studies in patients with extreme PSA values should therefore be performed with standard assays.

By using PSA POC measurements, the regularly observed delay between PSA sampling, receipt of test results, and the information and discussion with the patient may be overcome for a large subgroup of patients. In a prospective study of 188 patients, Wilkinson et al. observed that 89 % of patients receiving a rapid result would prefer to have this method again in order to facilitate the discussion regarding their future management. However, no significant differences between stress and anxiety of patients receiving PSA test results within 15 min after the test, and 1–4 days after PSA testing were detected [18].

Handling of the POC system was favorable. While other one-step POC test systems, usually based on lateral flow chromatographic immunoassays, could demonstrate

Table 3 Comparison of receiver operator characteristic curves (*CI* confidence interval, *SE a* standard error, *PSA* prostate specific antigen)

	Difference between areas	Standard error	95 % CI	z statistic	Significance level
PSA Immulite® vs. PSA concile®	0.0333	0.0162	0.00165 to 0.0650	2062	P = 0.0392
PSA Centaur® vs. PSA concile®	0.026	0.0201	-0.0134 to 0.0654	1293	P = 0.1961

Table 5 Performance of different standard and POC assays at PSA cut-off 4 ng/ml (CI confidence interval, PC prostate cancer, PSA prostate specific antigen, [a] from chi-square test)

	PSA Immulite®				PSA Centaur®				Concile®			
	No PC	PC	PSA < 4	PSA ≥ 4	No PC	PC	PSA < 4	PSA ≥ 4	No PC	PC	PSA < 4	PSA ≥ 4
PSA < 4	20	5	25 (36.8 %)		25	7	32 (47.1 %)		22	5	27 (39.7 %)	
PSA ≥ 4	13	30		43 (63.2 %)	8	28		36 (52.9 %)	11	30		41 (60.3 %)
	33 (48.50 %)	35 (51.50 %)	68		33 (48.50 %)	35 (51.50 %)	68		33 (48.50 %)	35 (51.50 %)	68	
Significance level[a]	P = 0.0002				P < 0.0001				P < 0.0001			
		95 % CI				95 % CI				95 % CI		
Sensitivity	85.71 %	69.74 to 95.19 %			80.00 %	63.06 to 91.56 %			85.71 %	69.74 to 95.19 %		
Specificity	60.61 %	42.14 to 77.09 %			75.76 %	57.74 to 88.91 %			66.67 %	48.17 to 82.04 %		
Positive predictive value	69.77 %	53.87 to 82.82 %			77.78 %	60.85 to 89.88 %			73.17 %	57.06 to 85.78 %		
Negative predictive value	80.00 %	59.30 to 93.17 %			78.12 %	60.03 to 90.72 %			81.48 %	61.92 to 93.70 %		

Table 6 Comparison of different standard and POC assays at cut-off PSA 4 ng/ml

	PSA < 4 Concile®	PSA ≥ 4 Concile®	
PSA < 4 Centaur®	129	13	142 (71.7 %)
PSA ≥ 4 Centaur®	0	56	56 (28.3 %)
	129 (65.2 %)	69 (34.8 %)	198 (100.0 %)

	PSA < 4 Concile®	PSA ≥ 4 Concile®	
PSA < 4 Immulite®	127	4	131 (66.2 %)
PSA ≥ 4 Immulite®	2	65	67 (33.8 %)
	129 (65.2 %)	69 (34.8 %)	198 (100.0 %)

	PSA < 4 Centaur®	PSA ≥ 4 Centaur®	
PSA < 4 Immulite®	131	0	131 (66.2 %)
PSA ≥ 4 Immulite®	11	56	67 (33.8 %)
	142 (71.7 %)	56 (28.3 %)	198 (100.0 %)

practical feasibility and good correlation to routine PSA lab values [13, 19, 20], earlier studies with semi-quantitative strip tests for the evaluation of PSA in whole blood, failed to prove their clinical utility due to impaired test handling and interpretation [21].

Conclusions

POC measurement with the herein evaluated system allows rapid quantitative analysis of PSA and may help to circumvent limitations of ambulatory PSA testing for patients and physicians in need of an immediate test result.

Abbreviations
AUC: area under the curve; CCD: charged-couple device; PC: prostate cancer; POC: point-of-care; PSA: prostate specific antigen; ROC: receiver-operator characteristic.

Competing interests
The authors declare that they have no competing interests.

Authors' contributions
SR, JHen, and TT participated in the design of the study and performed the statistical analysis. AH, JHei, JW carried out the measurements. SR, JHen, TT, AS, and CS drafted the manuscript. All authors read and approved the final manuscript.

Acknowledgements
The study was financially supported by concile GmbH, Freiburg, Germany. SR is supported by a Ferdinand-Eisenberger-grant of the German Society of Urology (RaS1/FE14). TT is supported by a Mildred-Scheel-Postdoctoral fellow grant of the German Cancer Foundation (Deutsche Krebshilfe).

References
1. Wang MC, Valenzuela LA, Murphy GP, Chu TM. Purification of a human prostate specific antigen. Invest Urol. 1979;17(2):159–63.
2. Gui-Zhong L, Libo M, Guanglin H, Jianwei W. The correlation of extent and grade of inflammation with serum PSA levels in patients with IV prostatitis. Int Urol Nephrol. 2011;43(2):295–301.
3. Mochtar CA, Kiemeney LA, Laguna MP, van Riemsdijk MM, Barnett GS, Debruyne FM, et al. Prognostic role of prostate-specific antigen and prostate volume for the risk of invasive therapy in patients with benign prostatic hyperplasia initially managed with alpha1-blockers and watchful waiting. Urology. 2005;65(2):300–5.
4. Stancik I, Luftenegger W, Klimpfinger M, Muller MM, Hoeltl W. Effect of NIH-IV prostatitis on free and free-to-total PSA. Eur Urol. 2004;46(6):760–4.
5. Boccon-Gibod L, Djavan WB, Hammerer P, Hoeltl W, Kattan MW, Prayer-Galetti T, et al. Management of prostate-specific antigen relapse in prostate cancer: a European Consensus. Int J Clin Pract. 2004;58(4):382–90.
6. Roehrborn CG, McConnell JD, Lieber M, Kaplan S, Geller J, Malek GH, et al. Serum prostate-specific antigen concentration is a powerful predictor of acute urinary retention and need for surgery in men with clinical benign prostatic hyperplasia. PLESS Study Group. Urology. 1999;53(3):473–80.
7. Roehrborn CG, Boyle P, Gould AL, Waldstreicher J. Serum prostate-specific antigen as a predictor of prostate volume in men with benign prostatic hyperplasia. Urology. 1999;53(3):581–9.
8. Lintz K, Moynihan C, Steginga S, Norman A, Eeles R, Huddart R, et al. Prostate cancer patients' support and psychological care needs: survey from a non-surgical oncology clinic. Psychooncology. 2003;12(8):769–83.
9. Brouwer N, van Pelt J. Validation and evaluation of eight commercially available point of care CRP methods. Clin Chim Acta. 2015;439:195–201.
10. Syal K. Point of care testing for measurement of white blood cell count and C-reactive protein levels in blood. Clin Chim Acta. 2014;437:218.
11. Knaebel J, Irvin BR, Xie CZ. Accuracy and clinical utility of a point-of-care HbA1c testing device. Postgrad Med. 2013;125(3):91–8.
12. Sanchez-Mora C, S Rodríguez-Oliva M, Fernández-Riejos P, Mateo J, Polo-Padillo J, Goberna R. Evaluation of two HbA1c point-of-care analyzers. Clin Chem Lab Med. 2011;49(4):653–7.
13. Karim O, Rao A, Emberton M, Cochrane D, Partridge M, Edwards P, et al. Point-of-care PSA testing: an evaluation of PSAwatch. Prostate Cancer Prostatic Dis. 2007;10(3):270–3.
14. Slev PR, La'ulu SL, Roberts WL. Intermethod differences in results for total PSA, free PSA, and percentage of free PSA. Am J Clin Pathol. 2008;129(6):952–8.
15. Heidenreich A, Bastian PJ, Bellmunt J, Bolla M, Joniau S, van der Kwast T, et al. EAU guidelines on prostate cancer. Part II: Treatment of advanced, relapsing, and castration-resistant prostate cancer. Eur Urol. 2014;65(2):467–79.
16. Shen S, Lepor H, Yaffee R, Taneja SS. Ultrasensitive serum prostate specific antigen nadir accurately predicts the risk of early relapse after radical prostatectomy. J Urol. 2005;173(3):777–80.
17. Thompson IM, Pauler DK, Goodman PJ, Tangen CM, Lucia MS, Parnes HL, et al. Prevalence of prostate cancer among men with a prostate-specific antigen level < or =4.0 ng per milliliter. N Engl J Med. 2004;350(22):2239–46.
18. Wilkinson S, Warren K, Ramsden A, Matthews A, Chodak G. Do "rapid" PSA assays reduce anxiety and stress of prostate cancer patients undergoing regular review? A prospective evaluation. Urology. 2008;71(4):567–72.
19. Miano R, Mele GO, Germani S, Bove P, Sansalone S, Pugliese PF, et al. Evaluation of a new, rapid, qualitative, one-step PSA Test for prostate cancer screening: the PSA RapidScreen test. Prostate Cancer Prostatic Dis. 2005;8(3):219–23.
20. Oh SW, Kim YM, Kim HJ, Kim SJ, Cho JS, Choi EY. Point-of-care fluorescence immunoassay for prostate specific antigen. Clin Chim Acta. 2009;406(1-2):18–22.
21. Oberpenning F, Hetzel S, Weining C, Brandt B, De Angelis G, Heinecke A, et al. Semi-quantitative immunochromatographic test for prostate specific antigen in whole blood: tossing the coin to predict prostate cancer? Eur Urol. 2003;43(5):478–84.

20

Do African-American men need separate prostate cancer screening guidelines?

Divya Shenoy[1], Satyaseelan Packianathan[2], Allen M. Chen[3] and Srinivasan Vijayakumar[2,4*]

Abstract

Background: In 2012, the United States Preventative Services Task Force issued new guidelines recommending that male U.S. residents, irrespective of race, no longer be screened for prostate cancer. In African American men, the incidence of prostate cancer is almost 60 % higher and the mortality rate is two to three times greater than in Caucasians. The purpose of this study is to reduce African American men's prostate cancer burden by demonstrating they need separate screening guidelines.

Methods: We performed a PubMed search using the keywords: African American, Prostate cancer, Outcomes, Molecular markers, Prostate-specific Antigen velocity, PSA density, and to derive data relevant to our hypothesis.

Results: In our literature review, we identified several aspects of prostate cancer that are different in Caucasian and African American men. These included prostate cancer incidence and outcome, the clinical course of the disease, serum PSA levels, genetic differences, and social barriers. It's also important to note that the USPSTF guidelines were based on two studies, one of which reported that only 4 % of its participants were African American. The other did not report demographic information, but used participants from seven European countries with small African American populations.

Conclusion: Given the above, we conclude that separate prostate cancer screening guidelines are greatly necessary to help save the lives of African Americans.

Keywords: Prostate cancer, African Americans, Screening guidelines

Background

Prostate cancer represents the most common male visceral cancer in the United States. The estimated number of annual new diagnoses and mortality in 2015 is 220,800 and 27,540, respectively [1]. The life time risk of a diagnosis of prostate cancer is 15.9 % while the life time risk of death is 2.8 % [2]. In African-American men, however, the incidence of prostate cancer is almost 60 % higher and the mortality rate is two- to three-times greater than that of Caucasian men. These numbers have remained remarkably constant for more than 20 years [3].

A commonly held perception about prostate cancer in the lay public and even within the scientific community is that prostate cancer is generally an indolent disease

and therefore not as deadly because individuals who are diagnosed with prostate cancer often die of other causes unrelated to the cancer. Although this view may be true to a certain extent when the at-risk U.S. population is taken as a whole, it is our contention that it should not apply to all prostate cancer patients, especially to those of African-American descent. Because of differences in the natural course of the disease and because of social issues that differentially impact African Americans, many of these patients may face a greater health burden than their Caucasian counterparts once they have been diagnosed [4–6]. Hence, a diagnosis that is made as early as possible in this population may improve overall prostate cancer outcomes. In this regard, we believe that the current prostate cancer screening guidelines promulgated by the U.S. Preventative Services Task Force (USPSTF) do not adequately take into account ethnic/racial differences in the impact of prostate cancer on the population. Separate screening guidelines for African

* Correspondence: svijayakumar@umc.edu
[2]University of Mississippi Medical Center, 2500 North State Street, 39216-4505 Jackson, MS, USA
[4]UMMC Cancer Institute, Department of Radiation Oncology, 2500 North State Street, 39216-4505 Jackson, MS, USA
Full list of author information is available at the end of the article

American men would facilitate earlier diagnosis and thereby reduce their mortality rate from the disease.

Hypothesis

African American men need separate screening guidelines to help decrease their prostate cancer burden.

Methods

We performed a "Pubmed search" using the following keywords:

African American
Prostate cancer
Outcomes
Molecular markers
Prostate-specific antigen (PSA) velocity
PSA density

We did not place any time restrictions. Specifically, we used the word "African American" and then one of the other five words listed above to create a total of four combinations total. The articles derived from the initial search were culled to identify peer-reviewed publications that were relevant to the clinical, social, and health policy aspects of the diagnosis and treatment of prostate cancer in African American men. These manuscripts were then analyzed closely to derive other sources of information and data that were relevant to our hypothesis.

In our review of the literature, we identified several aspects of prostate cancer that are different in Caucasian and African-American males. These included prostate cancer incidence and outcomes, the clinical course of the disease itself, serum PSA levels, and social barriers/behaviors. These are discussed in more detail in subsequent sections below.

Results/Discussion

In 2012, the USPSTF issued new guidelines recommending that U.S. male residents, irrespective of their race, no longer be screened for prostate cancer using PSA. In early 2015, the American Cancer Society recommended men who are considering being screened for prostate cancer should make an informed decision only after discussing their prostate cancer specific risk factors and general clinical situation, considering variables such as overall health, performance status, and the presence or absence of medical comorbidities, with their physician. There are several differences between African American and Caucasian men that make such guidelines ineffective for African Americans.

Incidence of prostate cancer among African Americans

The incidence of prostate cancer among African American males is higher than in any ethnic/racial group in the United States. In fact, worldwide, those men with West African ancestry have a disproportionately larger burden of prostate cancer [3]. In the United States, the incidence of prostate cancer in African American males has been 60 % higher than the incidence in Caucasians [3]. Furthermore, there are sociological aspects that adversely affect the incidence of prostate cancer in African American males. These will be discussed in sections below.

Clinical course of prostate cancer in African Americans

The course of prostate cancer has been shown to be different in African American men; for instance, prostate cancer volume is greater in African American men and advanced metastatic prostate cancer occurs at a 4:1 ratio in black and white men, respectively [7]. While clinical characteristics do not differ by race at an early age, prostate cancer transforms earlier in black men (from indolent to aggressive). Therefore, one can surmise that the growth or transformation rate of prostate cancer is greater in black men. Because of this augmented growth rate, African American men likely present at a later stage of disease than Caucasians at a similar age. Additionally, among African American patients who had prostate biopsies without histological evidence of prostate cancer, their PSA values were about 1.8-fold higher than those in whites, even when controlling for prostate volume [8]. Genetically, there seem to be differences between African American and white males as well. For example, it has been suggested that African American men may be more susceptible to prostate cancer because of differences in the expression of the androgen receptor genes [9]. Additionally, several risk-associated single nucleotide polymorphisms (SNPs), appear to be differentially overexpressed in African American men compared to control subjects [10].

Social Differences in the African American Population

African American men face several social barriers that Caucasian men may not, contributing further to their risk of poorer prognoses and outcomes. For example, when comparing men over the age of 50, only 81 % of African Americans are likely to have health insurance compared to nearly 90 % of Caucasians. This difference is statistically significant [4]. African American men have been noted to be less likely to be treated for prostate cancer when compared to white patients with a similar stage of disease [6]. Financial barriers associated with a lower socioeconomic status (SES) are also a major contributor to racial disparities in prostate cancer outcomes [10, 11]. Nonfinancial related barriers such as poor health seeking behaviors often can delay a prostate cancer diagnosis in African American men [5]. Thus, an inherent fear of a cancer diagnosis coupled with a mistrust of the health care system at large, can significantly affect the outcome of African-American men with prostate cancer [5].

Diets high in fat content have been associated with an increased risk of prostate cancer. Specifically, a diet higher in saturated fats is positively correlated to an increased risk of prostate cancer. When considering Caucasians, Asians, and African Americans, African Americans generally tend to consume more saturated fats and a greater number of calories in their daily diet [9]. This dietary discrepancy alone may account for almost 10 % of the difference in prostate cancer incidence between Caucasian and African American men [12].

PSA levels are higher among African Americans

In general, African American men present with higher PSA values when compared to white men [13]. Several studies have shown that African American men with nonmetastatic prostate cancer have higher serum PSA levels at diagnosis than Caucasian men with nonmetastatic prostate cancer, suggesting that perhaps African Americans have a higher tumor cell burden [13, 14]. Furthermore, African American men with or without evidence for prostate cancer have a higher PSA density (when the prostate is controlled for volume) than Caucasians [8, 13]. However, the differences between African Americans and Caucasians in PSA velocity is controversial (assuming there is any difference at all). In one study, Caucasians had higher PSA velocities than African American men of a similar age, despite the fact that African Americans had a higher baseline PSA value, age-for-age [15]. This finding could be attributed to laboratory test access as perhaps African American men may have had fewer PSA tests over time, thus impacting their velocity score despite higher individual PSA values. Another study, reported that PSA velocity is higher in Caucasians only in the 60–69 age bracket, whereas in the 40–49 age group, PSA velocity is higher in African Americans. Nonetheless, despite the fact that PSA levels, density, and velocity appear different in African-American men compared to Caucasians, the USPSTF has issued guidelines that are not race specific.

Mortality rate

An undeniable certainty is that regardless of previous screening recommendations, African American men have had a higher mortality rate from prostate cancer (two- to three-fold higher) and are carrying a larger prostate cancer burden than their Caucasian contemporaries [7]. African American men also are less likely to have health insurance and a higher proportion of them are of lower SES. In regards to SES, however, its impact on prostate cancer outcomes is controversial. For instance, Xu et al. reported that after adjusting for SES, the differences in prostate cancer mortality were eliminated. This is particularly relevant to screening because

even among African Americans, screening guidelines may differ based on SES [4, 10, 11].

USPSTF recommendation

In the past (2008), the USPSTF had stated there was insufficient evidence on the pros and cons of prostate cancer screening for men below age 75 (Grade I —insufficient knowledge of risks of the service), but that at and above age 75, screening should not be performed (Grade D — moderate or high risk of certainty that the service has no net benefit or the risks outweigh the benefits). The purpose of PSA screening is to reduce death rates directly linked to prostate cancer by intervening with treatment; however, screening and early treatment only benefited anywhere from 0 to 1 man per 1,000 men screened [16]. Currently, however, the USPSTF is against PSA based screening for male U.S. residents, regardless of ethnicity. It considers PSA screening to be "Grade D." Prostate cancer has a lifetime risk of diagnosis estimated to be 15.9 %, while the lifetime risk of dying from prostate cancer is 2.8 % [2]. Thus, the argument is that many cases of prostate cancer are likely to have a favorable outcome and unlikely to impact survival, even without treatment or a delayed diagnosis.

Another USPSTF argument against screening is that even asymptomatic cancer is detected by PSA screening; often, these tumors will not progress or will progress so slowly that men are unlikely to experience deleterious symptoms in their lifetime. This type of overdiagnosis or pseudo-diagnosis is estimated to occur about 17 % to 50 % of the time in prostate cancer screening [16].

The USPSTF guidelines were based on two key studies: The Prostate, Lung, Colorectal, and Ovarian Cancer Screening Trial (PLCO) and the European Randomized Study of Screening for Prostate Cancer (ERSPC). According to the USPSTF, the PLCO Trial reported that only 4 % of enrolled men were non-Hispanic black while the ERSPC study, based on populations in seven countries with low populations of men of African descent, did not report demographic statistics. From that one can surmise that the majority of the subjects were likely Caucasian [16].

Several studies examining the utility of screening have generated differing findings. For example, the ERSPC tried to answer the question of whether screening using PSA leads to an improvement in cancer specific survival. Remarkably, it noted that at 11 years of follow-up, 1,055 additional men would need to be screened and 37 extra cases of prostate cancer would need to be detected to prevent just one death from prostate cancer [17].

In the PLCO Trial, the men who underwent annual prostate cancer screening with PSA and digital rectal examination had a 12 % higher incidence of prostate cancer than men in the control group [18]. The rate of death due to prostate cancer, however, was equal amongst both groups of men [18]. This study also found negative consequences such as pain and bleeding being associated with follow-up and treatment of abnormal screening tests [18].

The Prostate Cancer Intervention Versus Observational Trial (PIVOT) study compared expectant management to radical prostatectomy [19]. Its findings indicated that there were no differences in outcomes of prostate cancer in black men compared to white men [19]. Despite this finding, however, black men have higher rates of mortality due to prostate cancer. Moreover, only 30 % of its participants were identified as African American; hence, the trial was likely under-powered due to selection bias and is not generalizable to the African American community [19]. Although the general prostate cancer population as a whole may have a strong proportion that is being over-treated, African American men generally appear to be facing undertreatment and thus, the higher mortality rates.

Molecular Markers

Evidence for differences between the course and outcome of prostate cancer in African American men also has been found in molecular markers. Several studies have been conducted regarding the location of SNPs and the differences in their rates of occurrence by race. Approximately 100 genes with SNPs are implicated in increasing men's susceptibility to prostate cancer [20, 21]. These are especially accurate because SNPs are stable throughout one's lifetime, so they cannot be affected by extraneous factors such as lifestyle [21]. Furthermore, several biomarkers appear to distinguish between aggressive and nonaggressive forms of prostate cancer; however, this information is not incorporated into conventional forms of prostate cancer screening [22]. The addition of genetic markers to current clinical parameters likely will detect the same number of prostate cancers without the need for a needle biopsy, making personalized medicine more effective and less invasive [23]. Unfortunately, African American men appear to be at an increased risk for developing prostate cancer in part because they possess several of these genetic variations. For instance, Xu et al. have reported that 17 of the 20 SNPs they have examined are more common in African American men and two of those 17 SNPs are associated with a higher risk of developing prostate cancer [24]. Other similar studies also have shown an association between African American men and specific genetic markers that appear to increase one's susceptibility for developing prostate cancer. For example, Freedman et al., noted there is a 3.8 MB interval on chromosome 8q24 that is associated with an increased risk of prostate cancer [25]. This chromosome interval is mainly found in African American men [25]. Individuals with a family history of allelic variants in this region are

9.46 times more likely to develop prostate cancer than someone without allelic variants [25].

Thus, despite the controversy associated with current prostate cancer screening, African American men need an updated set of screening guidelines that incorporate what is currently being used for screening with cutting edge molecular analyses to more successfully identify the patients who are at an increased risk of prostate cancer. Addressing the medical needs of such patients earlier will contribute significantly to reducing the burden of advanced disease, improve the chances of successful treatment, and lower the associated treatment costs.

Other considerations

In 2013, the American Urological Association mentioned that African American race is considered to be a risk factor for prostate cancer, and that screening with PSA should be individualized based on personal preference and an informed discussion with health care providers after weighing the costs versus the benefits associated with screening [26]. We believe that this statement is not robust enough for African Americans. The American Urological Association's stance has alluded to the fact that due to the difference in disease course, there ought to be some differences in the approach to screening for prostate cancer; however, we propose that this statement understates the necessity and importance of separate screening guidelines by failing to address the differences in disease course between African Americans and Caucasians.

The National Comprehensive Cancer Network and the American Cancer Society both also report that African American race is considered to be a risk factor for prostate cancer but they do not provide personalized screening guidelines [27, 28]. The American Cancer society goes one step further stating that African American men should begin discussions with their physician at age 45 (5 years earlier than men at average risk) [28]. However, neither the National Comprehensive Cancer Society nor the American Cancer Society have provided guidelines that meet the needs of African American men using an individualized approach.

It is also important to note that the lifetime risk of dying due to prostate cancer is approximately 3 % and men diagnosed with low to intermediate risk prostate cancer are unlikely to have a compromised lifespan due to said diagnosis [29]. Men with high risk prostate cancer do benefit from treatment if their projected life expectancy is greater than 10 years, but the majority of men who are diagnosed with high risk prostate cancer also have life expectancy of less than 10 years due to causes unrelated to their prostate cancer [27]. Hence, it is understandable that many individuals believe that prostate cancer is generally indolent and men who are diagnosed with prostate cancer often die of other causes unrelated to the cancer. However, it is our contention that this view is not generalizable to all prostate cancer patients as this data is derived from the entire male US population as opposed to considering just men of African American descent. Studies show that African American men with lower educational attainment have lower rates of prostate cancer screening; this discrepancy can in part be explained by a fatalistic attitude [30]. These fatalistic notions further highlight the importance of race specific guidelines for the African American community. By having separate screening guidelines, we can potentially overcome fatalism in African Americans regardless of their educational attainment and improve their survival.

It has been shown that African Americans have higher PSA levels in cancerous tumors [14, 31–35]. Even in non-cancerous prostates, African Americans have higher PSA levels [13, 36]. Furthermore, a large national cohort study found that African American veterans aged 40–54 were more likely to have 3 or more positive core biopsies yet they were less likely to be actively surveilled when compared to their white counterparts [36]. Indeed, African American veterans, aged 55–70, were more likely to have a higher grade and stage prostate cancer than African American veterans aged 40–54 [36]. There is new evidence, however, that highly undifferentiated tumors in African Americans may secrete less PSA [37]. This finding needs to be further explored, and the diversity of data available on this topic highlights the need for personalized guidelines.

Finally, it is crucial to consider that the current ad hoc approach to treatment of prostate cancer in African Americans is unreliable and needs to be better tailored. For example, Pietzak et al. found that the current criteria to evaluate which patients would benefit from active surveillance are not reliable in appropriately selecting African Americans when compared to Caucasians [38]. Kryvenko et al. found that over half of diagnosed prostate cancers considered to be insignificant (based on the Epstein criteria) were actually misclassified, in part due to a greater frequency of anterior tumors in African Americans compared to the tumors of white men [39]. Lastly, Sundi et al. have reported that African American men with very low risk prostate cancer at diagnosis still have a significantly higher prevalence of cancer at the anterior focus along with a higher grade and larger volume when compared to Caucasians [40].

Conclusion

We have shown that the general prostate cancer screening guidelines developed by the USPSTF may be inappropriate for African American men because the course of the disease is different for them due to social and genetic characteristics. Furthermore, African American men appear to intrinsically have a higher incidence of prostate cancer and higher rates of mortality. It is important to note that currently there is no cure for metastatic prostate cancer and unfortunately, African American men are the most likely individuals to present with aggressive prostate cancer at initial diagnosis that advances to metastatic prostate cancer [7]. At the same time, there are subsets of African American patients who may not need aggressive treatment at all, similar to the fair portion of the general population diagnosed with prostate cancer. Both these groups of patients are not readily identified and thus, the screening recommendations have to be examined separately from treatment recommendations [41]. Given the above, we conclude that separate prostate cancer screening guidelines are important if we are to improve outcomes and save the lives of of African American men. At this time, we are working towards developing such guidelines by conducting a survey among national prostate cancer specialists. These guidelines will be the subject of future correspondence.

Abbreviations
ERSPC: European Randomized Study of Screening for Prostate Cancer; PIVOT: Prostate Cancer Intervention versus Observational Trial; PLCO: Prostate, Lung, Colorectal, and Ovarian cancer screening trial; PSA: Prostate-Specific Antigen; SNP: Single Nucleotide Polymorphism; USPSTF: United States Preventive Services Task Force.

Competing interests
The authors declare that they have no competing interests.

Authors' contributions
DS participated in the background research and performed the initial draft for the manuscript. SP participated in the editing of the manuscript and incorporated the final research idea. AC participated in the editing of the manuscript. SV originated the idea for the manuscript, participated in the editing, and responsible for the overall outcome of the manuscript. All authors read and approved the final manuscript.

Acknowledgements
The authors are grateful to Cancer Institute Editor/Writer Cynthia Wall for help in editing this review.

Funding
N/A.

Author details
[1]University of Mississippi Medical School, Jackson, MS, USA. [2]University of Mississippi Medical Center, 2500 North State Street, 39216-4505 Jackson, MS, USA. [3]University of California, Los Angeles-David Geffen School of Medicine, Los Angeles, California, USA. [4]UMMC Cancer Institute, Department of Radiation Oncology, 2500 North State Street, 39216-4505 Jackson, MS, USA.

References
1. Siegel RL, Miller KD, Jemal A. Cancer Statistics 2015. CA Cancer J Clin. 2015;65(1):5–29.

2. SEER Cancer Statistics Review, 1975–2006. National Cancer Institute Web site. http://seer.cancer.gov/archive/csr/1975_2006/ Published 2009. Accessed 01 June 2015.

3. Odedina FT, Akinremi TO, Chinewundoh F, Roberts R, Yu D, Reams RR, et al. Prostate cancer disparities in Black men of African descent: a comparative literature review of prostate cancer burden among Black men in the United States, Caribbean, United Kingdom, and West Africa. Infect Cancer Agent. 2009;4(1):S2.

4. Behavioral Risk Factor Surveillance System Survey Data. Center for Disease Control and Prevention. http://www.cdc.gov/brfss/ Published 2009. Accessed 03 June 2015.

5. Powell IJ, Heilbrun L, Littrup PL, Franklin A, Parzuchowski J, Gelfand D, et al. Outcome of African American men screened for prostate cancer: the Detroit Education and Early Detection Study. J Urol. 1997;158(1):146–9.

6. Underwood W, De Monner S, Ubel P, Fagerlin A, Sanda MG, Wei JT. Racial/ethnic disparities in in the treatment of localized/regional prostate cancer. J Urol. 2004;171(4):1504–7.

7. Powell IJ, Bock CH, Ruterbush JJ, Sakr W. Evidence supports a faster growth rate and/or earlier transformation to clinically signifiant prostate cancer in black than in white American men, and influences racial progression and mortality disparity. J Urol. 2010;183(5):1792–6.

8. Henderson RJ, Eastham JA, Culkin DJ, Whatley T, Mata J, Venable D, et al. Prostate Specific Antigen (PSA) and PSA Density: Racial Differences in Men Without Prostate Cancer. J Natl Cancer Inst. 1997;89(2):134–8.

9. McIntosh H. Why Do African-American Men Suffer More Prostate Cancer? J Natl Cancer Inst. 1997;89(3):188–9.

10. Du XL, Fang S, Coker AL, Sanderson M, Aragaki C, Cormier JN, et al. Racial disparity and socioeconomic status in association with survival in older men with local/regional stage prostate carcinoma: findings from a large community-based cohort. Cancer. 2006;106(6):1276–85.

11. Ward E, Jemal A, Cokkinides V, Singh GK, Carinez C, Ghafoor A, et al. Cancer disparities by race/ethnic and socioeconomic status. CA Cancer J Clin. 2004;54(2):78–93.

12. Whittemore AS, Kolonel LN, Wu AH, John EM, Gallagher RP, Howe GR, et al. Prostate cancer in relation to diet, physical activity, and body size in blacks, whites, and Asians in the United States and Canada. J Natl Cancer Inst. 1995;87(9):652–61.

13. Abdalla I, Ray P, Ray V, Vaida F, Vijaykumar S. Comparison of serum prostate-specific antigen levels and PSA density in African-American, white, and Hispanic men without prostate cancer. Urology. 1998;51(2):300–5.

14. Vijayakumar S, Winter K, Sause W, Gallagher MJ, Michalski J, Roach M, et al. Prostatespecific antigen levels are higher in African-American than in white patients in a multicenter registration study: results of a RTOG 94–12. Int J Radiat Oncol Biol Phys. 1998;40(1):17–25.

15. Preston DM, Levin LI, Jacobson DJ, Jacobson SJ, Rubertone M, Holmes E, et al. Prostate specific antigen levels in young white and black men 20–45 years old. Urology. 2000;56(5):812–5.

16. Final Recommendation Statement: Prostate Cancer: Screening. U.S. Preventive Services Task Forcewebsite. http://www.uspreventiveservicestaskforce.org RecommendationStatementFinal/prostate-cancer-screening Published 2014. Accessed 04 June 2015.

17. Schröder FH, Hugosson J, Roobol MJ, Tammela TL, Ciatto S, Nelen V, et al. Prostate-cancer mortality at 11 years of follow-up. N Engl J Med. 2012;366(11):981–90.

18. Andriole GL, Crawford ED, Grubb 3rd RL, Buys S, Chia D, Church TR, et al. Prostate cancer screening in the randomized Prostate, Lung, Colorectal, and Ovarian Cancer Screening Trial: mortality results after 13 years of follow-up. J Natl Cancer Inst. 2012;104(2):125–32.

19. Wilt TJ, Brawer MK, Barry MJ, Jones KM, Kwon Y, Gingrich JR, et al. The Prostate cancer Intervention Versus Observation Trial:VA/NCI/AHRQ Cooperative Studies Program #407 (PIVOT): design and baseline results of a randomized controlled trial comparing radical prostatectomy to watchful waiting for men with clinically localized prostate cancer. Contemp Clin Trials. 2009;30(1):81–7.

20. Hicks C, Koganti T, Giri S, Tekere M, Ramani R, Sitthi-Amom J, et al. Integrative genomic analysis for the discovery of biomarkers in prostate cancer. Biomark Insights. 2014;29(9):39–51.

21. Helfand BT, Catalona WJ, Xu J. A genetic-based approach to personalized prostate cancer screening and treatment. Curr Opin Urol. 2015;25(1):53–8.

22. David S, Chan DW. Biomarkers in prostate cancer: what's new? Curr Opin Oncol. 2014;26(3):259–64.

23. Kader K, Sun J, Reck B, Newcombe PJ, Kim ST, Hsu FC, et al. Potential Impact of Adding Genetic Markers to Clinical Parameters in Predicting Prostate Biopsy Outcomes in Men Following an Initial Negative Biopsy: Findings from the REDUCE Trial. Eur Urol. 2012;62(6):953–61.

24. Xu J, Kibel AS, Hu JJ, Turner AR, Pruett K, Zheng SL, et al. Prostate cancer risk associated loci in African Americans. Cancer Epidemiol Biomarkers Prev. 2009;18(7):2145–9.

25. Freedman ML, Haiman CA, Patterson N, McDonald GJ, Tadon A, Waliszewsk A, et al. Admixture mapping identified 8q24 as a prostate cancer risk locus in African-American men. Proc Natl Acad Sci U S A. 2006;103(38):14068–73.

26. Carter HB, Albertson PC, Barry MJ, Etzioni R, Freedland SJ, Greene KL et al. Early Detection of Prostate Cancer: AUA Guidelines. https://www.auanet.org/ Published 2013. Accessed 04 Mar 2016.

27. National Comprehensive Cancer Network, Prostate Cancer. National Comprehensive Cancer Network website. http://www.nccn.org/patients/guidelines/prostate/ Published 2015. Accessed 03 Mar 2016.

28. Prostate Cancer Prevention and Early Detection. American Cancer society website. http://www.cancer.org/cancer/prostatecancer/moreinformation/prostatecancerearlydetection/prostate-cancer-early-detection-acs-recommendations. Accessed 03 Mar 2016.

29. Daskivich TJ. Life Expectancy and Treatment Choice for Men with High-risk Prostate Cancer. Eur Urol. 2015;68(1):59–60.

30. Hararah MK, Pollack CE, Garza MA, Yeh HC, Markakis D, Phelan-Emrick DF, et al. The Relationship Between Educational and Prostate-Specific Antigen Testing Among Urban African American Medicare Beneficiaries. J Racial Ethn Health Disparities. 2015;2(2):176–83.

31. Vijayakumar S, Karrison T, Weichselbaum RR, Quadri SF, Awan AM. Racial Differences in Prostate-specific Antigen Levels in Patients with Local-Regional Prostate Cancer. Cancer Epidemiol Biomarkers Prev. 1992;1(7):541–5.

32. Vijayakumar S, Weichselbaum RR, Vaida F, Dale W, Hellman S. Prostate-Specific Antigen Levels in African Americans Correlate with Insurance Status as an Indicator of Socioeconomic status. Cancer J Sci Am. 1996;2(4):225–33.

33. Asbell S, Vijayakumar S. Racial Differences in Prostate Specific Antigen Levels in Patients with Local-Regional Prostate Cancer. Prostate. 1997;31(1):42–6.

34. Vijayakumar S, Vaida F, Weichselbaum R, Hellman S. Race and the Will Rogers Phenomenon in Prostate Cancer. Cancer J Sci Am. 1998;4(1):27–34.

35. Abdalla I, Ray P, Vijayakumar S. Race and Serum Prostate-Specific Antigen Levels: Current Status and Future Directions. Semin Urol Oncol. 1998;16(4):207–313.

36. Saltzman AF, Luo S, Scherrer JF, Carson KD, Grubb III RL, Hudson MA. Earlier Prostate-specific antigen testing in African American men—Clinical support for the recommendation. Urol Oncol. 2015;33(7):330e9–17.

37. Kryvenko ON, Balise R, Soodana Prakash N, Epstein JI. African American Men with Gleason Score 3 + 3 = 6 Prostate Cancer Produces Less Prostate Specific Antigen than Caucasian Men: A Potential Impact on Active Surveillance. J Urol. 2016;195(2):301–6.

38. Pietzak EJ, Van Arsdalen K, Patel K, Malkowica SB, Wein AJ, Guzzo TJ. Impact of Race on Selecting Appropriate Patients for Active Surveillance with Seemingly Low-risk Prostate Cancer. Urology. 2015;85(2):436–40.

39. Kryvenko ON, Carter HB, Trock BJ, Epstein JI. Biopsy Criteria for Determining Appropriateness for Active Surveillance in the Modern Era. Urology. 2014;83(4):869–74.

40. Sundi D, Kryvenko ON, Carter HB, Ross AE, Epstein JI, Schaeffer EM. Pathological Examination of Radical Prostatectomy Specimens in Men with Very Low Risk Disease at Biopsy Reveals Distinct Zonal Distribution of Cancer in Black American Men. J Urol. 2014;191(1):60–7.

41. Adams LK, Ferrington LS. New recommendations in prostate cancer screening and treatment. JAAPA. 2014;27(8):14–20.

21

Do men regret prostate biopsy: Results from the PiCTure study

Catherine Coyle[1*], Eileen Morgan[2], Frances J. Drummond[3,4], Linda Sharp[3,5†] and Anna Gavin[2†]

Abstract

Background: Understanding men's experience of prostate biopsy is important as the procedure is common, invasive and carries potential risks. The psychological aspects of prostate biopsy have been somewhat neglected. The aim of this study was to explore the level of regret experienced by men after prostate biopsy and identify any associated factors.

Methods: Men attending four clinics in Republic of Ireland and two in Northern Ireland were given a questionnaire to explore their experience of prostate biopsy. Regret was measured on a Likert scale asking men how much they agreed with the statement "It [the biopsy] is something I regret."

Results: Three hundred thirty-five men responded to the survey. The mean age was 63 years (SD ±7 years). Three quarters of respondents (76%) were married or co-habiting, and (75%) finished education at primary or secondary school level. For just over two thirds of men (70%) their recent biopsy represented their first ever prostate biopsy. Approximately one third of men reported a diagnosis of cancer, one third a negative biopsy result, and the remaining third did not know their result. Two thirds of men reported intermediate or high health anxiety. 5.1% of men agreed or strongly agreed that they regretted the biopsy.

Conclusions: Level of regret was low overall. Health anxiety was the only significant predictor of regret, with men with higher anxiety reporting higher levels of regret than men with low anxiety (OR = 3.04, 95% CI 1.58, 5.84). Men with high health anxiety may especially benefit from careful counselling before and after prostate biopsy.

Keywords: Prostate, Biopsy, Regret

Background

Prostate biopsy is an invasive test that involves rectal insertion of an ultrasound probe to diagnose cancer of the prostate. It is usually prompted by a raised Prostate Specific Antigen (PSA), prostatic symptoms, an abnormal digital rectal examination (DRE) or a combination of these. The incidence of prostate cancer has until recently increased in most developed countries [1] and has the potential to increase further in future decades [2]. While acknowledging that predictions can be uncertain and that the ongoing debate about the benefits of screening for prostate cancer may also affect incidence, given population growth and the growing proportion of older people in the population, it is possible that the absolute

number of biopsies will increase further. Prostate biopsy can be difficult for men to tolerate, and commonly results in physical side effects [3, 4] including bleeding, pain, urinary retention and infection. While the physical side effects have been well investigated, the psychological impact of prostate biopsy has been somewhat neglected [5, 6].

Decision-related regret is a negative emotion associated with thinking about a choice one has made or is about to make [7]. Evidence has grown which shows that men who choose different treatment options for prostate cancer report differing levels of regret, and the factors which predict regret have become a focus of investigation [8]. Previous studies of men with prostate cancer suggest that the demographic factors of: older age [8], being single [8–10] and lower educational attainment [10, 11] were associated with higher levels of treatment regret. Clinically, those experiencing treatment-related complications/side effects [8], with better pre-operative

* Correspondence: catherine.coyle@hscni.net
†Equal contributors
[1]Public Health Agency, Belfast, Northern Ireland
Full list of author information is available at the end of the article

erectile function, post-operative incontinence, longer time from surgery to survey [8], and trait anxiety [9], were associated with higher levels of treatment regret. Decisional regret with respect to prostate biopsy does not appear to have been investigated.

The aim of this study was to investigate, for the first time, levels of decisional regret in men undergoing prostate biopsy and the factors associated with this. The hypothesis was that regret would be low and would not represent a significant burden for men undergoing prostate biopsy. The rationale for this was that men are likely to feel reassurance irrespective of the biopsy result; a negative biopsy result provides relief, and a positive result justifies the decision to proceed with biopsy.

Methods

Setting

The study took place on the island of Ireland, which comprises the Republic of Ireland (RoI) and Northern Ireland (NI). Four of the eight rapid access clinics (RAC) in the RoI public healthcare system agreed to take part in the study. In NI, two of the five Health and Social Care Trusts which are part of the public-funded NHS participated.

Ethical approval for the study was obtained for the four participating RoI hospitals and from the office for Research Ethics in Northern Ireland.

Recruitment

Men were recruited between November 2012 and December 2013. They were eligible to participate if they were undergoing prostatic biopsy as a result of a raised PSA level and/or an abnormal DRE, were over eighteen years of age, could understand English, were usually resident in either the RoI or NI, and were deemed well enough by their medical teams to complete a questionnaire, and in particular, had no cognitive impairment. They were ineligible if they had a previous diagnosis of prostate cancer.

Two methods of recruitment were used due to differing ethical and data protection requirements in the participating hospitals. In two hospitals in the RoI, a study information leaflet was sent to all men with their prostate biopsy appointment. Between four and six weeks post-biopsy these men were sent a questionnaire pack, with two reminder letters sent to non-responders at fortnightly intervals.

In the remaining hospitals all men, when attending for their prostate biopsy result, were given a questionnaire pack by nurse specialists. These men received no written reminders. In total 811 men were given/sent a questionnaire.

Questionnaire

The questionnaire captured socio-demographic information including date of birth, marital status, and educational attainment.

Men were asked about their urinary symptoms prior to first PSA test, and also questions about their route to PSA testing. They were also asked if, prior to biopsy, they had experienced urinary symptoms or erectile dysfunction. Information was requested regarding preparation for biopsy and number of cores taken.

Eighteen statements about men's feelings about prostate biopsy (both positive and negative) were developed based on discussions with prostate cancer survivor groups. Men were asked to record their level of agreement, on a 4-point Likert scale ranging from "strongly agree" to "strongly disagree", with each of the statements. Regret was measured with the statement "It [the biopsy] is something I regret."

Information was sought on the biopsy result. Men were asked questions about their experience of specific physical side effects following their most recent biopsy (fever, bleeding, pain, erectile dysfunction and urinary retention). Questions enquired about the severity, duration and need for treatment where these occurred.

The questionnaire was pretested with 24 men attending three prostate cancer groups in the RoI, and modified accordingly.

A copy of the questionnaire is included as Additional file 1.

Statistical analysis

As there is limited literature on regret of biopsy, the factors investigated were chosen based on the literature on regret after cancer treatment decisions, and are largely explorative. These included socio-demographic variables, health anxiety, clinical variables and physical side effects.

Ordinal logistic regression was used to explore relationships between these variables and regret. An initial univariate analysis was conducted. Physical side effects (fever, bleeding, pain, erectile dysfunction and urinary retention) were analysed as both 'any side effect', and also individually for an association with regret. Variables significant at $p < 0.10$ were added simultaneously to a multivariate model and likelihood ratio tests obtained to assess whether each variable should be included in the final model ($p \leq 0.05$). The proportional odds assumption was checked using a likelihood ratio test.

Chi-squared tests were used to investigate differences in characteristics between those who responded to the question on regret and those who did not.

Statistical analyses were conducted using STATA release 11 (StataCorp, College Station, TX).

Results

Three hundred thirty-five men responded to the survey (response rate 41%). The demographic features of respondents are shown in Table 1. The mean age was 63 years. Three-quarters of respondents (76%) were married or co-habiting, and 75% finished education at

Table 1 Socio-demographic and clinical characteristics of participants

	Frequency n (%)
Total	335 (100.0)
Socio-demographic variables	
Age at questionnaire completion	
< 65 years	192 (57.3)
≥ 65 years	140 (41.8)
Missing	3 (0.9)
Marital status	
Married/partnership	254 (75.8)
Other	80 (23.9)
Missing	1 (0.3)
Highest education level completed	
Primary/ secondary school	250 (74.6)
Third level	78 (23.3)
Missing	7 (2.1)
Employment status	
Working	128 (38.4)
Retired	130 (38.8)
Other	66 (19.7)
Missing	11 (3.3)
Health anxiety	
Low	112 (33.4)
Intermediate	148 (44.2)
High	74 (22.1)
Missing	1 (0.3)
Clinical variables	
Given choice of first PSA	
Yes	243 (72.5)
No	63 (18.8)
Missing	29 (8.7)
Pre-biopsy symptoms	
Incontinence	
None/mild	244 (72.8)
Moderate/severe	53 (15.8)
Missing	38 (11.3)
Erectile dysfunction	
None/mild	239 (71.3)
Moderate/severe	75 (22.4)
Missing	21 (6.3)
Symptoms at time of PSA test	
Asymptomatic	188 (56.1)
Symptomatic	119 (35.5)
Other/Missing	28 (8.4)

Table 1 Socio-demographic and clinical characteristics of participants *(Continued)*

Enough information pre-biopsy	
Yes received enough	270 (80.6)
Yes but would have liked more	25 (7.5)
No but did not want/need any	6 (1.8)
No but would have liked some	13 (3.9)
Missing	21 (6.3)
Biopsy result	
Negative	109 (32.5)
Positive	118 (35.2)
Don't know	108 (32.2)
Expectations of side-effects	
Same as expected	117 (34.9)
Worse than expected	46 (13.7)
Not as bad as expected	62 (18.5)
Did not have side-effects	97 (29.0)
Missing	13 (3.9)
Number of previous biopsies (including most recent biopsy)	
One	234 (69.9)
More than one	83 (24.8)
Missing	18 (5.4)
Physical Side-effects from biopsy	
Any side-effectZ[a]	
Yes	295 (88.1)
No	38 (11.3)
Missing	2 (0.6)

[a]Fever, bleeding, pain, erectile dysfunction and urinary retention

primary or secondary school level. 38% were working and 39% retired at the time of survey completion. For just over two thirds (70%) of men, their recent biopsy represented their first ever biopsy. Approximately one third of men reported a diagnosis of cancer, one third a negative biopsy result, and the remaining third did not know their result. 88% of men reported experiencing one or more physical side effects, most commonly bleeding (reported by 80%). Just over half (53.4%) of respondents reported that these were the same or better than expected. Two thirds of men reported high or intermediate health anxiety.

Of the 335 men, 11.9% did not respond to the question on regret and thus were excluded from further analysis. More of the men who completed the regret question were married or in a partnership (77.9% vs 62.5%, $p = 0.03$) and had third level education (26.7% vs. 2.5%, $p = 0.01$) compared to those who did not.

Of the 295 men who answered the regret question, 5.1% agreed (1.4%) or strongly agreed (3.7%) with the statement "It [the biopsy] is something I regret". 37.6% of men disagreed, and 57.3% strongly disagreed.

The univariate analysis found significant associations between health anxiety ($p < 0.01$) and number of previous prostate biopsies (including the most recent biopsy) ($p = 0.03$) with regret (Table 2). There was no association with individual physical side effects and regret, or with 'any physical side effect'. In multivariate analyses, the significant association between increasing health anxiety and biopsy regret remained after adjusting for number of biopsies. After adjusting for health anxiety, the number of biopsies was no longer significantly associated with regret (Table 3).

Discussion

This study found that overall levels of regret were low (5%) among men following prostate biopsy. A higher level of regret following prostate cancer treatment decisions (11–12%) has been reported in a number of published studies [8, 10, 12] suggesting the possibility of differences in how men view the decisions around biopsy and treatment. Further suggestion of the difference between biopsy and treatment regret is reflected in the different predictor variables significantly associated with regret in this study compared with the existing literature on regret following prostate cancer treatment. One theory to explain this difference and supported by our results is that these men may have received better pre-procedure counselling for prostate biopsy. This is based on more than 80% of men reporting that they received enough information before the biopsy, and less than one fifth of men had side effects worse than expected. Also, at this point more than one-third of these men did not have cancer, a fact for which they may be grateful that they had the biopsy. Further research is needed to clarify if and how predictors of regret in biopsy and treatment differ with the aim of ensuring men are appropriately prepared and counselled at each point in the prostate cancer diagnosis and treatment pathway.

The evidence base for PSA testing as a screening tool for prostate cancer – the route by which many men are referred for a prostate biopsy - includes conflicting results which has not as yet made a clear case for widespread PSA testing. However its use in Ireland [13] and elsewhere is widespread. Ransohoff and McNaughton Collins argue that this widespread use is because the system acts to make PSA attractive through positive feedback mechanisms [14]. A patient will be grateful for a negative PSA result or suspicious result followed by a negative biopsy; furthermore a positive PSA result followed by a cancer diagnosis makes the patient grateful for early detection. The clinician is also affected by positive feedback resulting from PSA testing and subsequent biopsy; we have previously shown that GPs who detect an asymptomatic prostate cancer via PSA testing were 3-times more likely to PSA test other asymptomatic men [15]. Additionally, litigation will usually only follow a cancer detected too late, not the one detected too early or which would never have caused harm.

This theory may explain why the level of regret reported by respondents in this survey was generally low; a negative biopsy result provides reassurance, and a positive result provides positive feedback that the test was worth it as the cancer has been detected.

Health anxiety was the only variable significantly associated with regret. Health anxiety can be thought of as a continuum, with hypochondriasis at the extreme. It is characterised by attentional biases towards illness-related information and cognitive biases leading to the misinterpretation of information as personally threatening and catastrophic [16]. Miles et al. [16] examined health anxiety in the context of screening for colorectal cancer and found that people with high health anxiety were less reassured following screening. In this study we found that men with higher health anxiety report higher levels of regret and, following from Miles et al. [16], it may be that men with high health anxiety were less reassured following prostate biopsy, and therefore were more likely to regret the procedure.

This study does have some limitations. The questionnaire designed to collect this data was in effect a new instrument. However it was tested for face validity and comprehension with 24 men in the RoI, and available validated tools were used within the questionnaire such as the Health Anxiety Questionnaire by Lucock and Morley, 1996. The limited sample size coupled with the low level of regret may explain in part why so few variables were associated with regret. The response rate is another limitation and we do not have any information on the characteristics of responders and non-responders, so we cannot assess participation bias. Respondents who answered the question on regret were more likely to be married or in a partnership and to have third level education than those who did not. The literature cited previously on regret after treatment decisions indicates that being married or in a partnership, and higher levels of educational attainment are associated with lower levels of regret. This suggests we may have somewhat underestimated regret in the current study.

The major strength of the study is that we were able to test a wide variety of variables for an association with regret. The inclusion of men from two jurisdictions with differing health systems increases generalizability.

The study overall can be viewed as a pilot study into regret among men following prostate biopsy and associated factors. This should raise the profile of this issue among researchers and the health community which may in turn lead to further research to explore this in other populations.

Table 2 Results of univariate ordinal logistic regression testing for association of predictor variables with regret post-biopsy: odds ratios (OR) with 95% confidence intervals (CI) and p- values

	Frequency	Univariate Analysis	
	n (%)	OR (95% CI)[a]	p-value*
Total	295 (100.0)		
Socio-demographic variables			
Age at questionnaire completion			
<65 years	174 (59.0)	1.00	
≥65 years	118 (40.0)	0.89 (0.56, 1.42)	0.64
Missing	3 (1.0)		
Marital status			
Married/ partnership	229 (77..6)	1.00	
Other	65 (22.0)	0.99 (0.57, 1.71)	0.96
Missing	1 (0.3)		
Highest education level completed			
Primary/secondary school	211 (71.5)	1.00	
Third level	77 (26.1)	0.67 (0.40, 1.14)	0.14
Missing	7 (2.4)		
Employment status			
Working	114 (38.6)	1.00	
Retired	117 (39.7)	0.72 (0.43, 1.22)	
Other	55 (18.6)	1.17 (0.62, 2.19)	0.27
Missing	9 (3.1)		
Health anxiety			
Low	100 (33.9)	1.00	
Intermediate	132 (44.8)	1.80 (1.05, 3.10)	
High	63 (21.4)	3.18 (1.68, 6.02)	0.001
Missing	0 (0.0)		
Clinical variables			
Given choice of first PSA			
Yes	215 (72.9)	1.00	
No	57 (19.3)	0.86 (0.48, 1.53)	0.60
Missing	23 (7.8)		
Pre-biopsy symptoms			
Incontinence			
None/mild	222 (75.3)	1.00	
Moderate/severe	45 (15.3)	1.12 (0.59, 2.11)	0.73
Missing	28 (9.5)		
Erectile dysfunction			
None/mild	213 (72.2)	1.00	
Moderate/ severe	65 (22.0)	1.08 (0.62, 1.89)	0.77
Missing	17 (5.8)		
Symptoms at time of PSA test			
Asymptomatic	166 (56.3)	1.00	
Symptomatic	106 (35.9)	1.34 (0.83, 2.17)	0.23
Other/Missing	23 (7.8)		

Table 2 Results of univariate ordinal logistic regression testing for association of predictor variables with regret post-biopsy: odds ratios (OR) with 95% confidence intervals (CI) and p- values *(Continued)*

Enough information pre-biopsy			
Yes received enough	238 (80.7)	1.00	
Yes but would have liked more	24 (8.1)	1.84 (0.81, 4.19)	
No but did not want/need any	5 (1.7)	2.84 (0.47, 17.27)	
No but would have liked some	12 (4.1)	1.10 (0.34, 3.54)	0.36
Missing	16 (5.4)		
Biopsy result			
Negative	106 (35.9)	1.00	
Positive	97 (32.9)	1.45 (0.84, 2.51)	
Don't know	92 (31.2)	1.34 (0.76, 2.35)	0.38
Expectations of side-effects			
Same as expected	108 (36..6)	1.00	
Worse than expected	41 (13.9)	1.97 (0.98, 3.96)	
Not as bad as expected	54 (18.3)	1.39 (0.72, 2.68)	
Did not have side-effects	83 (28.1)	1.08 (0.60, 1.93)	0.24
Missing	9 (3.1)		
Number of biopsies			
One	209 (70.9)	1.00	
More than one	72 (24.4)	0.62 (0.36, 1.07)	0.08
Missing	14 (4.8)		
Physical Side-effects from biopsy			
Any side-effect[b]			
Yes	263 (89.2)	1.00	
No	32 (10.9)	0.88 (0.42, 1.84)	0.74
Missing	0 (0.0)		

*p-values obtained from the likelihood ratio test
[a]The OR for ordinal logistic regression shows the likelihood of having an increased level of the outcome variable (regret) within each category of the predictor variable compared to a reference category in the predictor variable
[b]Fever, bleeding, pain, erectile dysfunction and urinary retention

Table 3 Results of multivariate ordinal logistic regression: multivariate model including predictor variables which had p-value <0.10 in univariate ordinal logistic regression - odds ratios (OR) with 95% confidence intervals (CI) and p- values

Variable	OR (95% CI)	p-values*
Number of previous biopsies (including most recent biopsy)		
One	1.00	
More than one	0.68 (0.39, 1.19)	0.17
Health anxiety		
Low	1.00	
Intermediate	1.87 (1.07, 3.26)	<0.01
High	3.04 (1.58, 5.84)	

*p-values obtained from the likelihood ratio test

Conclusions

In conclusion, regret is low overall shortly after a prostate biopsy. Men with high health anxiety are more likely to report higher levels of regret. These men may especially benefit from careful counselling before and after biopsy. Given the potential for the number of biopsies being performed to increase and the limited evidence-base, further research on different aspects of men's views and experiences of biopsy would be of value.

Abbreviations
DRE: Digital rectal examination; NI: Northern Ireland; PSA: Prostate specific antigen; RAC: Rapid access clinics; RoI: Republic of Ireland

Acknowledgements
The authors thank the clinical teams; Mr Garrett Durkan, Mr David Galvin, Mr Gordan Smyth, Ms Sheila Keily, Ms Sara White, Ms Eimear Dunne, Moya Power and Ms Rosaleen Padin, who facilitated recruitment of men to this study. The authors thank Dr Heather Kinnear for work in the design and administration of the survey.

Funding
Prostate Cancer UK, the Health Research Board and the R&D office of NI Public Health Agency funded the study. The NI Cancer Registry is funded by the NI Public Health Agency and the National Cancer Registry Ireland by the Department of Health. None of the funding bodies had a role in the design, data collection, analysis or interpretation of the data contained within this manuscript.

Availability of data and materials
The data are not available at this time because the study team are currently working on other papers based on these. The questionnaire is provided as Additional file 1.

Authors' contributions
AG and LS obtained the initial funding for the study, and AG, LS and FJD obtained additional funding for the study. AG, LS and FD contributed to study design and questionnaire development. FD undertook data collection. EM and LS provided statistical advice and EM and CC analysed the data. All authors contributed to the interpretation of the results and drafting the manuscript. All authors have approved the final manuscript.

Competing interests
LS held an unrestricted project grant, 2011–2012, from Sanofi-Aventis for research into patterns of treatment and survival for prostate cancer. The remaining authors have no competing interests.

Ethics approval and consent to participate
Ethical approval for the study was obtained for the participating RoI hospitals:
Beaumont Hospital 19/1/12
Mater Misericordiae University Hospital 2/5/13
University Hospital Galway 4/1/12
University Hospital Limerick 11/10/12
Ethical approval was granted in August 2012 from the Office for Research Ethics in Northern Ireland (ORECNI) (Ref 12/NI/0106). Potential participants received a pack either by post or in person depending on their study area, which included a study information sheet, questionnaire and consent form.

Those who chose to take part in the study were requested to return, by post, a completed and signed consent form together with the completed questionnaire.

Author details
[1]Public Health Agency, Belfast, Northern Ireland. [2]Northern Ireland Cancer Registry, Queen's University, Belfast, Northern Ireland. [3]National Cancer Registry Ireland, Cork, Ireland. [4]Department of Epidemiology and Public Health, University College Cork, Cork, Ireland. [5]Institute of Health & Society, Newcastle University, Newcastle, UK.

References
1. Wong MCS, Goggins WB, Wang HHX, Fung FDH, Leung C, Wong SYS, Ng CF, Sung JJY. Global incidence and mortality for prostate cancer: Analysis of temporal patterns and trends in 36 countries. Eur Urol. 2016; 70:862–74.
2. Maddams J, Utley M, Møller H. Projections of cancer prevalence in the United Kingdom, 2010–2040. Br J Cancer. 2012;107:1195–202.
3. Nobrega de Jesus CM, Correa LA, Padovani CR. Complications and risk factors in transrectal ultrasound-guided prostate biopsies. Sao Paulo Med J. 2006;124(4):198–202.
4. Jeon SS, Woo SH, Hyun JH, Choi HY, Chaie SE. Bisacodyl rectal preparation can decrease infectious complications of transrectal ultrasound-guided prostate biopsy. Urology. 2003;62:461–6.
5. De Sio M, D'armiento M, Di Lorenzo G, Damiano R, Perdona S, De Placido S, et al. The need to reduce patient discomfort during transrectal ultrasonography-guided prostate biopsy: what do we know? BJU Int. 2005; 96:977–83.
6. Wade J, Rosario DJ, Macefield RC, Avery KNL, Salter E, Goodwin ML, et al. Psychological Impact of Prostate Biopsy: Physical Symptoms, Anxiety, and Depression. J Clin Oncol. 2013;31(33):4235–41.
7. Connolly T, Reb J. Regret in cancer-related decisions. Health Psychol. 2005; 24 Suppl 4:29–34.
8. Lavery HJ, Levinson AW, Hobbs AR, Sebrow D, Mohamed NE, Diefenbach MA, et al. Baseline functional status may predict decisional regret following robotic prostatectomy. J Urol. 2012;188:2213–8.
9. Berry DL, Wang Q, Halpenny B, Hong F. Decision preparation, satisfaction and regret in a multi-center sample of men with newly diagnosed localized prostate cancer. Patient Educ Couns. 2012;88:262–7.
10. Sidana A, Hernandez DJ, Feng Z, Partin AW, Trock BJ, Saha S, et al. Treatment decision-making for localized prostate cancer: what younger men choose and why. Prostate. 2012;72(1):58–64.
11. Hu JC, Kwan L, Saigal CS, Litwin MS. Regret in men treated for localized prostate cancer. J Urol. 2003;169:2279–83.
12. Morris BB, Farnan L, Song L, Addington EL, Chen RC, Nielsen ME, et al. Treatment decisional regret among men with prostate cancer: Racial differences and influential factors in the North Carolina Health Access and Prostate Cancer Treatment Project (HCaP-NC). Cancer. 2015;121(12): 2029–35.
13. Drummond FJ, Barrett E, Burns R, O'Neill C, Sharp L. The number of tPSA tests continues to rise and variation in testing practices persists: a survey of laboratory services in Ireland 2008–2010. Ir J Med Sci. 2014;183(3):369–75.
14. Ransohoff DF, McNaughton Collins M, Fowler FJ. Why is prostate cancer screening so common when the evidence is so uncertain? A system without negative feedback. Am J Med. 2002;113:663–7.
15. Drummond FJ, Carsin AE, Sharp L, Comber H. Factors prompting PSA-testing of asymptomatic men in a country with no guidelines: a national survey of general practitioners. BMC Fam Pract. 2009. doi:10.1186/1471-2296-10-3.
16. Miles A, Wardle J. Adverse psychological outcomes in colorectal cancer screening: does health anxiety play a role? Behav Res Ther. 2006;44:1117–27.

22

Degarelix therapy for prostate cancer in a real-world setting: experience from the German IQUO (Association for Uro-Oncological Quality Assurance) Firmagon® registry

Götz Geiges[1*], Thomas Harms[2], Gerald Rodemer[3], Ralf Eckert[4], Frank König[5], Rolf Eichenauer[6] and Jörg Schroder[5]

Abstract

Background: We investigated the use of the gonadotropin-releasing hormone (GnRH) antagonist degarelix in everyday clinical practice using registry data from uro-oncology practices in Germany.

Methods: Data were analysed retrospectively from the IQUO (Association for uro-oncological quality assurance) patient registry. Data were prospectively collected from all consecutive PCa patients treated with degarelix ($n = 1010$) in 138 uro-oncology practices in Germany between May 2009 and December 2013.

Results: Median overall survival had not yet been reached in the all-patient group or in subgroups who had or had not received prior hormonal therapy (HT). Cox regression analysis showed that patients who had received prior HT ($n = 542$) had a 58 % increased mortality risk (hazard ratio 1.58, 95 % CI 1.20–2.09) versus patients who had not ($n = 468$) ($p = 0.001$). Also, in patients who had received prior luteinizing hormone-releasing hormone (LHRH) analogue therapy (LHRH agonists or GnRH antagonists), median time to PSA progression was shorter (209 weeks) than in those who had not received prior LHRH analogues ($n = 555$; median PSA progression-free survival not yet reached). Degarelix was generally well tolerated.

Conclusions: Degarelix was effective and well tolerated in everyday clinical practice, confirming observations from clinical studies. Patients who received prior HT appeared to have a significantly higher mortality risk.

Keywords: Degarelix, Prostate cancer, Registry

Background

The gonadotropin-releasing hormone (GnRH) antagonist, degarelix, is an effective and well tolerated treatment for advanced prostate cancer (PCa) [1–3]. As an antagonist, degarelix benefits from a direct mechanism of action that inhibits GnRH without causing an initial surge in gonadotropins or consequently testosterone [4]. Degarelix displays similar efficacy to the luteinizing hormone-releasing hormone (LHRH) agonist, leuprolide, for testosterone suppression in PCa [1]. However, testosterone reduction was more rapid with degarelix and,

unlike leuprolide, occurred without a testosterone surge or microsurges; in advanced disease, the testosterone surge associated with LHRH agonists can produce symptom flare [5]. Degarelix also displayed superior prostate-specific antigen (PSA) progression-free survival (PFS) compared with leuprolide [6] and in metastatic disease was associated with better control of the bone formation marker serum alkaline phosphatase (S-ALP), suggesting that it might offer prolonged control of skeletal metastases [7].

While degarelix has been well studied in clinical trials, it is important to examine its efficacy and tolerability in everyday clinical practice. Clinical trials give important data about treatment effects in controlled conditions,

* Correspondence: goetz.geiges@freenet.de
[1]Arztpraxis für Urologie (Partnerpraxis der Charité), Berlin, Germany
Full list of author information is available at the end of the article

but patient registries offer additional data from a wide population (with few excluded patients), allowing evaluation of care as actually provided [8]. Consequently, registry data are likely to provide a more representative indication of the real-world patient experience with degarelix. Therefore, the current study investigated the use of degarelix in patients from uro-oncology practices in Germany by analysing data from the IQUO (Association for uro-oncological quality assurance) Firmagon® patient registry.

Methods

Data were analysed retrospectively from the IQUO (Association for uro-oncological quality assurance) patient registry records using the QuaSi-URO® documentation system, a live system based on data from IQUO members. Data from the Firmagon® Registry (The Electronic Therapy Documentation [ETD] Firmagon® – Urology) were prospectively collected from all consecutive patients with PCa treated with degarelix in 138 uro-oncology practices in Germany between 27 May 2009 and 10 December 2013. All patients with PCa receiving degarelix who were entered into ETD Firmagon® were documented and all patients with at least one fully documented entry in the registry were included. The only criterium for inclusion into the registry was prescription of degarelix, thus everyday usage should be mirrored by this register. The decision to treat patients with degarelix was taken by the treating physician before the decision for inclusion into the registry.

The underlying data collection for this publication was performed in accordance with the principles of the Declaration of Helsinki. The data collection did not take place in a study environment but utilized electronic data capture according to the documentation system and documentation guidelines of the IQUO. Within the electronic data capture there is no personal or patient identifying information; data were collected anonymously and pseudonymised. Identification of patients is possible only by the physician and the documentation staff. Therefore, according to three independent legal opinions there was no need for ethics committee approval or a patient consent form.

Study variables

The data repository was reviewed for information on the following variables: tumour response to degarelix; overall survival (OS); PSA PFS; percentage change in median PSA and testosterone over time; percentage of patients with PSA ≤ 4 ng/ml over time; percentage change in median S-ALP over time; change in mean prostate volume. These variables were measured for patient subgroups as summarized in Table 1. Prior hormonal therapy (HT) included LHRH agonists, GnRH antagonists or antiandrogens. Prior LHRH analogue therapy included LHRH agonists or GnRH antagonists. Recording of the testosterone, S-ALP and prostate volume at the time of documentation was optional.

Tumour response (objective progression or stabilization, complete or partial remission) was assessed using the Response Evaluation Criteria In Solid Tumors [RECIST] guidelines [9] and measured at 6-month intervals up to a total duration of 3 years. Median time to PSA progression was defined according to Prostate Cancer Clinical Trials Working Group [PCWG2] criteria: a ≥ 25 % increase and an absolute increase of ≥ 2 ng/ml from the nadir, confirmed by a second value ≥ 3 weeks later [10]. At the time of PSA progression, patients were also required to have testosterone levels < 0.5 ng/ml [castration level]. The date of PSA progression was the date of the first PSA test value.

Percentage change in median PSA, testosterone and S-ALP, and mean prostate volume were measured monthly during the first year of treatment and thereafter in 3-monthly intervals for up to 39 months. Percentage change in median PSA and percentage of patients with PSA ≤ 4 ng/ml are presented for 3-month intervals for up to 36 and 24 months, respectively. Longer term data is not shown due to the smaller patient numbers towards the end of the evaluation period, especially in subgroups. Since collection of testosterone, ALP and prostate volume data was optional, patient numbers are smaller and therefore percentage change in median testosterone is presented for up to 2 years (1 year in metastatic disease subgroup), S-ALP for up to 1 year and mean prostate volume for up to 6 months.

The first data point in the registry refers to the time of the first administration of degarelix (baseline). In ongoing treatments, the last data point refers to the time of the last documented administration of a degarelix dose.

Statistics

Change in PSA, S-ALP, and prostate volume are summarized using descriptive statistics (percentage change, percentage change in median, mean). OS and PSA PFS were analysed using the Kaplan–Meier method. Survival was calculated from the date of first treatment until the date of any cause of death.

Results

Patients

A total of 1,010 patients received degarelix and were included. Baseline demographic and disease characteristics of the registry population are summarized in Table 2. Around two-thirds of patients had localized ($n = 469$) or locally advanced ($n = 201$) disease (340 had metastatic disease) and almost half had a Gleason score of 8–10.

Table 1 Summary of efficacy evaluations according to patient subgroup

Evaluation	Patient subgroup						
	All patients	Patients with metastatic disease	Prior HT[a]	No prior HT	Baseline PSA ≥20 ng/ml	Prior LHRH analogue therapy[b]	No prior LHRH analogue therapy
Tumour response	√						
Overall survival	√		√	√		√	√
PSA progression-free survival	√	√				√	√
Percentage change in median PSA	√	√	√	√			
Percentage change in median testosterone	√	√	√	√			
Percentage change in median S-ALP		√		√			
Mean prostate volume	√						
Percentage of patients with PSA ≤ 4 ng/ml	√	√			√		

[a]LHRH agonists, GnRH antagonists or antiandrogens; [b]LHRH agonists or GnRH antagonists

A total of 542 patients had received prior HT, predominantly LHRH agonists (53.7 %); of these, 455 had received prior LHRH analogue therapy (LHRH agonists or GnRH antagonists). Baseline PSA (median 14.27 ng/ml) was ≥20 ng/ml in 43.6 % of patients.

At the time of this report, a total of 401, 158 and 44 patients had received degarelix for 12, 24 and 36 months, respectively; only two patients had received treatment for 48 months, reflecting entry to the register over time, at the time of this analysis.

Reasons for discontinuation of degarelix in patients with documented answers (n = 479) included change in therapy (30.7 %), patient request/others (22.8 %), death (14.2 %), PSA progression (14.4 %), clinical progression (7.5 %), adverse event (6.1 %) or lost to follow-up (4.4 %).

Tumour response

After 1 year of treatment, among patients with a documented response (n = 221), 19.9 % (n = 44) had complete remission, 19.5 % (n = 43) partial remission, 27.6 % (n = 61) objective stabilization and 21.7 % (n = 48) objective progression; 11.3 % (n = 25) were not evaluable. After 24 months (n = 80), these values were 18.8 % (n = 15), 22.5 % (n = 18), 25.0 % (n = 20), 22.5 % (n = 18) and 11.3 % (n = 9), respectively. After 36 months, (n = 23), these values were 34.8 % (n = 8), 17.4 % (n = 4), 21.7 % (n = 5), 26.1 % (n = 6) and 0 % (n = 0), respectively. Patient responses over time are summarized in Fig. 1.

Overall survival

In total, 212 of 1,010 patients died and 51 were lost to follow-up. The median OS (all patients) had not yet been reached; the 75th percentile value (i.e. where 25 % of patients had reached event) was 148.9 weeks.

While the median OS had also not yet been reached in patients with or without prior HT, the 75th percentile value was longer for those without prior HT (176.4 weeks) compared with those with prior HT (131.7 weeks). A Cox regression analysis showed patients who received prior HT (n = 542) had a 58 % increased mortality risk (hazard ratio 1.58, 95 % CI 1.20–2.09) compared with patients who had not received prior HT (n = 468) (p = 0.001).

Similarly, median OS had not been reached in patients with or without prior LHRH analogue therapy (LHRH agonist/GnRH antagonist), however, the 75th percentile value was shorter (123.1 weeks) in those who received prior LHRH analogues compared with those who had not (167.4 weeks).

PSA PFS

Of the 1,010 patients in this study, 200 (20 %) experienced PSA progression, 137 patients died, 41 were lost to follow-up and 632 were alive and PSA progression-free. Median PSA PFS was not yet reached; the 75th percentile value for PSA PFS was 59.6 weeks.

Of the 340 patients with metastatic disease, 91 (27 %) experienced PSA progression. Median time to PSA progression (PSA PFS) was 141.4 weeks (75th percentile value 32.4 weeks).

In patients who received prior LHRH analogue therapy (n = 455), median time to PSA progression was shorter (209 weeks [75th percentile value 30.4 weeks]) than in those who had not received prior LHRH analogues (n = 555) where median PSA PFS was not reached (75th percentile value 88.4 weeks). Also, a greater proportion of patients who received prior LHRH analogue therapy (25.05 %; n = 114) experienced PSA progression compared with those who had not (15.5 %, n = 86).

Table 2 Baseline patient characteristics

Characteristic	$N = 1,010$ (100)
Mean (SD) age,[1] years	70.29 (8.55)
Mean (SD) BMI,[1] kg/m^2	26.88 (3.81)
Median (range) PSA ng/ml	14.27 (0–6131)
Median (range) testosterone ng/ml ($n = 266$)[a]	0.52 (0–34.45)
Testosterone categories n, % ($n = 266$)	
<0.1 ng/ml	26 (9.8)
0.1– ≤0.2 ng/ml	54 (20.3)
0.2–0.5 ng/ml	48 (18.1)
> 0.5 ng/ml	138 (51.9)
Disease stage n (%)	
Localized[b]	469 (46)
Locally advanced[c]	201 (20)
Metastatic[d]	340 (34)
Gleason score n, %	$N = 868$
2–4	13 (1.5)
5–6	130 (15.0)
7	290 (33.4)
8–10	416 (47.9)
Not classified	19 (2.2)
PSA categories n, %	
< 10 ng/ml	438 (43.4)
10– ≤20 ng/ml	133 (13.1)
20–50 ng/ml	160 (15.8)
> 50 ng/ml	279 (27.6)
Previous treatment	
Watchful waiting (%)	
N	829 (82.1)
Y	181 (17.9)
External radiotherapy (%)	
N	783 (77.5)
Y	227 (22.5)
Brachytherapy (%)	
N	990 (98.0)
Y	20 (2.0)
High-intensity focused ultrasound(%)	
N	1002 (99.2)
Y	8 (0.8)
Radical prostatectomy (%)	
N	764 (75.6)
Y	246 (24.4)
Hormone therapy (%)	
N	468 (46.3)
Y	542 (53.7)
LHRH agonists	309 (57.0)

Table 2 Baseline patient characteristics (Continued)

GnRH antagonist	146 (26.9)
Antiandrogen	87 (16.1)
Palliative therapy (%)	
N	766 (75.8)
Y	244 (24.2)

Baseline is defined as the beginning of degarelix therapy. [a]Documentation of the testosterone value was optional; [b]Localized disease: T1/T2, NX or N0, and MX or M0; [c]Locally advanced disease: T3/T4, NX or N0, and MX or M0; [d]Metastatic disease: N1 or M1, any T
[1]Recorded at the time of initial diagnosis of PCa

PSA

Overall, degarelix produced a rapid and profound PSA reduction, sustained for up to 36 months (Fig. 2a). A similar PSA profile was observed in patients with baseline metastatic disease (Fig. 2b). PSA suppression was greater and more rapid, and maintenance of PSA suppression more effective, in patients who had not received prior HT compared with those who had received prior HT (Fig. 2c–d).

Overall, PSA reduction to ≤ 4 ng/ml was achieved in 65 % of patients at 12 months and 71 % of patients at 24 months (Fig. 3a). These values were lower in patients with metastatic disease (41 % and 63 %, respectively) and patients with baseline PSA ≥20 ng/ml (41 % and 44 %, respectively); (Fig. 3b–c).

Testosterone

Overall, degarelix produced a rapid and profound reduction in testosterone (an optional measurement), falling to 0.19 ng/mL after 1 month ($n = 217$). Testosterone suppression <20 ng/mL was sustained for the first 24 months in the all-patient group (median testosterone 0.13 ng/mL at 24 months [$n = 18$]). Testosterone was also suppressed in patients with baseline metastatic disease: median testosterone level was 0.2 ng/mL after 1 month ($n = 92$) and 0.13 ng/mL at 12 months ($n = 20$).

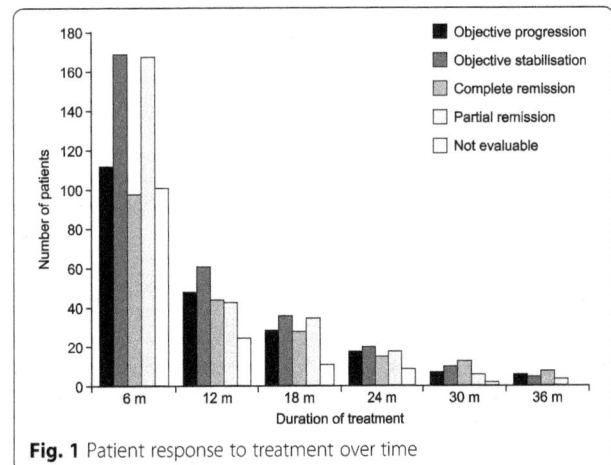

Fig. 1 Patient response to treatment over time

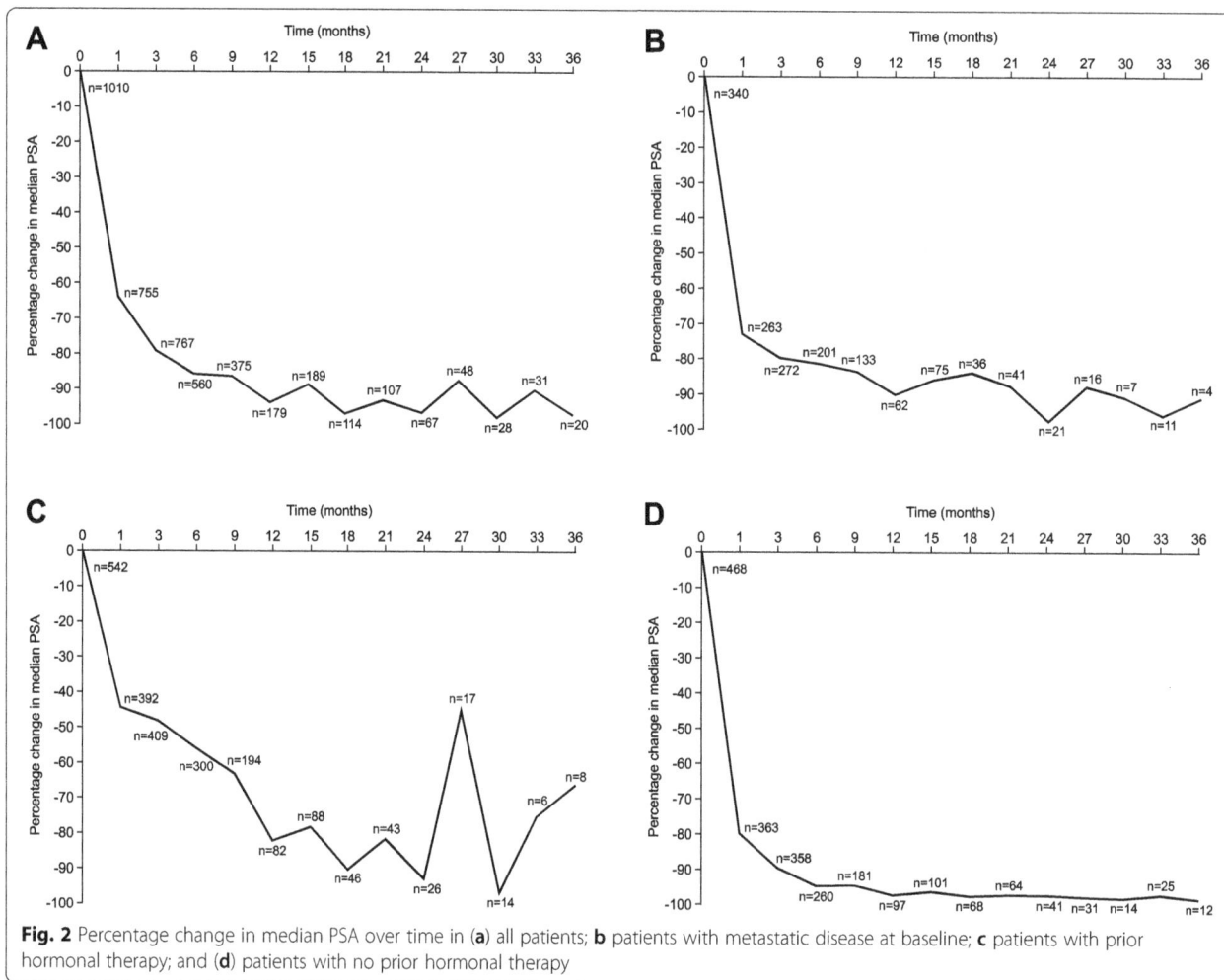

Fig. 2 Percentage change in median PSA over time in (**a**) all patients; **b** patients with metastatic disease at baseline; **c** patients with prior hormonal therapy; and (**d**) patients with no prior hormonal therapy

S-ALP

Changes in S-ALP (an optional measurement) over time for patients with metastatic disease ($n = 70$ at 0 months and $n = 11$ at 12 months) and those without prior HT ($n = 53$ at 0 months and $n = 11$ at 12 months) are summarized in Fig. 4. In the metastatic cohort, S-ALP was suppressed after 6–12 months of treatment. S-ALP suppression was observed after 1 month in patients with no prior HT and this was maintained for up to 12 months.

Prostate volume

Mean prostate volume decreased from 36.83 ml at baseline ($n = 85$ patients) to 30.32 ml ($n = 25$) after 3 months and to 26.38 ml after 6 months ($n = 16$).

Tolerability

The most frequent adverse events recorded in patients included hot flushes (12.9 %), injection site erythema (8.5 %), fatigue (5.2 %) and pain (4.2 %). Adverse events experienced by patients at the first and last data points during degarelix therapy are summarized in Table 3.

Apart from a slight increase in the incidence of hot flushes, there were no significant changes in frequency of adverse events between the first and last data points.

Discussion

Patient registries offer a unique and powerful tool for the collection of observational and clinical data, helping provide a clearer understanding of a therapy's impact on patients in a real-world context. While patient populations in clinical trials are tightly controlled, with rigorous selection criteria, registries generally have much broader inclusion criteria and fewer exclusion criteria which can lead to greater generalizability [11].

Degarelix is a GnRH antagonist for the first-line treatment of androgen-dependent advanced PCa. However, comparison of patient populations in the Firmagon registry versus clinical trials shows that while degarelix trials excluded patients with previous hormonal management of PCa (except those who underwent localized therapy of curative intent in which neoadjuvant or adjuvant HT for ≤ 6 months was accepted) [1, 3, 12, 13], over half the patients in the current registry had received

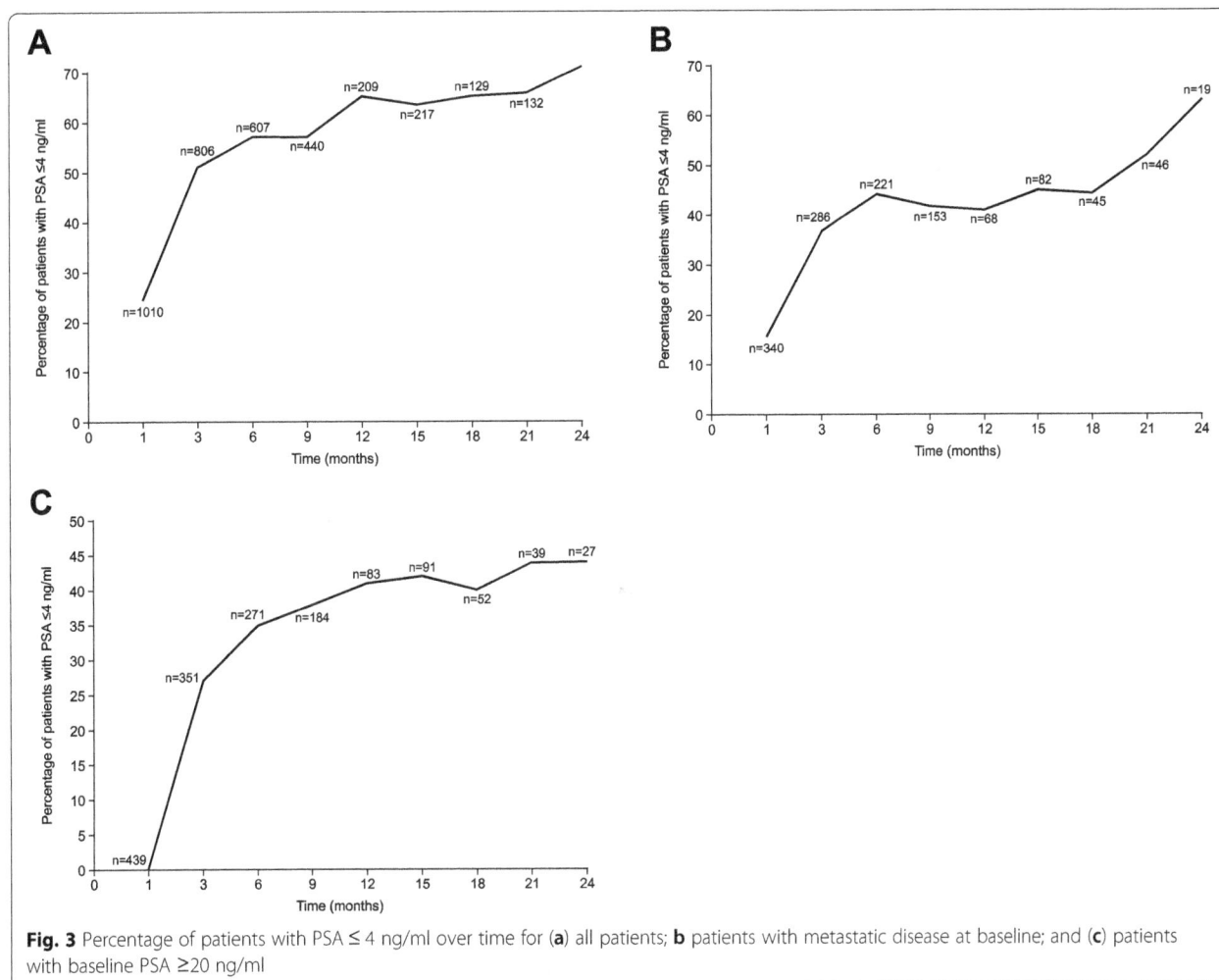

Fig. 3 Percentage of patients with PSA ≤ 4 ng/ml over time for (**a**) all patients; **b** patients with metastatic disease at baseline; and (**c**) patients with baseline PSA ≥20 ng/ml

prior HT (30 % of the total population had received prior LHRH agonists). It was observed that, in this study of real-world experience with degarelix therapy, of those with documented answers, degarelix was discontinued in 30.7 % of patients due to a change in therapy and in 22.8 % as a result of patient request/other reasons compared with 14.4 % of patients discontinuing due to PSA progression and 7.5 % due to clinical progression. Information regarding the reasons for patients changing therapy was not collected in the current analysis; reasons for changing treatment may possibly include higher expectations regarding efficacy and/or lowering side effects.

Also, 34 % of the registry population had baseline metastastic disease compared with around 20 % [1, 12, 13] to 23 % [3] in clinical trials. Interestingly, in our registry, 46 % of patients who received degarelix had localised disease and over half had PSA ≤20 ng/mL. In the community setting, ADT has been used commonly as primary therapy for localised prostate cancer [14] particularly in the elderly [15]. However, European Association of Urology guidelines consider androgen suppression to be unsuitable as

primary therapy for low-risk prostate cancer and consider that, in patients with non-metastatic localised disease not suitable for curative treatment, immediate ADT should be used only in patients requiring symptom palliation [16].

In the current study, degarelix achieved a complete response in 20 % of patients after 1 year and 19 % after 2 years; although this value rose to 35 % at 3 years, patient numbers at this time were small. Partial responses were noted in 20 %, 22.5 % and 17 % of patients, after 1, 2 and 3 years, respectively. In the degarelix trial of Ozono et al. [3], the best overall response (complete response [3.6 %] + partial response [67.9 %]) was 71.4 % in the 240/80 mg group.

In our registry study, patients with prior HT appeared to have a significantly higher mortality risk (hazard ratio 1.58) compared with those who had not received prior HT. Castration resistance and concomitant progression is inevitable in these patients and it is not surprising that prior HT shortens the observed remission time for every other androgen deprivation therapy, such as degarelix, that commences thereafter. Also, in the subgroup who

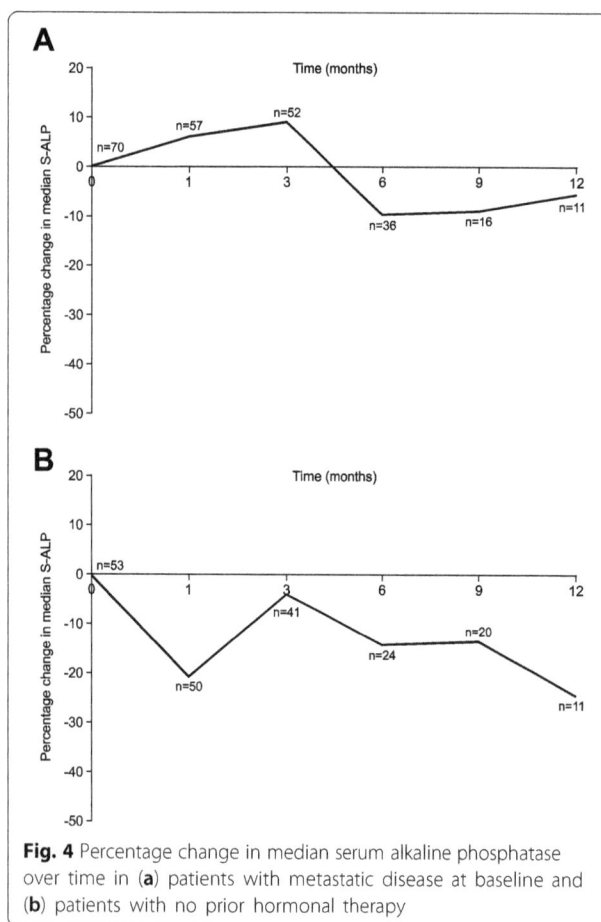

Fig. 4 Percentage change in median serum alkaline phosphatase over time in (**a**) patients with metastatic disease at baseline and (**b**) patients with no prior hormonal therapy

Table 3 Adverse events at first and last data points during degeralix therapy

Adverse event n,%	First data point[a]	Last data point[b]
Total[c]	276 (27.3)	380 (37.6)
Hot flushes	80 (7.9)	130 (12.9)
Erythema at the injection site	61 (6.0)	86 (8.5)
Fatigue	41 (4.1)	53 (5.2)
Pain	29 (2.9)	42 (4.2)
Weight gain	20 (2.0)	20 (2.0)
Back pain	10 (1.0)	18 (1.8)
Hypertension	12 (1.2)	6 (0.59)
Cardiac arrhythmia	3 (0.3)	3 (0.3)
Thromboembolism	0	0
Heart attack	2 (0.2)	1 (0.1)
Arteriosclerosis	0	1 (0.1)
Osteoporosis	0	1 (0.1)
Others	18 (1.8)	19 (1.9)

[a]At the time of the first degarelix dose; [b]at the final degarelix dose;
[c]percentages are stated as a percentage of the total patient population

had received prior LHRH analogues (LHRH agonist/GnRH antagonist), the 75th percentile value for OS was shorter than in those not pre-treated with LHRH analogues. Similarly, a higher percentage of patients who had received prior LHRH analogues experienced PSA progression compared with those who had not, and median time to PSA progression was shorter (209 weeks) in the subgroup who had received prior LHRH analogues versus those who had not (median PSA PFS not reached). These results appear to compare favourably with earlier studies of ADT. One large study of ADT in previously untreated PCa patients showed a median PFS of 16.5 months and 13.9 months, with LHRH agonists with and without antiandrogen, respectively [17]. In other studies in previously hormone-naïve patients, similar times to progression have been noted with LHRH agonists with/without antiandrogens (in the range of 12 to 23 months) [18–22].

Data from clinical studies show that degarelix displayed superior PSA PFS compared with leuprolide over 1 year [6], and there was an improvement in PSA PFS in patients who crossed over from leuprolide to degarelix in a long-term extension trial [2]. Furthermore, a pooled analysis also showed improved PSA PFS and longer OS (likely due to a decreased risk of cardiovascular disease) with degarelix compared with LHRH agonists [23]. Indeed, compared to LHRH agonists, GnRH antagonists appear to halve the number of cardiac events experienced by men with pre-existing cardiovascular disease during the first year of ADT [24]. Improvements in PSA PFS are indicative of delayed progression to castration-resistant disease with degarelix. Interestingly, since over half of the registry patients had received prior HT, it was not expected to achieve the same efficacy as in controlled studies which generally excluded patients who had prior HT. Nevertheless, the current registry data indicate that degarelix provides some benefit in patients who were pre-treated with HT (e.g. LHRH-agonists), while most benefit was observed in hormone-naïve patients.

PSA suppression in registry patients with no prior HT was more rapid and effective than those pre-treated with HT; moreover, the hormone-naïve cohort showed a PSA suppression profile similar to that observed with degarelix in clinical trials where previous hormonal management of PCa was excluded.

In the registry patients, PSA reduction to ≤ 4 ng/ml was achieved in 65 % of patients at 12 months and 71 % at 24 months. In the pivotal phase III degarelix clinical trial (CS21), the proportion of patients achieving PSA suppression < 4 ng/ml was 83 % after 1 year [6]. The difference most likely reflects the fact that patients in the registry had a higher risk compared to the registration trial, CS21. Over time, the proportion of registry patients with metastatic disease who achieved PSA suppression < 4 ng/ml was lower than the overall registry population; similarly, the proportion of patients with metastatic disease in the CS21 trial achieving PSA suppression < 4 ng/ml was also lower than the overall study population. Southwest Oncology Group trial S9346 data showed that PSA ≤ 4 ng/ml after ADT is a strong predictor of survival [25]. After controlling for prognostic factors, patients with PSA ≤ 4 to > 0.2 ng/ml had less than one-third the risk of death versus those with PSA > 4 ng/ml; median survival was 13 months for patients with PSA > 4 ng/ml versus 44 months for patients with PSA > 0.2 to ≤ 4 ng/ml.

The registry data also showed that overall, degarelix produced a rapid and profound testosterone suppression that was sustained for up to 24 months. Testosterone was also suppressed in patients with baseline metastatic disease. Testosterone measurement was optional and so, over time, patient numbers were small.

S-ALP is a marker of bone formation and baseline levels are high in metastatic disease, indicative of skeletal metastases [7]. Therefore, we examined the effect of degarelix in the cohort of patients with metastatic disease and found that S-ALP was suppressed after 6–12 months with degarelix. This compares with S-ALP suppression below baseline levels in the metastatic cohort after only 2 months of degarelix therapy in the CS21 trial [7]. A decrease in bone turnover marker levels may delay progression of bone metastases and improve survival.

Neo-adjuvant ADT can reduce prostate volume before radiotherapy. The registry data showed a decrease in prostate volume of almost 18 % at 3 months (and ~28 % at 6 months). This is slightly below the reported reductions (37–42 %) in prostate volume achieved with degarelix in clinical studies [26, 27]. As well as facilitating more effective delivery of radiotherapy, rapid and pronounced reduction of total prostate volume may also provide additional benefit for patients with obstructive lower urinary tract symptoms.

Degarelix was well tolerated in registry patients, with similar adverse event profiles for patients at the first and last data points. Moreover, the adverse event profile (based on adverse events at the last data point) was as expected for this patient population and similar to that of patients receiving degarelix in the 1-year phase II and III clinical trials, with the most frequent adverse events typically comprising injection-site reactions, hot flushes, and fatigue [1, 12, 13].

Some limitations of registry-based cohort studies may include limited availability of treatment data and under-reporting of outcomes if a patient leaves the registry or is not adequately followed up [11]. In the current registry, over time, patient numbers for some parameters (especially e.g. testosterone, prostate volume, and S-ALP where recording was optional) became quite small in some patient subgroups (e.g. metastatic patients) which may affect the reliability of measurements towards the end of the observation period in these cases. Missing data are a common phenomenon in healthcare research projects; not all data provided are complete due to the non-interventional nature of this study type. The uncertainty based on this will be relativized by the collection and generation of more data. Where there is a significant quantity of missing data, this may bias or impact on the study finding. One reason for the reduced number of patients is that some patients at the time of the analysis had not yet reached the full follow-up period.

Conclusion

This analysis of registry data showed degarelix to be effective and well tolerated in this real-world setting, confirming observations from controlled clinical studies. PSA-PFS appeared to be more favourable in comparison to earlier studies with other ADT treatments. Patients who had received prior HT appeared to have a significantly higher mortality risk than those who had not received prior HT.

Abbreviations
ADT: androgen deprivation therapy; GnRH: gonadotropin-releasing hormone; HT: hormonal therapy; IQUO: association for uro-oncological quality assurance; LHRH: luteinizing hormone-releasing hormone; OS: overall survival; PCa: prostate cancer; PCWG: Prostate Cancer Clinical Trials Working Group; PFS: progression-free survival; PSA: prostate-specific antigen; RECIST: Response Evaluation Criteria In Solid Tumors; S-ALP: serum alkaline phosphatase.

Competing interests
G. Geiges: None.
T. Harms: None.
G. Rodemer: None.
R. Eckert: None.
F. König: Advisory board Bayer, Lilly, Sanofi, Ferring, Berlin-Chemie.
R. Eichenauer: board member/consultant and received travel support/honoraria for lectures from: Astellas, AstraZeneca, Bayer Health Care, Ferring, Ipsen, Janssen-Cilag, Medacs, Novartis, Pfizer, Sanofi-Aventis, Takeda and Teva.
J. Schroder: honoraria as advisory board meeting participant for Ferring.

Authors' contributions
All authors were involved in the conception and design of the study; all authors made substantial contributions to the acquisition of data; all authors were involved in revising the manuscript critically for important intellectual content. All authors read and approved the final manuscript.

Acknowledgements
This study was funded by Ferring Pharmaceuticals. Medical writing assistance (funded by Ferring Pharmaceuticals) was provided by Thomas Lavelle of Bioscript Medical.

Author details
[1]Arztpraxis für Urologie (Partnerpraxis der Charité), Berlin, Germany. [2]Gemeinschaftspraxis Urologikum, Köln, Germany. [3]Praxisgemeinschaft für Onkologie und Urologie, Wilhelmshaven, Germany. [4]Urologische Arztpraxis, Lutherstadt Eisleben, Germany. [5]ATURO – Praxis für Urologie, Berlin, Germany. [6]Urologikum Hamburg, Hamburg, Germany.

References

1. Klotz L, Boccon-Gibod L, Shore ND, Andreou C, Persson BE, Cantor P, et al. The efficacy and safety of degarelix: a 12-month, comparative, randomized, open-label, parallel-group phase III study in patients with prostate cancer. BJU Int. 2008;102(11):1531–8.

2. Crawford ED, Tombal B, Miller K, Boccon-Gibod L, Schroder F, Shore N, et al. A phase III extension trial with a 1-arm crossover from leuprolide to degarelix: comparison of gonadotropin-releasing hormone agonist and antagonist effect on prostate cancer. J Urol. 2011;186(3):889–97.

3. Ozono S, Ueda T, Hoshi S, Yamaguchi A, Maeda H, Fukuyama Y, et al. The efficacy and safety of degarelix, a GnRH antagonist: a 12-month, multicentre, randomized, maintenance dose-finding phase II study in Japanese patients with prostate cancer. Jpn J Clin Oncol. 2012;42(6):477–84.

4. Van Poppel H. LHRH agonists versus GnRH antagonists for the treatment of prostate cancer. Belgian J Med Oncol. 2010;4:18–22.

5. Thompson IM. Flare associated with LHRH-agonist therapy. Rev Urol. 2001;3 Suppl 3:S10–14.

6. Tombal B, Miller K, Boccon-Gibod L, Schroder F, Shore N, Crawford ED, et al. Additional analysis of the secondary end point of biochemical recurrence rate in a phase 3 trial (CS21) comparing degarelix 80 mg versus leuprolide in prostate cancer patients segmented by baseline characteristics. Eur Urol. 2010;57(5):836–42.

7. Schroder FH, Tombal B, Miller K, Boccon-Gibod L, Shore ND, Crawford ED, et al. Changes in alkaline phosphatase levels in patients with prostate cancer receiving degarelix or leuprolide: results from a 12-month, comparative, phase III study. BJU Int. 2010;106(2):182–7.

8. Gliklich RE, Dreyer NA. Registries for Evaluating Patient Outcomes: A User's Guide. (Prepared by Outcome DEcIDE Center [Outcome Sciences, Inc. dba Outcome] under Contract No. HHSA290200500351 TO1), AHRQ Publication No. 07-EHC001-1. Rockville: Agency for Healthcare Research and Quality; 2007.

9. Therasse P, Arbuck SG, Eisenhauer EA, Wanders J, Kaplan RS, Rubinstein L, et al. New guidelines to evaluate the response to treatment in solid tumors. European Organization for Research and Treatment of Cancer, National Cancer Institute of the United States, National Cancer Institute of Canada. J Natl Cancer Inst. 2000;92(3):205–16.

10. Scher HI, Halabi S, Tannock I, Morris M, Sternberg CN, Carducci MA, et al. Design and end points of clinical trials for patients with progressive prostate cancer and castrate levels of testosterone: recommendations of the Prostate Cancer Clinical Trials Working Group. J Clin Oncol. 2008;26(7):1148–59.

11. Gliklich RE, Dreyer NA. Registries for Evaluating Patient Outcomes: A User's Guide. 2nd ed. (Prepared by Outcome DEcIDE Center [Outcome Sciences, Inc. d/b/a Outcome] under Contract No. HHSA290200500351 TO3). Rockville, MD, USA: Agency for Healthcare Research and Quality; 2010.

12. Gittelman M, Pommerville PJ, Persson BE, Jensen JK, Olesen TK, Degarelix Study G. A 1-year, open label, randomized phase II dose finding study of degarelix for the treatment of prostate cancer in North America. J Urol. 2008;180(5):1986–92.

13. Van Poppel H, Tombal B, de la Rosette JJ, Persson BE, Jensen JK, Kold Olesen T. Degarelix: a novel gonadotropin-releasing hormone (GnRH) receptor blocker–results from a 1-yr, multicentre, randomised, phase 2 dosage-finding study in the treatment of prostate cancer. Eur Urol. 2008;54(4):805–13.

14. Perlmutter MA, Lepor H. Androgen deprivation therapy in the treatment of advanced prostate cancer. Rev Urol. 2007;9 Suppl 1:S3–8.

15. Lu-Yao GL, Albertsen PC, Moore DF, Shih W, Lin Y, DiPaola RS, et al. Fifteen-year survival outcomes following primary androgen-deprivation therapy for localized prostate cancer. JAMA Intern Med. 2014;174(9):1460–7.

16. Mottet N, Bellmunt J, Briers E, van den Bergh RCN, Bolla M, van Casteren NJ, et al. Guidelines on prostate cancer. European Association of Urology 2015. Available from: http://uroweb.org/wp-content/uploads/EAU-Guidelines-Prostate-Cancer-2015-v2.pdf Accessed August 2015

17. Crawford ED, Eisenberger MA, McLeod DG, Spaulding JT, Benson R, Dorr FA, et al. A controlled trial of leuprolide with and without flutamide in prostatic carcinoma. N Engl J Med. 1989;321(7):419–24.

18. Di Silverio F, Serio M, D'Eramo G, Sciarra F. Zoladex vs. Zoladex plus cyproterone acetate in the treatment of advanced prostatic cancer: a multicenter Italian study. Eur Urol. 1990;18 Suppl 3:54–61.

19. Bono AV, DiSilverio F, Robustelli della Cuna G, Benvenuti C, Brausi M, Ferrari P, et al. Complete androgen blockade versus chemical castration in advanced prostatic cancer: analysis of an Italian multicentre study. Italian Leuprorelin Group. Urol Int. 1998;60 Suppl 1:18–24.

20. Ferrari P, Castagnetti G, Ferrari G, Baisi B, Dotti A. Combination treatment versus LHRH alone in advanced prostatic cancer. Urol Int. 1996;56 Suppl 1:13–7.

21. Du Plessis DJ. Castration plus nilutamide vs castration plus placebo in advanced prostate cancer. A review. Urology. 1991;37(2 Suppl):20–4.

22. Lin GW, Yao XD, Zhang SL, Dai B, Ma CG, Zhang HL, et al. Prostate-specific antigen half-life: a new predictor of progression-free survival and overall survival in Chinese prostate cancer patients. Asian J Androl. 2009;11(4):443–50.

23. Klotz L, Miller K, Crawford ED, Shore N, Tombal B, Karup C, et al. Disease control outcomes from analysis of pooled individual patient data from five comparative randomised clinical trials of degarelix versus luteinising hormone-releasing hormone agonists. Eur Urol. 2014;66(6):1101–8.

24. Albertsen PC, Klotz L, Tombal B, Grady J, Olesen TK, Nilsson J. Cardiovascular morbidity associated with gonadotropin releasing hormone agonists and an antagonist. Eur Urol. 2014;65(3):565–73.

25. Hussain M, Tangen CM, Higano C, Schelhammer PF, Faulkner J, Crawford ED, et al. Absolute prostate-specific antigen value after androgen deprivation is a strong independent predictor of survival in new metastatic prostate cancer: data from Southwest Oncology Group Trial 9346 (INT-0162). J Clin Oncol. 2006;24(24):3984–90.

26. Anderson J, Al-Ali G, Wirth M, Gual JB, Gomez Veiga F, Colli E, et al. Degarelix versus Goserelin (+ Antiandrogen Flare Protection) in the relief of lower urinary tract symptoms secondary to prostate cancer: results from a phase IIIb study (NCT00831233). Urol Int. 2013;90(3):321–8.

27. Axcrona K, Aaltomaa S, da Silva CM, Ozen H, Damber JE, Tanko LB, et al. Androgen deprivation therapy for volume reduction, lower urinary tract symptom relief and quality of life improvement in patients with prostate cancer: degarelix vs goserelin plus bicalutamide. BJU Int. 2012;110(11):1721–8.

23

Infrarenal high intra-abdominal testis: fusion of T2-weighted and diffusion-weighted magnetic resonance images and pathological findings

Seiji Hoshi, Yuichi Sato, Junya Hata, Hidenori Akaihata, Soichiro Ogawa, Nobuhiro Haga and Yoshiyuki Kojima[*]

Abstract

Background: Several recent reports have demonstrated that the preoperative sensitivity and accuracy of identifying and locating non-palpable testes increases with the use of conventional MRI, in addition to diffusion-weighted imaging (DWI). Therefore, pre-operative prediction of the presence and location of testes using imaging techniques may guide management of intra-abdominal testis. Fowler-Stephens orchiopexy is effective for treating patients with intra-abdominal testis; however, long-term testicular function after this procedure has not been clarified. We present a case of a high intra-abdominal testis located below the kidney, and discuss the usefulness of fusion view with T2-weighted and DWI images to make a diagnosis of high intra-abdominal testis and the pathological findings to predict future fertility potential.

Case presentation: A 10-month-old boy was referred to the urology department for the management of non-palpable testis. We employed not only conventional MRI, but also DWI, to improve the diagnostic accuracy of non-palpable testes by MRI examination. The high-intensity mass-like structure below the kidney on the T2-weighted image and the markedly high signal intensity mass on the DWI image completely matched, which suggested that the mass below the kidney was the right testis. The patient underwent diagnostic and therapeutic laparoscopy. A testis was found under the ascending colon, 1 cm below the right kidney. We performed 2-stage Fowler-Stephens orchiopexy. The testis could be delivered to the scrotum without any tension. We examined expression patterns of the stem cell marker, undifferentiated embryonic cell transcription factor 1 (UTF1) in the testicular biopsy sample, and demonstrated that the UTF1-positive Ad spermatogonia / negative Ad spermatogonia ratio was lower in this patient than in boys his age with descended and inguinal undescended testes, indicating that spermatogonial stem cell activity may decrease remarkably in this boy.

Conclusions: Fusion view with T2-weighted and DWI images may be a useful diagnostic modality for high intra-abdominal testes. Fowler-Stephens orchiopexy may provide blood supply to the testis but that might not be enough to achieve spermatogenesis.

Keywords: Cryptorchidism, Intraabdominal testis, MRI, Stem cell, Case report

* Correspondence: ykojima@fmu.ac.jp
Department of Urology, Fukushima Medical University School of Medicine, 1,
Hikarigaoka, Fukushima 960-1295, Japan

Background

The advent of laparoscopy has dramatically changed the diagnosis and treatment of non-palpable testis in children. Laparoscopy is an accepted procedure to investigate the presence and location, and to perform subsequent treatment, of intra-abdominal testis. Several recent reports have demonstrated that the preoperative sensitivity and accuracy of identifying and locating non-palpable testes increases with the use of conventional MRI, in addition to diffusion-weighted imaging (DWI) [1, 2]. Therefore, pre-operative prediction of the presence and location of testes using imaging techniques may guide management of intra-abdominal testis. Fowler-Stephens orchiopexy is effective for treating patients with intra-abdominal testis; however, long-term testicular function after this procedure has not been clarified. We present a case of a high intra-abdominal testis located below the kidney, and discuss the usefulness of fusion view, with T2-weighted and DWI images, to make a diagnosis of high intra-abdominal testis and the pathological findings to predict future fertility potential.

Case presentation

A 10-month-old boy was referred to the urology department for the management of non-palpable testis. There was no significant familial or past history. A clinical examination demonstrated a left, well-positioned testis, 16 × 11 × 11 mm in size, and an empty right scrotum. No abnormality of the external genitalia was found. Physical examination could not confirm the presence of the right testis.

Ultrasonography could not identify the right testis in the abdomen or inguinal region. We employed not only conventional MRI, but also DWI, to improve the diagnostic accuracy of non-palpable testes by MRI examination. The T2-weighted image showed a high-intensity mass-like structure, which was difficult to distinguish from the surrounding fat tissue, below the right kidney. Furthermore, DWI showed a mass, at that position, of markedly high signal intensity. The T2-weighted image was fused with the DWI image, using medical image viewer software (EV Insite R, PSP Co., Tokyo, Japan), to identify the anatomical location. The high-intensity

mass-like structure on the T2-weighted image and the markedly high signal intensity mass on the DWI image completely matched (Fig. 1), which suggested that the mass below the kidney was the right testis.

The patient underwent diagnostic and therapeutic laparoscopy. The 5-mm 0-degree camera, introduced through the umbilicus, showed an opened right inguinal ring, with vas deferens. Two more trocars were introduced and a testis was found under the ascending colon, 1 cm below the right kidney. We decided to perform 2-stage Fowler-Stephens orchiopexy. The spermatic vessels were ligated with nonabsorbable 2–0 sutures with the expectation that this would allow collateral blood supply to develop more fully. Ten months after the first surgery, the second stage of the 2-stage laparoscopic Fowler-Stephens procedure was performed. Because the vessel derived from the inferior epigastric artery had developed enough, as a feeding vessel, to provide blood supply to the right testis, retroperitoneal dissection was carried down from the level of the testis to the internal ring to create a wide peritoneal pedicle. The 15 × 10 × 6 mm testis could be delivered to the scrotum without any tension from the radially dilating system. After delivery of the testis, we performed testicular biopsy to compare pathological findings between the present patient and inguinal undescended testis, because we routinely do testicular biopsy during orchiopexy to predict future testicular function. For biopsy, the tunica albuginea was exposed and iris scissors were used to remove a small piece of the testicular parenchyma. Pathological findings in the biopsies taken at stage 2 of the operation showed that median seminiferous tubule diameter and median number of spermatogonia per tubular cross section were comparable to those in inguinal undescended testes of boys his age (*n* = 5; Fig. 2). We also examined expression patterns of the stem cell marker, undifferentiated embryonic cell transcription factor 1 (UTF1) [3–5], and demonstrated that the UTF1-positive Ad spermatogonia / UTF1-negative Ad spermatogonia ratio was lower in this patient than in boys of his age with descended testes (*n* = 5) and in inguinal undescended testes (the same biopsy samples used in the pathological

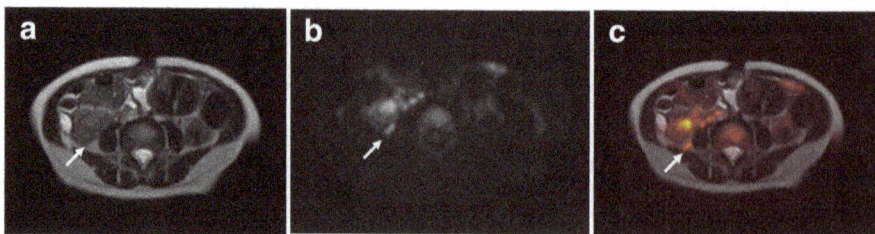

Fig. 1 MRI findings. **a** T2-weighted image. **b** DWI. (**c**) T2-weighted image and DWI fusion image using medical image viewer software (EV Insite R, PSP Co., Tokyo, Japan). *Arrows*: intra-abdominal testis located below right kidney

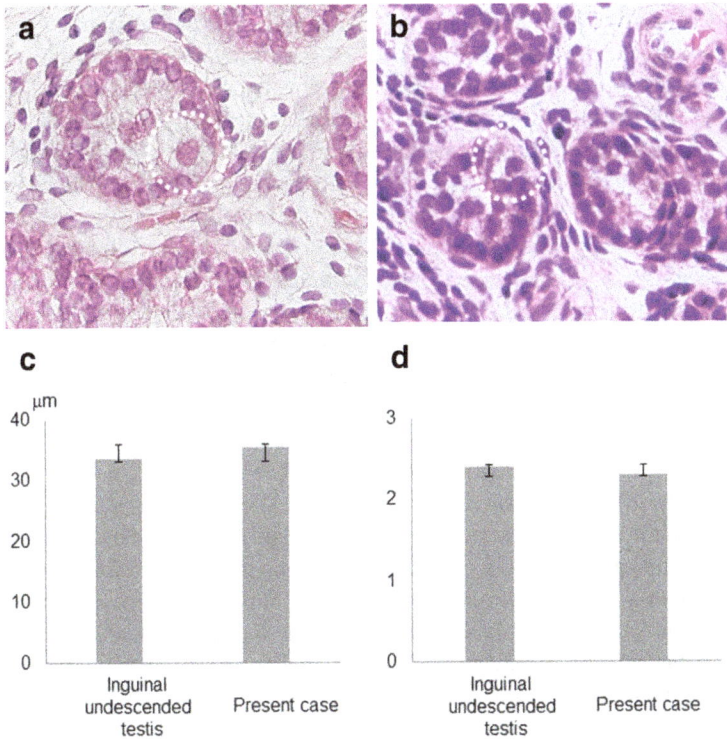

Fig. 2 Histopathological findings of testicular tissue (hematoxylin-eosin staining; × 400) in inguinal undescended testis (**a**) and the present case (**b**). *Dotted circle*: spermatogonia. Median seminiferous tubule diameter (**c**) and median number of spermatogonia per tubular cross section (**d**) in inguinal undescended testis cases and the present case. *Error bars*: standard deviation

study) (Fig. 3). This was part of a study examining the histopathological findings and stem cell activity of undescended testes, which was approved by the ethics committee of Fukushima Medical University School of Medicine. Informed consent was obtained from the patients before the study, after explaining its purpose and methods.

Ten months after the second surgery, the right testis, 13 × 8 × 7 mm in size, was located in the scrotum, and good vascularization was detected on echo color Doppler ultrasound.

Discussion

Diagnostic modalities, such as ultrasound and MRI, are nonspecific in the intra-abdominal testis, and the accuracy of these examinations was not satisfactory. The only effective diagnostic procedure is considered to be laparoscopy. However, there is a possibility of being unable to locate a testis on diagnostic laparoscopy [6]. An accurate preoperative diagnosis is usually useful to determine the surgical approach for non-palpable testes management, particularly for high intra-abdominal cases. Kanrarci reported that identifying and locating non-palpable testes was improved by

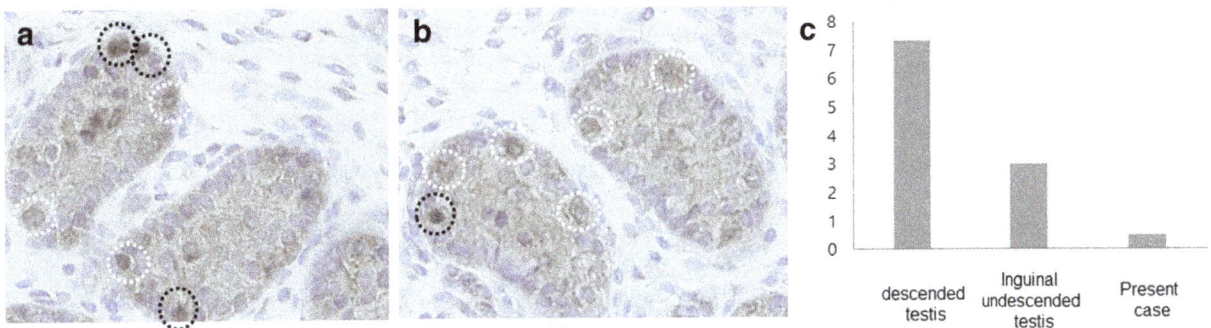

Fig. 3 Comparison of UTF1 expression patterns in the testis between inguinal undescended testis (**a**) and the present case (**b**). *White dotted circle*: UTF1-negative Ad spermatogonia. *Black dotted circle*: UTF1-positive Ad spermatogonia. **c** The ratio of UTF1-negative Ad spermatogonia to UTF1-positive Ad spermatogonia in the testis among descended testis, inguinal undescended testis, and the present case

160   Clinical Andrology

using the combination of DWI and conventional MRI, with about 90% sensitivity and accuracy [1]. Kato et al. also reported that preoperative combined assessment using T1- and T2-weighted imaging, fat-suppressed T2-weighted imaging, and DWI enabled the identification of intra-abdominal or intra-canalicular testes preoperatively and facilitated an accurate diagnosis of non-palpable testes [2]. They demonstrated that combined MRI assessments had an accuracy of 92.3% in the diagnosis of intra-abdominal testes; however, high intra-abdominal testes located over the pelvis, as in the present case, were not included in their reports [2]. In the present case, we could predict the presence and location of the intra-abdominal testis, below the kidney, preoperatively by fusion view with T2-weighted and DWI images. At our center, we usually perform MRI in patients who have a non-palpable testis without contralateral testicular hypertrophy and if ultrasonography fails to demonstrate a testis, because MRI improves the accuracy of diagnosing non-palpable testis and can be useful for identifying the presence and location of a testis. However, as described in the AUA guideline, although MRI is being used more widely due to greater sensitivity and specificity, it has the problems of higher cost, low availability, and need for anesthesia [7]. In addition, no imaging method can confirm absence of the testis with 100% accuracy [7]. Therefore, the AUA guideline recommends surgical exploration, such as diagnostic laparoscopy (or open exploration), rather than MRI [7]. Despite this recommendation, it would have been quite difficult to find the right testis at laparoscopy in our patient without the information obtained by MRI. Although it is hard to be dogmatic about the situations in which MRI is beneficial, examination of fusion views with T2-weighted and DWI images may be useful for preoperative localization of high intra-abdominal testes or for postoperative assessment in the rare cases where the testis cannot be identified by laparoscopy.

Previous reports demonstrated that the success rate of Fowler-Stephens orchiopexy, which was assessed by whether the testis was returned to the scrotum or the testicular size, was 69–95% [8, 9]. A recent report suggested that the testicular blood supply after Fowler-Stephens orchiopexy was preserved in most cases [10]; however, testicular function after Fowler-Stephens orchiopexy has not been clarified. Rosito et al. reported that ligation of the spermatic vessels during the first stage of orchiopexy for intra-abdominal testis was associated with a significant reduction of spermatogonia, although no significant changes were observed in the volumetric characteristics of the testes [11]. Kamisawa et al. also reported, in their animal study, that Fowler-Stephens orchiopexy may not significantly contribute to the improvement of spermatogenesis [12]. In our case, we examined the histological findings and expression pattern of the stem cell marker, UTF1, in the testicular biopsy specimen, during the second stage of a 2-stage

Fowler-Stephens orchiopexy. A previous animal study demonstrated that the differentiation from gonocytes into early A spermatogonia and the stem cell activity of early A spermatogonia were disturbed during the early stage of spermatogenesis, suggesting that the loss of spermatogonial stem cell activity results in disturbances in spermatogenesis and may make fertility difficult in cryptorchidism [13]. In our patient, although good vascularization was detected on echo color Doppler ultrasound, and median seminiferous tubule diameter and median number of spermatogonia per tubular cross section were comparable to those in inguinal undescended testis cases, the UTF1-positive Ad spermatogonia (actual stem cells) / UTF1-negative Ad spermatogonia (potential stem cells) ratio was lower than in descended testes and inguinal undescended testes. This implies that spermatogonial stem cell activity was markedly reduced, and that development of collateral vessels after the first stage of 2-stage Fowler-Stephens orchiopexy may provide enough blood to maintain testicular viability but might not be sufficient to achieve spermatogenesis, although it is unclear if the testicular findings were attributable to the intra-abdominal location of the testis or were caused by ligation of the primary testicular vessels and the 10-month collateralization period.

Conclusions
We presented a case of a high intra-abdominal testis located below the kidney. Fusion view with T2-weighted and DWI images may be a useful diagnostic modality for high intra-abdominal testes. Fowler-Stephens orchiopexy may provide blood supply to the testis but that might not be enough to achieve spermatogenesis; therefore, further studies are needed.

Abbreviations
DWI: Diffusion-weighted imaging; UTF1: Undifferentiated embryonic cell transcription factor 1

Acknowledgements
None.

Funding
None.

Availability of data and materials
The datasets generated during and/or analysed during the current study are not publicly available due to restrictions of our Institutional Review Board but are available from the corresponding author on reasonable request.

Authors' contributions
SH participated in the follow up care, performed literature review, carried out hematoxylin-eosin staining and evaluate the results, and drafted the manuscript. YS carried out the surgery, participated in the follow up care and drafted the manuscript. JH participated in the follow up care, and

drafted the manuscript. HA participated in the follow up care and edited the manuscript. SO participated in the surgery, participated in the follow up care, and edited the manuscript. NH performed literature review carried out the immunostaining and evaluate the results, and edited the manuscript. YK carried out the surgery and edited the manuscript. All authors read and approved the final manuscript.

Competing interests

The authors declare that they have no competing interests.

References

1. Kantarci M, Doganay S, Yalcin A, et al. Diagnostic performance of diffusion-weighted MRI in the detection of nonpalpable undescended testes: comparison with conventional MRI and surgical findings. AJR Am J Roentgenol. 2010;195:W268–73.
2. Kato T, Kojima Y, Kamisawa H, et al. Findings of fat-suppressed T2-weighted and diffusion-weighted magnetic resonance imaging in the diagnosis of non-palpable testes. BJU Int. 2011;107:290–4.
3. Liu A, Cheng L, Du J, et al. Diagnostic utility of novel stem cell markers SALL4, OCT4, NANOG, SOX2, UTF1, and TCL1 in primary mediastinal germ cell tumors. Am J Surg Pathol. 2010;34:697–706.
4. Kristensen DM, Nielsen JE, Skakkebaek NE, et al. Presumed pluripotency markers UTF-1 and REX-1 are expressed in human adult testes and germ cell neoplasms. Hum Reprod. 2008;23:775–82.
5. van Bragt MP, Roepers-Gajadien HL, Korver CM, et al. Expression of the pluripotency marker UTF1 is restricted to a subpopulation of early A spermatogonia in rat testis. Reproduction. 2008;136:33–40.
6. Kim C, Bennett N, Docimo SG. Missed testis on laparoscopy despite blind-ending vessels and closed processus vaginalis. Urology. 2005;65:1226 e7–8.
7. Kolon TF, Herndon CD, Baker LA, Baskin LS, et al. Evaluation and treatment of cryptorchidism: AUA guideline. J Urol. 2014;192:337–45.
8. Koff SA, Sethi PS. Treatment of high undescended testes by low spermatic vessel ligation: an alternative to the Fowler-Stephens technique. J Urol. 1996;156:799–803.
9. Clatworthy HW Jr, Hollabaugh RS, Grosfeld JL. The "long loop vas" orchidopexy for the high undescended testis. Am Surg. 1972;38:69–73.
10. Esposito C, Vallone G, Savanelli A, et al. Long-term outcome of laparoscopic Fowler-Stephens orchiopexy in boys with intra-abdominal testis. J Urol. 2009;181:1851–6.
11. Rosito NC, Koff WJ, da Silva Oliveira TL, et al. Volumetric and histological findings in intra-abdominal testes before and after division of spermatic vessels. J Urol. 2004;171:2430–3.
12. Kamisawa H, Kojima Y, Mizuno K, et al. Spermatogenesis after 1-stage fowler-stephens orchiopexy in experimental cryptorchid rat model. J Urol. 2010;183:2380–4.
13. Kamisawa H, Kojima Y, Mizuno K, et al. Attenuation of spermatogonial stem cell activity in cryptorchid testes. J Urol. 2012;187:1047–52.

24

A positive Real-Time Elastography (RTE) combined with a Prostate Cancer Gene 3 (PCA3) score above 35 convey a high probability of intermediate- or high-risk prostate cancer in patient admitted for primary prostate biopsy

Yngve Nygård[1,3*], Svein A. Haukaas[1,3], Ole J. Halvorsen[2,4], Karsten Gravdal[2], Jannicke Frugård[1], Lars A. Akslen[2,4] and Christian Beisland[1,3]

Abstract

Background: The standard of care in patients with suspected prostate cancer (PCa) is systematic prostate biopsies. This approach leads to unnecessary biopsies in patients without PCa and also to the detection of clinical insignificant PCa. Better tools are wanted. We have evaluated the performance of real-time elastography (RTE) combined with prostate cancer gene 3 (PCA3) in an initial biopsy setting with the goal of better identifying patients in need of prostate biopsies.

Methods: 127 patients were included in this study; three were excluded because of not measureable PCA3 score leading to 124 evaluable patients. A cut-off value of 35 was used for PCA3. All patients were examined with a Hitachi Preirus with an endfire probe for RTE, a maximum of five targeted biopsies were obtained from suspicious lesions detected by RTE. All patients then had a 10-core systematic biopsy performed by another urologist unaware of the RTE results. The study includes follow-up data for a minimum of three years; all available histopathological data are included in the analysis.

Results: There was a significant difference in PCA3 score: 26.6 for benign disease, 73.6 for cancer patients ($p < 0.001$). 70 patients (56 %) were diagnosed with prostate cancer in the study period, 21 (30 %) low-risk, 32 (46 %) intermediate-risk and 17 (24 %) high-risk. RTE and PCA3 were significant markers for predicting intermediate- and high-risk PCa ($p = 0.001$). The combination of RTE and PCA3 had a sensitivity of 96 % and a negative predictive value (NPV) of 90 % for the group of intermediate- and high-risk PCa together and a NPV for high-risk PCa of 100 %. If both parameters are positive there is a high probability of detecting intermediate- or high-risk PCa, if both parameters are negative there is only a small chance of missing prostate cancer with documented treatment benefit.

Conclusions: RTE and PCA3 may be used as pre-biopsy examinations to reduce the number of prostate biopsies.

Keywords: Prostate cancer, Ultrasound, Diagnosis, PCA3, Real-time elastography, RTE

* Correspondence: yngve_nygard@yahoo.no
[1]Department of Urology, Haukeland University Hospital, N-5021 Bergen, Norway
[3]Department of Clinical Medicine, University of Bergen, Bergen, Norway
Full list of author information is available at the end of the article

Background

The mainstay in the diagnosis of prostate cancer (PCa) is biopsy-driven by serum prostate-specific antigen (PSA) and digital rectal examination (DRE). There is really no level of PSA that excludes PCa, and many benign prostatic diseases may cause PSA elevation. The threshold value of PSA for prostate biopsy is arbitrarily chosen, which is dependent on the age of the patient, life expectancy and the size of the prostate. It is well recognized that PSA screening results in both the over-diagnosis and overtreatment of prostate cancer [1–3]. Furthermore, a lot of men with benign disease are going through prostate biopsy without any beneficial effects. There is also an increase in biopsy-related infections because of antibiotic resistant bacteria, and some of these infections can be lethal [4, 5]. There is a need to better identify those men not harboring PCa to avoid unnecessary biopsies and related complications.

Currently, there is little enthusiasm for population-based PSA screening, and in May 2012 the U.S. Preventive Services Task Force recommended against routine PSA screening [6]. Moreover, European Association of Urology (EAU) Guidelines (2013) do not support programmed mass PSA screening, while recommending early detection in well-informed men [7].

To assist in the decision to perform prostate biopsy, nomograms have been created. The US Food and Drug Administration has approved prostate cancer gene 3 (PCA3) as a predictive test prior to performing a repeat biopsy. PCA3 has shown to enhance the performance of nomograms based on initial biopsy results [8, 9].

Standard systematic prostate biopsy is performed by placing a biopsy needle in 10 to 12 prostate sectors of the peripheral zone under transrectal ultrasound (US) guidance. Cancer in the central or anterior part of the prostate may be overlooked, and insignificant cancer detected with such biopsy regimens [10].

Imaging techniques, specifically advanced US and multiparametric MRI (mpMRI), are evolving, and thereby making it possible to identify areas suspected of harboring PCa [11, 12]. Targeted biopsy guided by RTE detects high-grade cancer, although it misses some significant cancers compared with a systematic 10-core biopsy [13, 14]. mpMRI, together with fusion into real-time US, is practical for targeted biopsy but this approach also misses significant PCa [15].

In a prospective series of patients undergoing radical prostatectomy, the combination of RTE and PCA3 detected 97 % of significant PCa [16]. The present study was undertaken to evaluate prospectively the capability of RTE and PCA 3 to predict clinically significant PCa in patients admitted for initial prostate biopsy.

Methods

The study was carried out in the outpatient clinic of the Department of Urology at Haukeland University Hospital from February 2011 to June 2012. The Regional Committee for Medical and Health Research Ethics in Western Norway approved the study.

A total of 127 consecutive patients were included using active inclusion, with only a very small amount of patients declining to participate. The inclusion criteria were a PSA level 3 – 25 ng/ml, age ≤75 years and no prior biopsies within the last five years, in addition to the patients being amenable for radical treatment.

At first, DRE was performed in all patients to determine clinical stage (cT) and to perform the prostatic massage needed before urine sampling. Before further evaluation, the first stray urine was captured and transferred to the transportation tubes needed for the PCA3 analysis. We used Progensa™ PCA3 analysis, and the tests were analyzed at the Fürst Medical Laboratory in Oslo, Norway. After the urine test, all patients were given a single dose of Ciprofloxacin 1 g as an antibiotic prophylaxis. All patients were examined in the left decubital position, with the ultrasound procedures being thoroughly previously described [16]. In brief, all patients were examined using a Hitachi Preirus Ultrasound machine with software for RTE. They were first examined using a V53W transrectal end-fire probe for B-mode evaluation, determination of prostate volume (Pvol), RTE and targeted biopsies. The peripheral zone (PZ) of the prostate was divided in six region of interest (ROI), one at the base, one at the mid prostate and one at the apex on each side. All RTE-reproducible hard lesions of more than 5 mm were allocated to the corresponding ROI. Furthermore, two to four targeted biopsies were taken from suspicious ROIs. A CC531 transrectal simultaneous biplane probe was used for standard systematic biopsies. In the same setting a different urologist blinded for the RTE results performed a 10-core systematic biopsy from the six ROIs. The biopsies were fixated in formaldehyde and analyzed by two uro-pathologists. Total core length, as well as the length of cancer tissue and Gleason grade and score, was separately recorded for each biopsy core.

In the statistical analyses, we included not only the results and outcomes of the initial biopsy, but also at least three years of follow-up data for the patients. If there was a clinically persisting suspicion of PCa after the initial biopsies, patients were monitored closely (see Fig. 1). Repeat biopsies were performed in 38 patients within the next six months, while in 24 patients no repeat biopsy was performed. Sixteen patients with benign repeat biopsies went through a mpMRI of the prostate, and in 12 of these we performed targeted biopsies of suspicious areas by TRUS guided biopsies with a "cognitive fusion" of

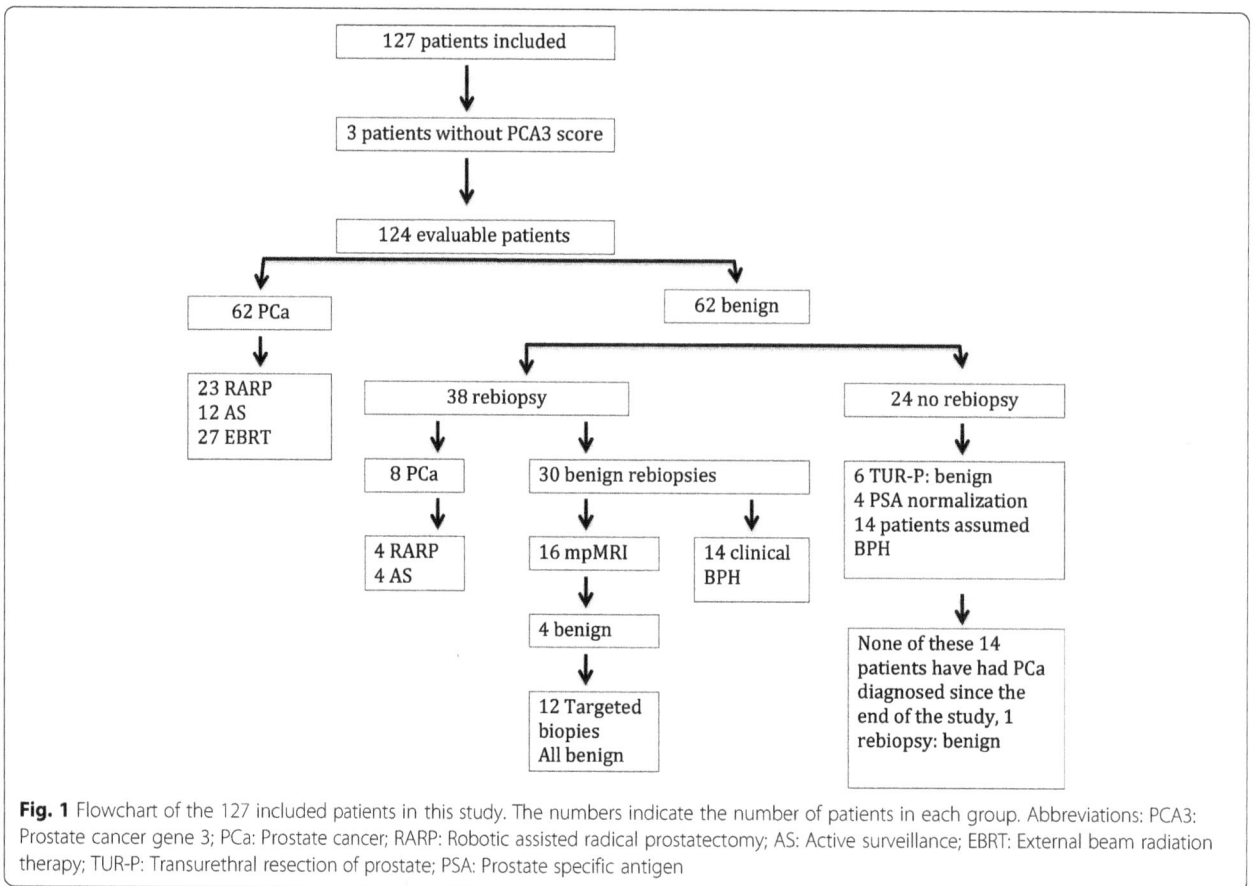

Fig. 1 Flowchart of the 127 included patients in this study. The numbers indicate the number of patients in each group. Abbreviations: PCA3: Prostate cancer gene 3; PCa: Prostate cancer; RARP: Robotic assisted radical prostatectomy; AS: Active surveillance; EBRT: External beam radiation therapy; TUR-P: Transurethral resection of prostate; PSA: Prostate specific antigen

mpMRI. Together with an uro-radiologist, a trained urologist performed such biopsies. All biopsy data were included in the analyses. Among those 24 patients with no repeat biopsy, four patients experienced a normalization of PSA levels at follow-up, six were admitted for TUR-P with a benign pathology, and in 14 patients benign prostatic hyperplasia was assumed as the reason for a slight elevation in PSA level. The medical records for these patients and the registry at our department of pathology were examined in October 2015 to identify whether PCa had been diagnosed since the end of inclusion. The mean observation time for these patients is 46.7 ± 1.5 months (median 44.4, range 41–55). The medical records for the 14 patients with benign repeat biopsies were also examined at the same time, though none have had PCa diagnosed in this period.

Statistical analyses

Standard descriptive statistics were used and presented as mean and median. A 95 % confidence interval (CI) was calculated. Negative predictive value (NPV), positive predictive value (PPV), sensitivity and specificity were calculated for RTE by ROI and by patient, for PCA3 using a cut-off value of 35 and for a combination of both. Different groups were compared using the exact

Chi-square test, a Mann–Whitney U-test and the t-test for categorical, ordinal and continuous data, respectively. A multiple logistic regression model was estimated entering the clinical parameters age, Pvol and PSA alone, or combined with a dichotomized PCA3 score of 35 and positive RTE by patient. DRE is commonly used in such clinical models but we excluded DRE from the model because DRE and RTE both are parameters expressing tissue stiffness. The performance of the calculations was expressed as the area under the curve (AUC) of the receiver operating curves (ROC). A 95 %CI was calculated for the AUC and displayed in parenthesis after AUC.

Results

In three patients the urine did not contain enough cells for the PCA3 analysis resulting in 124 evaluable patients.

A total of 70 (56 %) patients were diagnosed with PCa, of whom 62 were identified in the initial biopsy setting and eight patients at the repeat biopsy. The inclusion of these eight patients did not alter the diagnostic performance of RTE by ROI as the sensitivity, specificity, PPV and NPV were 43, 84, 49 and 80 %, respectively; the false positive rate was 16 % and the false negative rate 12 %.

According to the European Association of Urology (EAU) risk stratification, there were 21 (30 %) low-, 32

(46 %) intermediate- and 17 (24 %) high-risk cancers [7]. In the eight patients detected with PCa on the repeat biopsies six were low-risk and two were intermediate-risk cancers, there were no high-risk PCa in this group.

The distribution of PSA, PCA3 score, Pvol, age and proportion of positive DRE for all patients and for patients with and without PCa is found in Table 1. The p-values are calculated for the difference between the groups with PCa and without PCa. The clinical stage, biopsy Gleason grade and score and risk stratification according to EAU guidelines are also detailed in Table 1.

RTE was positive in 85 cases and negative in 39 . The average PCA3 score in patients with PCa was significantly higher compared with normal or benign disease (73.6 vs. 26.6, $p < 0.001$). For PSA, there were no statistical significant differences between those patients with- and those without PCa (9.7 vs. 8.3, $p = 0.09$).

The sensitivity, specificity, PPV and NPV of RTE by patient, PCA3 at score 35 and the combination of both for any PCa, for intermediate- and high-risk PCa together, and for high-risk PCa alone, are shown in Table 2.

In univariate logistic regression analysis a positive RTE was a highly significant predictor of intermediate- risk and high-risk PCa (Table 3).

Entering PCA3 and RTE in a clinical model encompassing age, PSA and Pvol; PSA, Pvol and PCA3 were independent predictors of intermediate-risk and high-risk PCa while RTE showed a tendency toward significance (Table 3).

The results of the logistic regression analyses were also expressed in a ROC curve that yielded an AUC of 0.826 (0.752-0.899) for the complete model and 0.787 (0.703-0.872) for the clinical model alone (Fig. 2).

To evaluate the clinical impact of the combination of PCA3 and RTE, we utilized the most commonly used cut-off value of 35 for PCA3, and allocated the patients into four groups.

Group 1 included patients for whom both RTE and PCA3 were positive. Patients with a positive RTE and negative PCA3 were put into Group 2, and RTE negative and PCA3 positive patients were allocated to Group 3. Finally, Group 4 encompassed patients negative for RTE,

Table 1 Patient characteristics of 124 patients of whom 70 were diagnosed with PCa

Variable		Total (n = 124)	PCa (n = 70)	No PCa (n = 54)	p-value*
PSA	Mean (Median; 95 %CI)	9.1 (7.2; 8.3-9.9)	9.7 (7.7; 8.5-11.0)	8.3 (6.7; 7.2-9.4)	0.090*
PCA3-score	Mean (Median; 95 %CI)	53.1 (33.5; 42.9-63.4)	73.6 (53.5; 57.7-89.6)	26.6 (19.0; 19.9-33-2)	<0.001*
Prostate volume	Mean (Median; 95 %CI)	60.0 (53.0; 54.7-65.4)	49.9 (43.5; 44.7-55.1)	73.2 (66.5; 63.8-82.5)	<0.001*
Age	Mean (Median; 95 %CI)	64.0 (65.1; 62.9-65.2)	64.9 (65.7; 63.5-66.2)	62.9 (63.0; 61.0-64.9)	0.094*
Positive DRE	Number (%)	31 (25 %)	22 (31 %)	9 (17 %)	0,060**
Clinical stage	Number (%)				
T1c			35 (50 %)		
T2a			12 (17 %)		
T2b			6 (9 %)		
T2c			11 (16 %)		
T3a			6 (9 %)		
Gleason score	Number (%)				
3 + 2 = 5			1 (1 %)		
3 + 3 = 6			21 (26 %)		
3 + 4 = 7a			15 (19 %)		
4 + 3 = 7b			9 (11 %)		
4 + 4 = 8			5 (6 %)		
4 + 5 = 9			4 (5 %)		
5 + 4 = 9			2 (2 %)		
EAU-risk	Number (%)				
Low-risk			21 (30 %)		
Intermediate-risk			32 (46 %)		
High-risk			17 (24 %)		

PCa prostate cancer, PSA prostate specific antigen, PCA3 prostate cancer gene 3, DRE digital rectal examination is considered positive if there was suspicion of PCa
*p-value is estimated for the difference of means between the group with PCa and the group without PCa using the t-test
**p-value is estimated for the difference of proportions between the group with PCa and the group without PCa using Chi-square test

Table 2 This table shows the diagnostic performance of RTE and PCA3 score with cut-off 35 for the group of any PCa, for the combined group of intermediate-and high-risk PCa, and for high-risk PCa

	Parameter	Sensitivity	Specificity	NPV	PPV
Any PCa	RTE	74 %	39 %	54 %	61 %
	PCA3	64 %	78 %	66 %	80 %
	Combination	91 %	26 %	70 %	62 %
IR and HR PCa	RTE	86 %	43 %	82 %	51 %
	PCA3	71 %	66 %	78 %	58 %
	Combination	96 %	24 %	90 %	55 %
HR PCa	RTE	88 %	35 %	95 %	18 %
	PCA3	82 %	57 %	95 %	23 %
	Combination	100 %	19 %	100 %	16 %

Abbreviations: PCa prostate cancer, IR intermediate-risk, HR high-risk, RTE real-time elastography, PCA3 prostate cancer gene 3, NPV negative predictive value, PPV positive predictive value

as well as PCA3. Group 1 encompassed 44 patients; 30 had a high- or intermediate-risk PCa, eight a low-risk PCa and six a benign prostate. If both tests were positive, we found a high (86 %) probability of PCa at biopsy. On the other hand, of 23 patients with a PCA3 below 35 and a negative RTE (Group 4), eight patients were diagnosed with PCa, including six with low-risk cancer and two with intermediate-risk cancer, while 15 patients did not have any cancer. There was no high-risk PCa in this group. Omitting a biopsy in this group would imply a 9 % likelihood of missing PCa of clinical importance. In Group 2, 14 patients were diagnosed with cancer and 27 without cancer. There were 16 patients with a PCA3 score equal to or higher than 35 and a negative RTE (Group 3); ten patients had cancer and no cancer was found in the other six. The results achieved from pre-biopsy PCA3 urinary tests and RTE assessments in both Group 1 and Group 4 are informative and may be of benefit in the decision-making process as to whether to perform a biopsy or not.

Out of 70 patients for whom PCa was diagnosed, 27 underwent radical prostatectomy, 27 received external radiotherapy and 16 opted for active surveillance.

Discussion

There is a changing wind in the way we detect and treat PCa as a consequence of the well-known over-diagnosis and overtreatment of PCa, in addition to the documented increasing rate of post-biopsy infections [4, 5]. There is an ongoing search for new biomarkers and the development of improved methods for identifying clinically significant PCa. Evolving evidences show the benefit of PCA3 in the decision-making process of performing repeat biopsies in men where the initial biopsy is negative.

Both RTE and mpMRI are capable of identifying PCa that is not visualized on B-mode ultrasound [17, 18].

To the best of our knowledge, the present paper is the first to present prospective data on the combination of pre-biopsy PCA3 and RTE by patient in predicting PCa in an unselected series of men admitted for an initial biopsy.

The most important findings are the high sensitivity as well as NPV in predicting intermediate-risk and high-risk PCa (Table 2). PCA3 and RTE appeared to be of benefit mostly in patients if both parameters were positive or negative. If both parameters are positive, there is good reason to perform a biopsy and there is a high probability of detecting aggressive disease. Additionally, avoiding a biopsy in which PCA3 and RTE are negative carries a small risk of missing patients harboring a clinically significant PCa. In this series we found 32 intermediate-risk PCa and 17 high-risk PCa. By using RTE and PCA3 as selection criteria for performing a biopsy, 23 patients would have been advised against having a biopsy; only two of these patients had intermediate-risk PCa and no patients had high-risk PCa. One could argue that the reduction of unnecessary biopsies is relatively small since only 23 patients (19 %) would have been advised against biopsy. On the other hand, these patients could safely be advised

Table 3 Logistic regression analyses for predicting high and intermediate risk prostate cancer (n = 124)

	Simple			Multiple					
	Unadjusted			Fully adjusted			Final model		
Variables	OR	95 % CI	p-value**	OR	95 % CI	p-value**	OR	95 % CI	p-value**
Age (cont. in years)	1.04	(0.98,1.10)	0.188	1.04	(0.96, 1.13)	0.287			
PSA (cont. in ng/ml)	1.18	(1.08, 1.29)	<0.001	1.19	(1.07, 1.34)	0.001	1.18	(1.03, 1.14)	0.001
Pvol. (cont. in ml)	0.98	(0.96, 0.99)	0.003	0.97	(0.95, 0.99)	0.005	1.04	(1.04, 1.07)	0.009
Positive RTE (Y/N)	4.46	(1.78, 11.22)	0.001	2.73	(0.96, 7.79)	0.052	2.56	(0.91, 7.23)	0.068
PCA3 (>35 vs. <35)	5.00	(2.28, 10.95)	<0.001	3.31	(1.27, 8.63)	0.013	4.12	(1.71, 9.91)	0.001

Abbreviations: RTE: real-time elastography, Cont continuous, Y/N yes/no, OR odds ratio, CI confidence interval, Pvol prostate volume
**p-value by the use of the Likelihood Ratio test

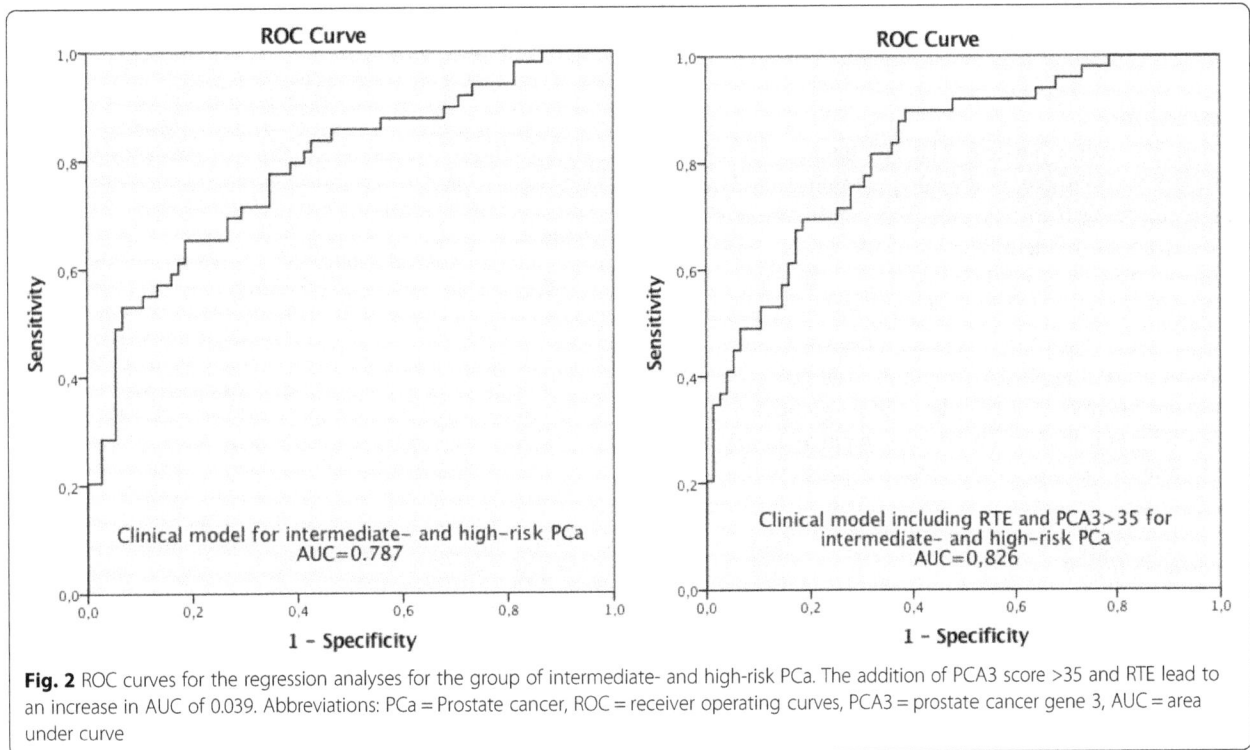

Fig. 2 ROC curves for the regression analyses for the group of intermediate- and high-risk PCa. The addition of PCA3 score >35 and RTE lead to an increase in AUC of 0.039. Abbreviations: PCa = Prostate cancer, ROC = receiver operating curves, PCA3 = prostate cancer gene 3, AUC = area under curve

against biopsy, as every reduction of unnecessary biopsies is a step in the right direction in reducing over-diagnosis and overtreatment of low-risk PCa. These findings are in line with our previous study of the combination of PCA3 and RTE in a smaller series of radically operated PCa patients [16].

In the logistic regression analysis PCA3 as well as a positive RTE contributed to the clinical model although RTE achieved a p-value close to significance (0. 068). In a ROC analysis, the full model with PCA3 and RTE achieved an AUC of 0.826. In univariate analysis a positive RTE is a highly significant predictor of PCa.

No definite threshold of PCA3 score has been agreed upon as yet, although a score of 35 is most frequently used as a cut-off value. In our study, we tested two different PCA3 score thresholds of 21 and 35, respectively. A threshold score of 35 provided the most optimal PPV of 80 %, which is the same figure found in a prospective randomized study by Wei et al., using a PCA3 score threshold of 60 in the initial biopsy setting [19]. In our analyses, we utilized a PCA3 score of 35 as the threshold value.

A strength of this study is that it includes histopathological data on initial biopsies, repeat biopsies as well as data of further follow-up, including mpMRI targeted biopsies of suspected lesions. No patients in the group diagnosed with a benign disease have been diagnosed with PCa in the period since the study inclusion was closed in June 2012. For all 14 patients with a presumably benign reason for an elevated PSA, both medical records and records for the regional pathology laboratory were checked. We believe that we are as close as possible to the true prevalence of PCa in the study population at the time of the examinations. This makes this study different from other studies investigating PCA3 [8, 20] and RTE [21, 22], in which the performance of these markers has been solely evaluated at the initial biopsy.

In this series of patients, a total of 70 patients were diagnosed with PCa, including 21 who were classified as low-risk and 49 as either high- or intermediate-risk.

Analyzing the group of PCa patients harboring either high- or intermediate-risk PCa, the combination of RTE and PCA3 correctly identified 47 of these patients. That means we correctly identified 96 % of the patients harboring PCa in need of treatment in a pre-biopsy setting. This result may be used to reduce the number of unnecessary biopsies at a small risk of missing PCa in need of treatment.

The present study has some limitations. Firstly, it is a single center, single investigator study. RTE like all US investigations are real-time examinations and are operator dependent and an inter-observer investigation would have been of value. As to the learning curve, it has been shown that after about 30 RTE the novice is achieving comparable results to experienced US operators [23]. Secondly, a relatively small number of patients are included. Thirdly, there is a limited number of patients with high-risk PCa, although the findings are in line with our previously published paper on patients planned for radical prostatectomy [16].

Conclusions

In patients with a positive RTE combined with a PCA3 score above 35 there is a high probability of detecting intermediate- or high-risk PCa. The combination of these markers correctly identified 47 of 49 (96 %) patients in need of a further diagnostic work-up. The high NPV of the combination of PCA3 and RTE makes it possible to avoid some 20 % of the prostate biopsies without missing high-risk PCa. If applied to the upper age group, in which a missing low-risk PCa may be seen as an advantage, the use of RTE and PCA3 may be implemented as pre-biopsy examinations to reduce the number of prostate biopsies.

Abbreviations

AUC, area under the curve; CI, confidence interval; DRE, digital rectal examination; EAU, European Association of Urology; mpMRI, multiparametric magnetic resonance imaging; NPV, negative predictive value; PCa, prostate cancer; PCA3, Prostate cancer gene 3; PPV, positive predictive value; PSA, prostate-specific antigen; Pvol, prostate volume; ROC, receiver operating curve; RTE, real-time elastography; TRUS, transrectal ultrasound; US, ultrasound

Acknowledgements

The authors acknowledge statistician Geir Egil Eide at the Center for Clinical Research, Haukeland University Hospital for his help in the preparation of the manuscript.

Funding

The study has been carried out with funding from the institutions mentioned on the title page and by a grant from the URO-BERGEN Research Foundation. This grant was used to purchase an endfire probe for the ultrasound machine. The Fürst Medical Laboratory in Oslo performed the PCA3 analyses at a reduced price since the results were used in a study setting. The funding body of the study had no part in the design, the data collection, the analysis, the interpretation of the study or in the writing of the manuscript.

Availability of data and materials

The approval from the ethical committee and the informed consent do not cover full open publication of the dataset. The raw data will be made available in unidentified form on request, if needed contact corresponding author.

Authors' contributions

YN: Project development, Data collection and analysis, Manuscript writing. SAH: Project development, Data Collection and analysis, Manuscript editing. OJH: Data collection and analysis, Manuscript editing. KG: Data collection and analysis, Manuscript editing. JF: Data collection and analysis, Manuscript editing. LAA: Data analysis, Manuscript editing. CB: Project development, Data analysis, Manuscript editing. All authors have read and approved the final manuscript.

Competing interests

The authors declare that they have no competing interests. The authors alone are responsible for the content and writing of the paper.

Author details

[1]Department of Urology, Haukeland University Hospital, N-5021 Bergen, Norway. [2]Department of Pathology, Haukeland University Hospital, N-5021 Bergen, Norway. [3]Department of Clinical Medicine, University of Bergen, Bergen, Norway. [4]Center for Cancer Biomarkers CCBIO, Department of Clinical Medicine, University of Bergen, Bergen, Norway.

References

1. Ilic D, Neuberger MM, Djulbegovic M, et al. Screening for prostate cancer. Cochrane Database Syst Rev. 2013;1:CD004720.
2. Chou R, Croswell JM, Dana T, et al. Screening for prostate cancer: a review of the evidence for the U.S. Preventive Services Task Force. Ann Intern Med. 2011;155:762–71.
3. Schroder FH, Hugosson J, Roobol MJ, et al. Screening and prostate cancer mortality: results of the European Randomised Study of Screening for Prostate Cancer (ERSPC) at 13 years of follow-up. Lancet. 2014;384:2027–35.
4. Carignan A, Roussy JF, Lapointe V, et al. Increasing risk of infectious complications after transrectal ultrasound-guided prostate biopsies: time to reassess antimicrobial prophylaxis. Eur Urol. 2012;62:453–9.
5. Loeb S, Vellekoop A, Ahmed HU, et al. Systematic review of complications of prostate biopsy. Eur Urol. 2013;64:876–92.
6. Moyer VA. Force USPST Screening for prostate cancer: U.S. Preventive Services Task Force recommendation statement. Ann Intern Med. 2012;157:120–34.
7. Heidenreich A, Bastian PJ, Bellmunt J, et al. EAU guidelines on prostate cancer. part 1: screening, diagnosis, and local treatment with curative intent-update 2013. Eur Urol. 2014;65:124–37.
8. Hansen J, Auprich M, Ahyai SA, et al. Initial prostate biopsy: development and internal validation of a biopsy-specific nomogram based on the prostate cancer antigen 3 assay. Eur Urol. 2013;63:201–9.
9. Nygard Y, Haukaas SA, Eide GE, et al. Prostate cancer antigen-3 (PCA3) and PCA3-based nomograms in the diagnosis of prostate cancer: an external validation of Hansen's nomogram on a Norwegian cohort. Scand J Urol. 2015;49:8–15.
10. Haas GP, Delongchamps NB, Jones RF, et al. Needle biopsies on autopsy prostates: sensitivity of cancer detection based on true prevalence. J Natl Cancer Inst. 2007;99:1484–9.
11. Walz J, Marcy M, Pianna JT, et al. Identification of the prostate cancer index lesion by real-time elastography: considerations for focal therapy of prostate cancer. World J Urol. 2011;29:589–94.
12. Rud E, Klotz D, Rennesund K, et al. Detection of the index tumour and tumour volume in prostate cancer using T2-weighted and diffusion-weighted magnetic resonance imaging (MRI) alone. BJU Int. 2014;114:E32–42.
13. Nygard Y, Haukaas SA, Halvorsen OJ, et al. A positive real-time elastography is an independent marker for detection of high-risk prostate cancers in the primary biopsy setting. BJU Int. 2014;113:E90–7.
14. Salomon G, Drews N, Autier P, et al. Incremental detection rate of prostate cancer by real-time elastography targeted biopsies in combination with a conventional 10-core biopsy in 1024 consecutive patients. BJU Int. 2014;113:548–53.
15. Filson CP, Natarajan S, Margolis DJ, et al. Prostate cancer detection with magnetic resonance-ultrasound fusion biopsy: The role of systematic and targeted biopsies Cancer 2016
16. Nygard Y, Haukaas SA, Waage JE, et al. Combination of real-time elastography and urine prostate cancer gene 3 (PCA3) detects more than 97% of significant prostate cancers. Scand J Urol. 2013;47:211–6.
17. Brock M, Loppenberg B, Roghmann F, et al. Impact of real-time elastography on magnetic resonance imaging/ultrasound fusion guided biopsy in patients with prior negative prostate biopsies. J Urol. 2015;193:1191–7.
18. Porpiglia F, Russo F, Manfredi M, et al. The roles of multiparametric magnetic resonance imaging, PCA3 and prostate health index-which is the best predictor of prostate cancer after a negative biopsy? J Urol. 2014;192:60–6.

19. Wei JT, Feng Z, Partin AW, et al. Can urinary PCA3 supplement PSA in the early detection of prostate cancer? J Clin Oncol. 2014;32:4066–72.
20. Ruffion A, Devonec M, Champetier D, et al. PCA3 and PCA3-based nomograms improve diagnostic accuracy in patients undergoing first prostate biopsy. Int J Mol Sci. 2013;14:17767–80.
21. Aigner F, Pallwein L, Junker D, et al. Value of real-time elastography targeted biopsy for prostate cancer detection in men with prostate specific antigen 1.25 ng/ml or greater and 4.00 ng/ml or less. J Urol. 2010;184:913–7.
22. Brock M, von Bodman C, Palisaar RJ, et al. The impact of real-time elastography guiding a systematic prostate biopsy to improve cancer detection rate: a prospective study of 353 patients. J Urol. 2012;187:2039–43.
23. Heinzelbecker J, Weiss C, Pelzer AE A learning curve assessment of real-time sonoelastography of the prostate World J Urol 2012

25

Thrombosed varicocele - a rare cause for acute scrotal pain

M. Raghavendran[1*†], A. Venugopal[2] and G. Kiran Kumar[3†]

Abstract

Background: Acute scrotal pain has various causes. Testicular torsion, torsion of appendages and Epididymo-orchitis are common causes, while varicocele thromboses are a rare cause. Varicocele thromboses can occur post operatively or spontaneously. Five cases of post-operative and five cases of spontaneous thromboses have been described till date. The traditional advice in the management of thrombosed varicocele has been to manage it conservatively in all patients by drugs and scrotal support with little description of the surgical treatment. Herein, we present an unusual sixth case of spontaneous thromboses of varicocele and discuss its presentation and surgical management. We would also like to highlight the differentiating points between spontaneous thrombosis and post operative in vitro clot formation in the varicoceles, as these two entities can often be confused for each other.

Case presentation: A 68 year-old man presented with excruciating scrotal pain of one week duration. Doppler study of scrotum revealed left varicocele with no evidence of Epididymo-orchitis. He was treated with intravenous antibiotics, analgesics and scrotal elevation. He had no relief and continued to have severe pain. Clinical examination was normal. Patient underwent exploratory surgery on a semi- emergent basis. Exploration revealed normal testis with thrombosed varicoceles. Patient underwent Varicocelectomy. Postoperatively patient had immediate pain relief. Histopathology revealed prominent thrombosed varicocele. A varicocelectomy specimen (done for primary infertility) was used for comparison. The differentiating points between the two entities were noted.

Conclusion: Spontaneous thrombosis of varicocele is a rare cause of acute scrotal pain. Pain out of proportion to clinical features is characteristic. Patients not responding to medical therapy may need varicocelectomy. Varicocelectomy may give immediate relief. Histopathology is useful in this disorder.

Keywords: Acute Orchialgia, Thrombosed varicocele, Acute Epididymo-Orchitis, Varicocelectomy, Testicular torsion, Post Varicocelectomy thrombosis

Background

Acute scrotal pain has multiple aetiologies. Torsion of testis or its appendages and Epididymo-orchitis are common [1], while Varicocele thrombosis is a rare cause [2]. Varicocele thromboses can occur post operatively (5 cases) or spontaneously (5 cases) [2–4]. Spontaneous thrombosis can occur due to trauma or in patients with coagulation abnormalities [5]. Kayes et al. had reported that vigorous sexual or sporting activity, infections, trauma, long hour flights and drugs could cause this condition [6]. There were no major predisposing

* Correspondence: maniyurr@yahoo.com
†Equal contributors
[1]Department Of Urology, Apollo BGS Hospitals, Adichunchunagiri Road, Kuvempunagar, Mysore, Karnataka 570009, India
Full list of author information is available at the end of the article

mechanisms for spontaneous thrombosis to occur in our patient, but it is possible that vigorous sexual activity could have caused this because patient developed pain after sexual intercourse. Varicocele thromboses (both spontaneous and post-operative) have been managed conservatively in all patients till date by means of drugs (antibiotics and anti-inflammatory agents) and scrotal support with no description of surgical treatment. There are contradictory reports with regards to the timing and requirement of surgery in thrombosed Varicocele patients. Roach et al. and El Hannawy et al. recommend conservative non-operative management, despite the fact that they subjected their patients to surgery. Hence the timing and requirement of surgery in thrombosed Varicocele patients becomes a hugely debatable point [7, 8]. Herein, we present a case of spontaneous Varicocele thromboses with special emphasis on its presentation and surgical management. Spontaneous in vivo thrombi has historically been mistaken for post varicocelectomy in vitro clot formations in veins. We would like to highlight the histopathological differentiation between these two distinct entities.

Case presentation

A 68 year-old man presented with excruciating left scrotal pain of one week duration. He had undergone Doppler study of the scrotum elsewhere, which revealed grade one varicocele with no evidence of Epididymo-orchitis. There was no other significant pathology in the Doppler. He was treated with intravenous antibiotics, parenteral and oral analgesics and scrotal elevation for around ten days. He had no relief and continued to have excruciating, severe pain. Pain was constant, continuous, with radiation from the scrotum to the inguinal region. Pain was not alleviated even with analgesics. There were no further aggravating factors. Clinical examination revealed normal looking scrotum with no features of inflammation. In view of pain out of proportion to clinical features, exploratory surgery was planned. Exploration revealed normal testis with blue prominent, tense and turgid varicoceles (red arrows in Fig. 1). Patient underwent left Varicocelectomy. Postoperatively patient had immediate pain relief. Histopathology showed prominent varicocele with lumen completely occluded by thrombi adherent to the wall with no retraction space (Fig. 2). A varicocelectomy specimen (done for primary infertility) was used for comparison and showed

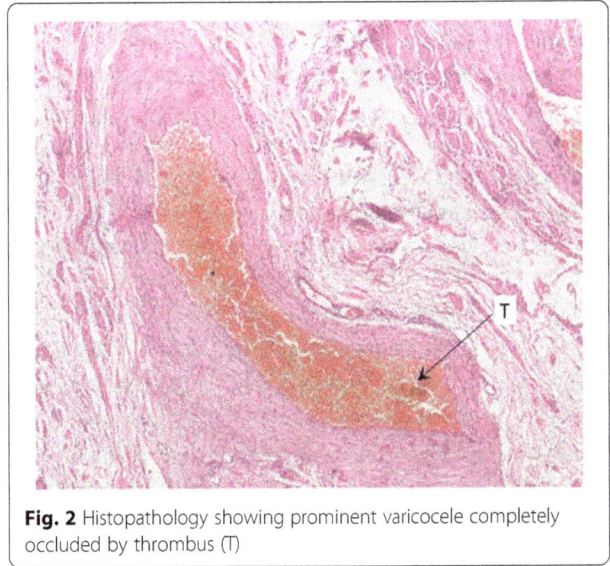

Fig. 2 Histopathology showing prominent varicocele completely occluded by thrombus (T)

veins with in- vitro clots. The clot was not attached to the wall and there was clear retraction space between the clot and wall (Fig. 3).

Discussion

Thrombosed varicoceles have been described as a rare cause of acute scrotal pain [2–4]. Postoperative thrombus in pampiniform plexuses have been managed conservatively with intravenous antibiotics, parenteral and oral analgesics, scrotal elevation with bed rest [3]. Spontaneously occurring thrombi have also been reported to have been managed medically in a previous case, though the exact details of medical treatment are unclear [2, 4]. As of date, all the cases mentioned in literature have been managed medically without any note of the surgical treatment needed in such cases. It is interesting to note the first report in literature by Roach et al. They had recommended conservative management. In their study of 2patients, both underwent surgical

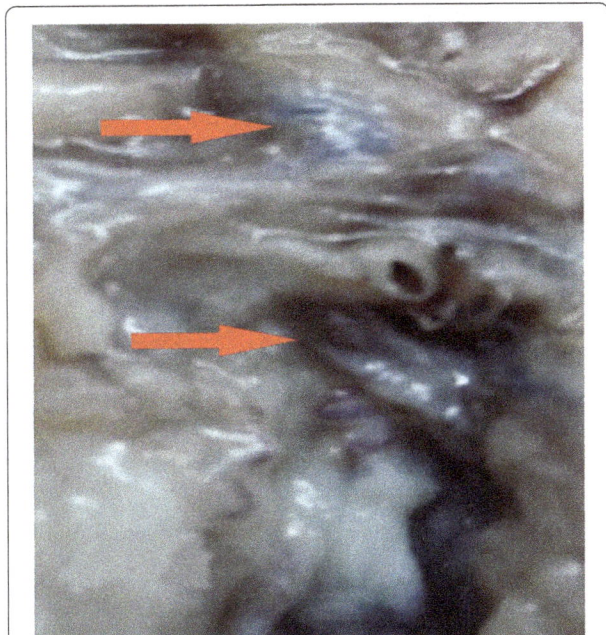

Fig. 1 Gross photograph showing prominent blue coloured varicoceles (red arrows)

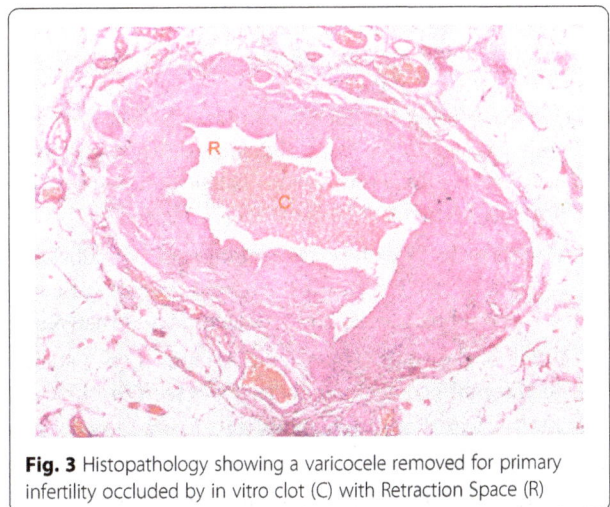

Fig. 3 Histopathology showing a varicocele removed for primary infertility occluded by in vitro clot (C) with Retraction Space (R)

ligation and excision of the thrombosed vein [7]. So their recommendations are contrary to their findings. Similarly El Hennawy et al. advice conservative management, when in their case they subjected the patient to surgery [8]. There are 2 other case reports which have reported that pain usually subsides with a week of non-steroidal anti-inflammatory medications and scrotal rest. Here also, Doerfler et al. recommend medical management, while their patient was subjected to surgery [2]. Kleinclauss et al. were the only ones who managed their patient successfully with medical management alone [4]. The other documentation of medical management is in that of post-operative Varicocelectomy patients. Summation of all the reports make us come to a conclusion that medical therapy may be successful if only a single superficial spermatic vein is involved, while in cases like ours where the majority of pampiniform plexus is thrombosed, surgical management will have a better outcome. This conclusion is similar to the one by Bolat et al. who opined that treatment can be started conservatively, with surgical intervention reserved for failed cases on an emergent basis [5]. Similarly Isenberg et al. advice that though venography, Doppler can be diagnostic, surgery should not be delayed in doubtful cases [9]. Hence, we feel that if severe pain persists in spite of adequate medical therapy (non-steroidal anti-inflammatory agents, scrotal elevation and rest for 7-10 days), as seen in our case, then these patients should be subjected to immediate surgical exploration. Varicocelectomy gives complete pain relief and should be considered as treatment of choice in this sub group of patients, who have failed medical management. Another controversial issue is whether to perform just ligation of the vein or to completely excise the segment of the thrombosed vein? Mallat et al. also reported a case where they had done complete excision of the thrombosed vein [10]. We also did surgical excision of the thrombosed vein as we felt that doing a simple ligation may not alleviate the pain completely. Another worrisome consideration is that delay in performing Varicocelectomy may probably lead to ischemic damage to the testis. Roach et al. had to perform orchiectomy due to severe venous congestion and testicular ischemia in one of their patients [7]. Hence, we postulate that in patients with severe scrotal pain not subsiding with 7 days of medical therapy, exploration and varicocelectomy should be immediately considered and may result in salvage of the testis. The second issue in these patients are do thrombi occur in varicoceles? As seen in our case, it is pretty clear that spontaneous thrombosis do occur in varicoceles. The histopathology can help in differentiating an in vivo thrombus from an in vitro post operative clot.

A long standing clot in Varicocelectomy specimen of infertility will remodel and have a retraction space, while the clot in thrombosed specimen may not have this space due to the acuteness of the episode.

Learning points

1. Spontaneous thrombosis of varicocele is a rare cause of acute scrotal pain.
2. Pain out of proportion to clinical features is characteristic of this condition.
3. Spontaneous thrombus in varicoceles not responding to adequate (7-10) medical therapy need varicocelectomy. Varicocelectomy produces immediate pain relief.
4. Histopathology can be useful in this disorder as it can help in differentiating a spontaneous complete thrombus in the acute thrombosed varicocele from an in vitro remodelled clot in a longer standing Varicocele.

Conclusion

Spontaneous thrombosis of varicocele is a rare cause of acute scrotal pain. Pain out of proportion to clinical features is characteristic. Patients not responding to medical therapy need varicocelectomy. Varicocelectomy gives immediate relief. Histopathology is useful in this disorder.

Authors' contributions
MR was involved in writing of the conception, design report, final draft critical review and revision. KK was also involved in the writing of the report, data collection, proof reading and appraisal. AV was involved in all the histopathology work and the interpretation of the specimens. All authors have read and approved the final manuscript.

Competing interests
The authors declare that they have no competing interests.

Author details
[1]Department Of Urology, Apollo BGS Hospitals, Adichunchunagiri Road, Kuvempunagar, Mysore, Karnataka 570009, India. [2]Apollo BGS Hospitals, Mysore, Karnataka, India. [3]Department Of Urology, Apollo Hospitals, Mysore, Karnataka, India.

References
1. Cavusoglu YH, Karaman A, Karaman I, et al. Acute scrotum—etiology and management. Indian J Pediatr. 2005;72(3):201–3.
2. Doerfler A, Ramadani D, Meuwly JY, Jichlinski P. Varicocele thrombosis:a rare etiology of testicular pain. Prog Urol. 2009;19(5):351–2.
3. Zampieri N, Castellani R, Mantovan A, et al. Thromboses of the pampiniform plexi after subinguinal varicocelectomy. Pediatr Surg Int. 2014;30(4):441–4.

4. Kleinclauss F, Della Negra E, Martin M, et al. Spontaneous thrombosis of left varicocele. Prog Urol. 2001;11(1):95–6.
5. Deniz Bolat, Bulent Gunlusoy,MD, , Serkan Yarimoglu, MD, et al. Isolated thrombosis of right spermatic vein with underlying factor V Leiden mutation. Can Urol Assoc J 2016; 10(9-10): E324–E327.
6. Kayes O, Patrick N, Sengupta AA. Peculiar case of bilateral, spontaneous thrombosis of the pampiniformplexi. Ann R Coll Surg Engl. 2010;92:22–3.
7. Roach R, Messing E, Starling J. Spontaneous thrombosis of left spermatic vein: report of 2 cases. J Urol. 1985;134(2):369–70.
8. El Hennawy HM, Abuzour ME, Bedair ESM. Surgical management of spontaneously thrombosed extratesticular varicocele presented with irreducible inguinal swelling: a case report. Eur. J Surg Sci. 2010;1(3):99–101.
9. Isenberg JS, Ozuner G, Worth MH, Ferzli G. Effort-induced spontaneous thrombosis of the left spermatic vein presenting clinically as a left inguinal hernia. J Urol. 1990;144(1):138.
10. Mallat F, Wissem H, Khaled BA, Sarra M, Faouzi M. Spontaneous spermatic vein thrombosis as a circumstance of discovery of the nutcracker syndrome: an exceptional entity. Int J Case Rep Images. 2014;5(7):519–23.

26

Abiraterone acetate in metastatic castration-resistant prostate cancer – the unanticipated real-world clinical experience

Darren M. C. Poon[1,7]*, Kuen Chan[2,7], S. H. Lee[3,7], T. W. Chan[4,7], Henry Sze[5,7], Eric K. C. Lee[6,7], Daisy Lam[1,7] and Michelle F. T. Chan[5,7]

Abstract

Background: There is much interest in confirming whether the efficacy of abiraterone acetate (AA) demonstrated within the trial setting is reproducible in routine clinical practice. We report the clinical outcome of metastatic castration-resistant prostate cancer (mCRPC) patients treated with AA in real-life clinical practice.

Methods: The clinical records of mCRPC patients treated with AA from all 6 public oncology centers in Hong Kong between August 2011 and December 2014 were reviewed. The treatment efficacy and its determinants, and toxicities were determined.

Results: A total of 110 patients with mCRPC were treated with AA in the review period, of whom 58 were chemo-naive and 52 had received prior chemotherapy (post-chemo). The median follow-up time was 7.5/11.4 months for chemo-naive/post-chemo patients. 6.9/15.4 % of chemo-naive/post-chemo patients had visceral metastases. The median overall survival (OS) and progression-free survival (PFS) were 18.1/15.5 months and 6.7/6.4 months for chemo-naive/post-chemo patients, respectively. Among chemo-naive patients, those with visceral diseases had significantly inferior OS (2.8 vs 18.0 $p = 0.0007$) and PFS (2.8 vs 6.8 months, $p = 0.0088$) than those without. Pain control was comparable in both groups of patients. The most common grade 3 or above toxicities were hypertension (6.9/5.8 %) and hypokalemia (3.4/3.8 %) in chemo-naive/post-chemo patients. In multivariate analysis, the presence of prostate-specific antigen (PSA) response (≥ 50 % drop of PSA from baseline) within the first 3 months of therapy was associated with favorable OS and PFS in both chemo-naive and post-chemo group.

Conclusions: In clinical practice outside the trial setting, OS after AA in our chemo-naive patient cohort (18.1 months) was considerably shorter than that reported in the COU-AA-302 trial (34.7 months), and the OS was particularly short in those with visceral metastases (2.8 months). Conversely, AA was efficacious in post-chemo patients. AA resulted in comparable pain control in both groups of patients. The presence of PSA response within the first 3 months of treatment was a significant determinant of survival.

Keywords: Castration-resistant prostate cancer, Abiraterone acetate, Chemo-naïve, Chemotherapy, PSA response

* Correspondence: mc_poon@clo.cuhk.edu.hk
[1]Department of Clinical Oncology, State Key Laboratory in Oncology in South China, Sir YK Pao Centre for Cancer, Hong Kong Cancer Institute and Prince of Wales Hospital, The Chinese University of Hong Kong, Hong Kong, Hong Kong
[7]Hong Kong Society of Uro-Oncology (HKSUO), Hong Kong, Hong Kong
Full list of author information is available at the end of the article

Background

Androgen deprivation therapy (ADT), either medical or surgical, is the backbone of first line treatment for metastatic prostate cancer [1]. While up to 80 % of patients will respond favorably to this therapy; metastatic castration-resistant disease (mCRPC), would be encountered ultimately [2].

Since 2004, docetaxel chemotherapy was the standard of care for patients with mCRPC [3, 4]. More recently, the treatment paradigm had been altered dramatically with the advent of several androgen receptor (AR) pathway targeted agents, new-generation chemotherapy, and immunotherapy [5]. Abiraterone acetate (AA), a potent and irreversible inhibitor of cytochrome-P (CYP)-17 that blocks androgen synthesis, has been shown in large-scale randomized trials to confer significant survival advantage over placebo in both chemo-naïve mCRPC patients and mCRPC patients with prior chemotherapy (post-chemo) [6, 7].

There is much interest in confirming whether the efficacy of AA demonstrated within the trial setting is reproducible in routine clinical practice, in consideration of possible differences in selection of patients, ethnic differences, and other factors in day-to-day practice. In fact, for the case of docetaxel for mCRPC patients, previous retrospective studies had shown unexpectedly higher incidence of febrile neutropenia and less favorable survival outcome compared to that in the trial setting [8, 9]. In the present study, we report on the clinical outcome of AA in patients with mCRPC from all 6 public oncology centers in Hong Kong.

Methods

Ethics statement

The study was approved by the institutional review board of the authors' institutions (Joint Chinese University of Hong Kong – New Territories East Cluster Clinical Research Ethics Committee/Ref no: CRE-2015.481). And permission to access the medical records through the inter-hospital computer network was granted by the aforementioned review board. Furthermore, the principles of the Helsinki Declaration were followed. Informed consent has been exempted by the review board as most of the patients in this study were dead when the data was collected.

Study population and treatment

In early 2011, AA was approved by the local health authority for use in patients with mCRPC who had received prior chemotherapy, and subsequently in 2012, also for chemo-naïve patients. The present review included mCRPC patients who were started on AA in 6 oncology centers between August 2011 and December 2014. All patients had metastatic prostate cancer which

had progressed despite achieving castration-level of testosterone. Enzalutamide, another AR pathway targeted agent, was not accessible during the study period and only be commercially available since October 2015 in our locality [10]. Patients with visceral disease who were medically unfit for, or who declined, chemotherapy, and treated with AA within the period were also included. Patients were treated with 1 g AA once daily in combination with 5 mg prednisone twice a day until disease progression, death or unacceptable toxicity. Clinical and biochemical follow-up with serum prostate-specific antigen (PSA), blood counts, liver and renal profile were regularly undertaken during the treatment period. Serum lactate dehydrogenase (LDH) was not a mandatory parameter to be regularly examined during the treatment. Regular imaging assessment was not mandatory unless clinical suspicion or biochemical progression was evident. Continuation of AA beyond disease progression and post-AA treatments were at the discretion of individual oncologists based on several factors including patient's preference, medical condition or affordability, physician's preference and availability of alternative treatment options.

Data collection and outcomes measures

The electronic clinical records of the patient cohort were retrieved by the inter-hospital computer network. The definition of clinical, biochemical and radiological progressive disease was according to the Prostate Cancer Clinical Trials Working Group (PCWG-2) criteria [11]. Overall survival (OS) and progression-free survival (PFS) were defined as time from first dose of AA to death, and to the first event of clinical, radiographic or PSA progression or death, respectively. Patients who had transient serum PSA level upsurge but not to the extent of biochemical progression (PCWG-2 criteria) followed by a drop, were defined as having PSA flare. PSA doubling time (PSA-DT) was calculated by determining the regression slope of the log PSA against time based on 3 consecutive PSA measurements prior to AA. Patients who had reduction or withdrawal of WHO class II or III analgesics according to the WHO analgesics ladder during or after AA was regarded as having improvement in pain control. Treatment-related toxicities were graded according to the National Cancer Institute Common Terminology Criteria for Adverse Events (CTCAE) 4.02 toxicity scale.

Statistical analysis

Statistical analysis was performed using the Statistical Package for the Social Sciences (Windows version 17.0.1.80; SPSS Inc, Chicago, US). The updated database as at 1 May 2015 was used for analysis. Kaplan-Meier plots of OS and PFS were obtained for subsets of patients segregated by various potential prognosticators. The log-rank test was employed to assess the difference in outcome between subsets. The variables were also subject to multivariate analyses using the Cox proportional hazards regression model. P values ≤ 0.05 were considered significant. The hazard ratio (HR) and the corresponding 95 % confidence interval were calculated.

Results
Characteristics of patients
Hundred and ten patients were reviewed, of whom 58 were chemo-naïve and 52 were post-chemo. Table 1 summarizes the characteristics of the patient cohort. The median follow-up duration was 7.5 (range, 1.0–24.6) and 11.43 (range, 1.2–30.2) months for chemo-naïve and post-chemo group respectively. Visceral diseases (non-nodal soft tissue metastases) were present in 4 (6.9 %) chemo-naïve and 8 (15.4 %) post-chemo patients. About 30 % of patients were symptomatic prior the initiation of AA.

Clinical efficacy
PSA response
The proportion of patients with PSA response (in about half of patients), PSA flare (about 30 % of patients), and eventual response after PSA flare (about two-thirds of patients with flare) were similar between the chemo-naïve and post-chemo groups (Table 2). All of the PSA response was present within the first 3 months of AA.

Duration of AA treatment and post-AA treatment
The median duration of AA treatment was 6.8 (range, 0.6–21.5) and 7.1 (0.5–25.0) months for chemo-naïve and post-chemo group respectively, with 27 chemo-naïve, and 13 post-chemo patients still under treatment at the time of last follow-up. Disease progression was the major reason of treatment discontinuation (Table 2). Continuation of AA treatment beyond disease progression and post-AA treatments were observed in 13/18 and 7/11 chemo-naïve/post-chemo group respectively.

Overall survival and progression-free survival
The median OS was 18.1 (95 % confidence interval (CI): 9.9–25) and 15.5 (95 % CI: 13.8–23.6) months for chemo-naïve and post-chemo group respectively (Fig. 1) whereas their respective median PFS was 6.7 (95 % CI: 4.5–14.7) and 6.4 (95 % CI: 5.4–8.3) months (Fig. 2). Chemo-naïve patients with visceral disease had significantly inferior OS and PFS than those without (OS, 2.8 vs 18.0 months, $p = 0.0007$, HR: 6.907, 95 % CI: 1.81–25.36; PFS, 2.8 vs 6.8 months, $p = 0.0088$, HR: 1.79, 95 % CI: 0.73–4.42). In contrast, the differences in OS and PFS were not significant between patients with or without visceral disease in the post-chemo group (Fig. 3).

Table 1 Patient's characteristics

	Chemo-naïve (n = 58)	Post-chemo (n = 52)
Age, years		
Median	77	66
Range	56–92	39–85
≥75 (%)	37 (63.8)	11 (21.2)
ECOG performance status, No. (%)		
0–1	36 (62.1)	45 (86.5)
2	18 (31.0)	7 (13.5)
3	4 (6.9)	0
4	0	0
Gleason score at time of initial diagnosis (%)		
<8	24 (41.4)	19 (36.5)
≥8	16 (27.6)	29 (55.8)
Unknown	18 (31.0)	4 (7.7)
Median PSA (range), ug/l	212 (6.22–3095)	191 (4.2–4694)
Median PSA doubling time (range), months	2.1 (0.5–9.0)	2.3 (0.7–13.4)
Symptomatic at presentation[a], No. (%)	19 (32.8)	16 (30.8)
Baseline Hb (g/dl), median (range)	12 (5.2–15.5)	11.7 (5.7–14.9)
Baseline ALP (IU/l), median (range)	116.5 (40–2960)	119 (45–1857)
Disease location, No. (%)		
Bone only	35 (60.3)	28 (53.8)
Bone	55 (94.8)	50 (96.2)
Lymph node	22 (37.9)	20 (38.5)
Lung	2 (3.4)[b]	3 (5.8)
Liver	3 (5.2)[b]	5 (9.6)
Co-morbidities, No (%)		
Diabetes Mellitus	16 (27.6)	8 (15.4)
Hypertension	32 (55.2)	20 (38.5)
Hyperlipidemia	0	4 (7.7)
Atrial fibrillation	1 (1.7)	1 (1.9)
Congestive heart failure	1 (1.7)	0
No. of previous cytotoxic regimen (%)		
1	0	44 (84.6)
2	0	7 (13.5)
3	0	1 (1.9)
Disease progression prior AA (%)		
Biochemical progression only	42 (72.4)	35 (67.3)
Clinical or radiographic progression	16 (27.6)	17 (32.7)

Abbreviations: ECOG Eastern Cooperative Oncology Group, PSA prostate specific antigen, Hb hemoglobin, ALP alkaline phosphatase, AA abiraterone acetate
[a]presence of pain prior abiraterone acetate and require WHO level II or above analgesics
[b]One patient with both liver and lung metastases

Table 2 Treatment details

	Chemo-naïve (n = 58)	Post-chemo (n = 52)
Median duration of AA treatment, month (range)	6.8 (0.6–21.5)	7.1 (0.5–25.0)
PSA response (%)		
≥50 % PSA decline from baseline	36 (62.1)	26 (50.0)
≥90 % PSA decline from baseline	16 (27.6)	8 (15.4)
Median time to PSA nadir, month (range)	3.1 (0.9–15.0)	2.8 (0.5–15.3)
PSA flare (%)		
No. of patients	17 (29.3)	15 (28.8)
Presence of eventual PSA response (≥50 % PSA decline from baseline)	12 (70.6)	10 (66.7)
Pain alleviation during or after AA[a] (%)	11 (57.9 %)	11 (68.8 %)
Reasons of discontinuing AA (%)		
Disease progression	24 (41.4)	36 (69.2)
Treatment-related complication	3 (5.2)	1 (1.9)
Patient's decision	3 (5.2)	2 (3.8)
Unknown	1 (1.7)	0
Continuation of AA beyond PD		
No. of patients (%)	13 (22.4)	18 (34.6)
Median time, month (range)	2.8 (1.0–5.8)	2.0 (1.2–16.2)
Subsequent therapy after PD (%)		
Docetaxel	5 (8.6)	2 (3.8)
Cabazitaxel	2 (3.4)	7 (13.5)
Mitoxantrone	0	1 (1.9)
Ketoconazole	0	1 (1.9)

Abbreviations: PSA prostate specific antigen, AA abiraterone acetate, PD disease progression
[a]Withdrawal or reduction of level II or III analgesics according to WHO analgesics ladder

Pain control
Improvement in pain control was observed in more than half of the patients (Table 2).

Adverse events
Table 3 shows the treatment-related toxicities in patients treated with AA. In chemo-naïve group, hypokalemia (3.4 %), hypertension (6.9 %) and peripheral edema (5.2 %) were the commonest grade 3 complications, whereas hypertension (5.8 %), hypokalemia (3.8 %) and elevation of liver enzymes (1.9 %) were the commonest grade 3 toxicities in post-chemo group. There was no grade 4 toxicity or treatment-related death among them.

Univariate and multivariate analysis
Chemo-naïve group
In univariate analysis, 6 variables, including the presence of visceral disease (HR 6.907, 95 % CI 1.881–25.357, $p = 0.0007$), were significantly determinants of the OS (Table 4). In multivariate analysis, presence of visceral disease (HR 4.8, 95 % CI 1.026–22.465, $p = 0.0015$), presence of PSA response (HR 0.104, 95 % CI 0.025–0.387, $p = 0.0001$), short (<10 months) response to prior ADT (HR 2.656, 95 % CI 1.061–6.648, $p = 0.0336$), ECOG 2 or above (HR 4.907, 95 % CI 1.648–14.612, $p = 0.0001$), and low hemoglobin level (HR 2.696, 95 % CI 0.912–7.7971, $p = 0.0409$) were determinants of OS. Presence of PSA response (HR 0.186, 95 % CI 0.079–0.439, $p < 0.0001$) and presence of visceral disease (HR 5.891, 95 % CI 1.43–24.267, $p = 0.0126$) were determinants of PFS.

Post-chemo group
In multivariate analysis, presence of PSA response (HR 0.213, 95 % CI 0.076–0.592, $p = 0.0001$), Gleason score of ≥ 8 (HR 2.658, 95 % CI 1.13–6.251, $p = 0.0186$) and PSA-DT of < 2 months (HR 3.006, 95 % CI 1.278–7.07, $p = 0.0289$) were determinants of OS, while presence of PSA response (HR 0.403, 95 % CI 0.203–0.797, $p = 0.0007$) was a determinant of PFS (Table 5).

Discussion
In the current study, we reported the efficacy and toxicity of AA in mCRPC patients from an unselected patient population in a non-trial setting. The inclusion of all AA-treated patients in all public oncology centers during a defined period serves to provide a representative picture of the efficacy of AA in clinical service setting. The clinical efficacy, notably the OS and PFS, and tolerability of AA in our post-chemo patients was similar to that of the COU-AA-301 study (Table 6), thus reproducing the efficacy of AA in the post-chemotherapy setting. However, unexpectedly, the median OS of chemo-naïve patients in our cohort (of 18.1 months) was remarkably much shorter than that reported in COU-AA-302 study (of 34.7 months). It is noted that our chemo-naïve patients with visceral disease, the patient group that was excluded in the COU-AA-302 study, had significantly inferior survival. If this small subset of poor-prognosis patients was excluded, the OS and PFS of the chemo-naïve patients without visceral metastases were still unfavorable, being similar to the whole group. Thus inclusion of patients with visceral disease in our study cannot entirely explicate the unfavorable survival outcome of chemo-naïve patients. It is also unlikely that the infrequency of post-AA treatment contributes to the unfavorable survival, as the subset of patients given post-AA treatment did not have more favorable survival than those without in the multivariate analysis. We postulate that the inferior survival outcome of our chemo naïve patients could be attributable to a relatively high tumor burden in this patient cohort, compared to that in the COU-302 study. This is supported by a higher baseline PSA level (median: 212 ug/l) in our patients as

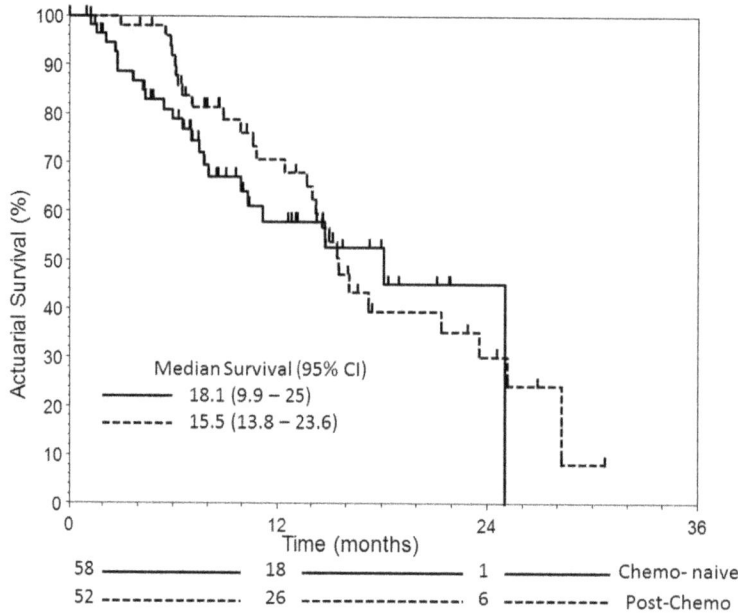

Fig. 1 The overall survival for mCRPC patients with (post-chemo) or without prior chemotherapy (chemo-naïve) treated with AA

compared to that in the COU-AA-302 study (median: 42 ug/l). Besides, the inclusion of chemo-naïve patients with poor prognostic features in our study could also account for the unsatisfactory survival results. For example, our patient cohort included symptomatic patients (only asymptomatic or mildly symptomatic patients were included in COU-AA-302 study) and patients with ECOG 2 (patients with ECOG 2 or above were excluded in COU-AA-302

study), and a higher proportion of elderly patients: 63.8 % of patients were age above 75 in our cohort, compared to 34 % in COU-AA-302 study.

It is worth noting that despite the somewhat disappointing survival outcome in chemo-naïve patients treated with AA; nearly 60 % of symptomatic patients had pain alleviation. In fact, such a rate of pain control is similar to that in post-chemo patients, and was also comparable to that in the COU-AA-301 study,

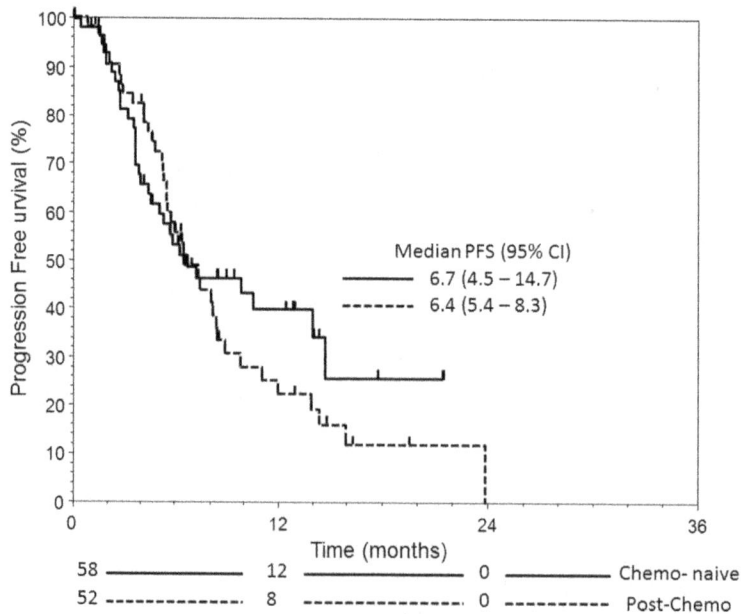

Fig. 2 The progression-free survival for mCRPC patients with (post-chemo) or without prior chemotherapy (chemo-naïve) treated with AA

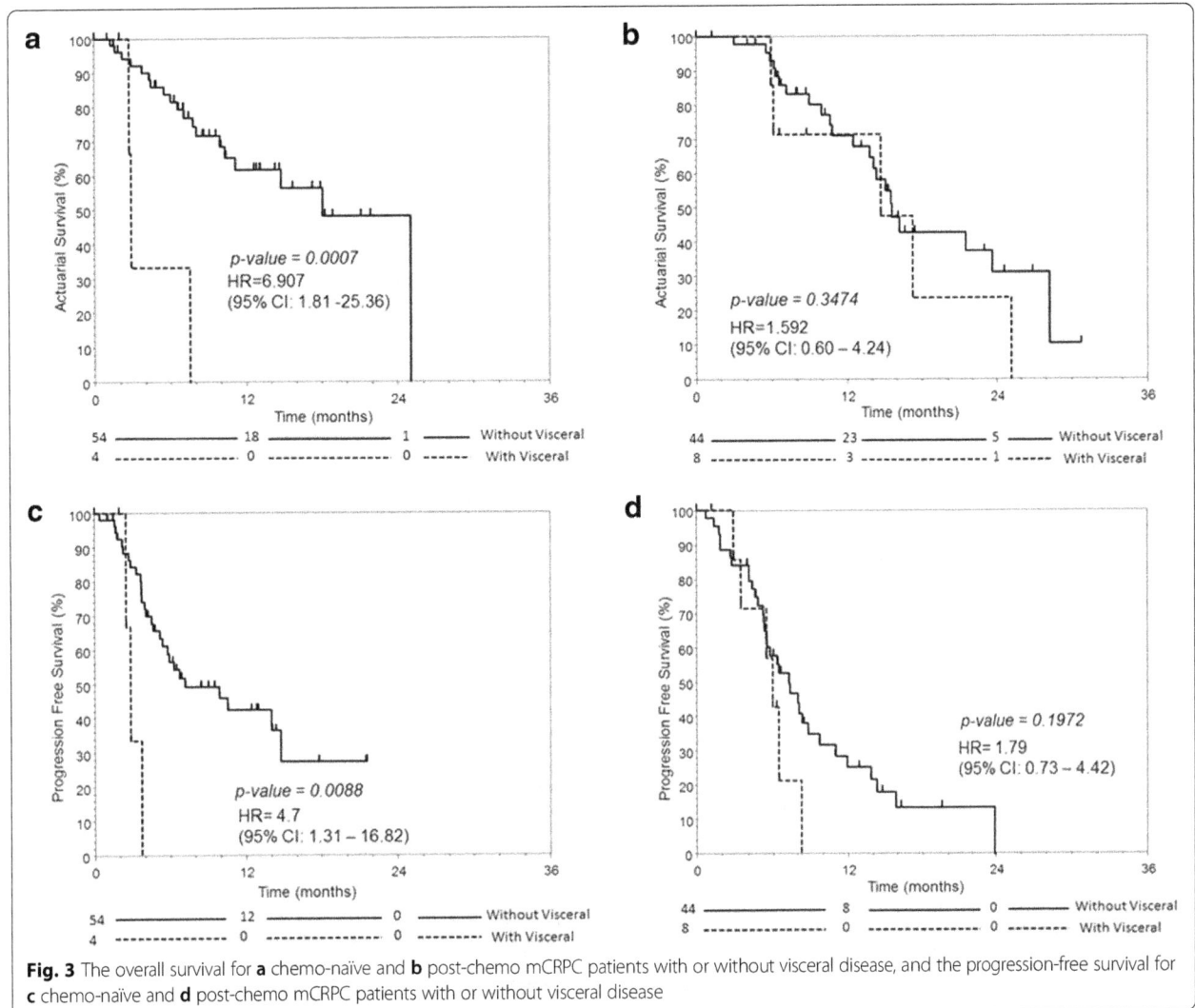

Fig. 3 The overall survival for **a** chemo-naïve and **b** post-chemo mCRPC patients with or without visceral disease, and the progression-free survival for **c** chemo-naïve and **d** post-chemo mCRPC patients with or without visceral disease

despite the pain assessment tools were not identical between ours and the pivotal studies (Table 6). To our knowledge, the present study is the first one to report on efficacy of pain control for symptomatic chemo-naïve patients with AA.

While data on efficacy of AA on chemo-naive patients with visceral metastases or symptomatic disease is being awaited, the present study suggests that patients with high tumor burden, visceral metastases and symptomatic disease may have inferior outcome with AA. An

Table 3 Adverse events during treatment

	Chemo-naïve (%)				Post-chemo (%)			
	Grade 1	Grade 2	Grade 3	Grade 4	Grade 1	Grade 2	Grade 3	Grade 4
Peripheral edema	6 (10.3)	0	3 (5.2)	0	2 (3.8)	1 (1.9)	0	0
Elevation of liver enzymes	7 (12.1)	0	0	0	3 (5.8)	0	1 (1.9)	0
Hypokalemia	15 (25.9)	1 (1.7)	2 (3.4)	0	9 (17.3)	2 (3.8)	2 (3.8)	0
Hypertension	9 (15.5)	7 (12.1)	4 (6.9)	0	17 (32.7)	3 (5.8)	3 (5.8)	0
Fatigue	1 (1.7)	0	0	0	1 (1.9)	0	0	0
Arthralgia	0	0	0	0	1 (1.9)	0	0	0
Diarrhoea	0	0	0	0	1 (1.9)	0	0	0
Dyspepsia	1 (1.7)	0	0	0	0	0	0	0

Table 4 Univariate and multivariate analysis of overall survival and progression-free survival – Chemo-naive group

Factors	Univariate analysis						Multivariate analysis					
	Progression-free survival			Overall survival			Progression-free survival			Overall survival		
	P value	HR	95 % CI	P value	HR	95 % CI	P value	HR	95 % CI	P value	HR	95 % CI
Time from ADT to CRPC (<10 vs ≥ 10 months)	0.0306	2.191	1.057–4.542	0.0002	4.566	1.913–10.898	0.816	1.104	0.49–2.489	0.0336	2.656	1.061–6.648
ECOG (2–3 vs 0–1)	0.273	1.51	0.718–3.176	0.0034	3.392	1.426–8.071	N.A.	N.A.	N.A.	0.0001	4.907	1.648–14.612
Age (<75 vs ≥75)	0.2687	0.664	0.319–1.381	0.8875	1.068	0.43–2.653	N.A.	N.A.	N.A.	N.A.	N.A.	N.A.
Gleason score (≥8 vs <8)	0.9539	1.023	0.471–2.225	0.9549	0.973	0.376–2.515	N.A.	N.A.	N.A.	N.A.	N.A.	N.A.
Visceral met (yes vs no)	0.0088	4.7	1.313–16.82	0.0007	6.907	1.881–25.357	0.0126	5.891	1.43–24.267	0.0015	4.8	1.026–22.465
Symptomatic (yes vs no)	0.6554	1.183	0.565–2.476	0.1193	1.966	0.826–4.682	N.A.	N.A.	N.A.	N.A.	N.A.	N.A.
PSA doubling time (<2 months vs ≥2 months)	0.1667	1.651	0.804–3.393	0.4794	1.573	0.568–3.319	N.A.	N.A.	N.A.	N.A.	N.A.	N.A.
Baseline PSA (≥200 vs <200 ug/l)	0.0014	3.26	1.513–7.021	0.0365	2.558	1.028–6.364	0.0686	2.15	0.933–4.954	0.6339	1.313	0.428–4.038
Baseline ALP (≥120 vs <120 IU/l)	0.1464	1.69	0.825–3.466	0.0535	2.459	0.987–6.13	N.A.	N.A.	N.A.	N.A.	N.A.	N.A.
Baseline Hb (<12 vs ≥12 g/dl)	0.1618	1.676	0.805–3.488	0.023	2.712	1.109–6.631	N.A.	N.A.	N.A.	0.0409	2.696	0.912–7.7971
PSA response (yes vs no)	<0.0001	0.135	0.061–0.299	0.0001	0.176	0.067–0.459	<0.0001	0.186	0.079–0.439	0.0001	0.104	0.025–0.387
PSA flare (yes vs no)	0.0623	0.471	0.209–1.06	0.0652	0.373	0.125–1.111	N.A.	N.A.	N.A.	N.A.	N.A.	N.A.
Continuation of AA beyond progression (yes vs no)	N.A.	N.A.	N.A.	0.9863	0.992	0.382–2.574	N.A.	N.A.	N.A.	N.A.	N.A.	N.A.
Post-AA treatment (yes vs no)	N.A.	N.A.	N.A.	0.3604	0.51	0.117–2.219	N.A.	N.A.	N.A.	N.A.	N.A.	N.A.

Abbreviations: HR hazard ratio, *95 % CI* 95 % confidence interval, *ADT* androgen deprivation treatment, *CRPC* castration-resistant prostate cancer, *ECOG* Eastern Cooperative Oncology Group, *Symptomatic* presence of pain prior abiraterone acetate and require WHO level II or above analgesics, *PSA* prostate-specific antigen, *ALP* alkaline phosphatase, *Hb* haemoglobin, *PSA response*, ≥50 % drop of PSA from baseline, *PSA flare*, PSA upsurge but not to the extent of biochemical progression, *AA* abiraterone acetate, *N.A.* not applicable

exploratory analysis of the visceral disease subgroup in the COU-AA-301 study [6] has demonstrated that the presence of visceral disease is prognostic but not predictive of the response to AA [12]. Nonetheless, there are growing evidences that the efficacies of therapies are different in chemo-naïve patients and post-chemo patients [13]. In contrast, the presence of symptomatic or visceral metastasis did not confer inferior clinical outcome to docetaxel-based chemotherapy, as reflected by the subgroup analysis in the TAX 327 study [14]. With the lack of randomized trial specifically addressing AA efficacy in chemo-naive patients with visceral or symptomatic disease, the practice of advocating AA in this particular subgroup should be further scrutinized in the context of clinical trial. Indeed, the data in the present study may support a treatment paradigm of offering AA to mCRPC patients with relatively low tumor burden, and chemotherapy for patients with high tumor burden, and visceral disease. Besides, based on the present study's data, patients with symptomatic disease may also be considered for AA to help pain control, though the survival outcome is less than favorable.

The achievement of PSA response after AA as a favorable prognosticator is in consistency with prior experience based on the data from COU-AA-302 and 301 studies, in which substantial correlation between survival and PSA kinetics was established [15]. Conversely, the absence of PSA response could potentially be used as a biomarker to select patients earlier for alternative or additional treatment in future clinical trial.

In our study, more than half of patients with initial PSA flare had ultimate PSA response to AA and, furthermore, there was no substantial difference in clinical outcome in patients with or without PSA flare. Consequently, in view of the not uncommon occurrence of PSA flare in some patients, PSA response is better determined at least 12 weeks after treatment, as recommended by the PCWG-2 and the premature discontinuation of AA when encountering initial PSA flare is not suggested [11]. In contrast, the practice of further continuation of AA beyond progression is not advised as the meta-analysis in our study has exemplified that there was no additional enhancement of survival with extended AA.

Short duration of response to prior ADT (<10 months) was associated with an unfavorable survival in chemo-naïve patients with AA in this study. Our finding substantiates the other reports that the short response to

Table 5 Univariate and multivariate analysis of overall survival and progression-free survival – Post-chemo group

Factors	Univariate analysis						Multivariate analysis					
	Progression-free survival			Overall survival			Progression-free survival			Overall survival		
	P value	HR	95 % CI	P value	HR	95 % CI	P value	HR	95 % CI	P value	HR	95 % CI
Time from ADT to CRPC (<10 vs ≥ 10 months)	0.4867	0.788	0.4–1.549	0.0649	0.476	0.213–1.063	N.A.	N.A.	N.A.	N.A.	N.A.	N.A.
ECOG (2–3 vs 0–1)	0.4084	0.648	0.229–1.832	0.7205	1.248	0.371–4.198	N.A.	N.A.	N.A.	N.A.	N.A.	N.A.
Age (<75 vs ≥75)	0.2988	0.649	0.285–1.478	0.0136	0.303	0.103–0.886	N.A.	N.A.	N.A.	0.3685	0.559	0.155–2.008
Gleason score (≥8 vs <8)	0.0528	1.922	0.98–3.77	0.0236	2.559	1.117–5.846	N.A.	N.A.	N.A.	0.0186	2.658	1.13–6.251
Visceral metastasis (yes vs no)	0.1972	1.793	0.727–4.42	0.3474	1.592	0.598–4.237	N.A.	N.A.	N.A.	N.A.	N.A.	N.A.
Symptomatic (yes vs no)	0.7678	1.112	0.549–2.253	0.637	1.227	0.524–2.87	N.A.	N.A.	N.A.	N.A.	N.A.	N.A.
PSA doubling time (<2 months vs ≥2 months)	0.251	1.459	0.762–2.794	0.0319	2.337	1.054–5.18	N.A.	N.A.	N.A.	0.0289	3.006	1.278–7.07
Baseline PSA (≥200 vs <200 ug/l)	0.3603	1.356	0.703–2.615	0.422	1.367	0.636–2.938	N.A.	N.A.	N.A.	N.A.	N.A.	N.A.
Baseline ALP (≥120 vs <120 IU/l)	0.6113	0.848	0.448–1.605	0.7189	1.151	0.536–2.471	N.A.	N.A.	N.A.	N.A.	N.A.	N.A.
Baseline Hb (<12 vs ≥12 g/dl)	0.2146	1.538	0.774–3.056	0.0811	2.143	0.892–5.149	N.A.	N.A.	N.A.	N.A.	N.A.	N.A.
PSA response (yes vs no)	0.0007	0.336	0.174–0.648	0.0001	0.207	0.089–0.493	0.0007	0.403	0.203–0.797	0.0001	0.213	0.076–0.592
PSA flare (yes vs no)	0.0130	0.38	0.172–0.838	0.2531	0.609	0.257–1.438	0.0987	0.505	0.222–1.149	N.A.	N.A.	N.A.
Refractory to prior chemotherapy (yes vs no)	0.3883	1.376	0.663–2.857	0.2234	1.659	0.729–3.773	N.A.	N.A.	N.A.	N.A.	N.A.	N.A.
Continuation of AA beyond progression (yes vs no)	N.A.	N.A.	N.A.	0.064	0.481	0.218–1.060	N.A.	N.A.	N.A.	N.A.	N.A.	N.A.
Post-AA treatment (yes vs no)	N.A.	N.A.	N.A.	0.3224	0.65	0.275–1.535	N.A.	N.A.	N.A.	N.A.	N.A.	N.A.

Abbreviations: HR hazard ratio, 95 % CI 95 % confidence interval, ADT androgen deprivation treatment, CRPC castration-resistant prostate cancer, ECOG Eastern Cooperative Oncology Group, Symptomatic presence of pain prior abiraterone acetate and require WHO analgesic class II or III analgesics, PSA prostate-specific antigen, ALP alkaline phosphatase, Hb haemoglobin, PSA response, ≥50 % drop of PSA from baseline, PSA flare PSA upsurge but not to the extent of biochemical progression, AA abiraterone acetate, N.A. not applicable

ADT was associated with poorer efficacy with AR-pathway targeted therapy, in particular AA, in mCRPC patients [16, 17]. And this echoed the statement made in the latest European consensus that short duration of response to ADT could be used to identify patients with increased risk of primary resistance to AR-pathway targeted agents [18].

Limitations existed in the present study, which include the typical shortcomings of retrospective study such as under-reporting of adverse events, incompleteness of data collection and selection bias etc. However, we consider these limitations would not affect the ability to capture the survival outcome of AA in this study. And the inadequate sample size, difference in follow-up

Table 6 Clinical outcome in the present study and the AA pivotal trial

Survival outcome	Present study (Chemo-naïve)	COU-AA-302 study	Present study (Post-chemo)	COU-AA-301 study
Median OS, months	18.1	34.7	15.5	15.8
Median PFS, months	6.7[a]	16.5[b]	6.4[a]	8.5[c]
				5.6[d]
PSA response, %	62.1	62	50.0	29
Pain control, %	57.9[e]	–	68.8[e]	44[f]

Abbreviations: OS overall survival, PFS progression-free survival, PSA response ≥50 % decline of PSA from baseline, PSA prostate-specific antigen
[a]Prostate Cancer Clinical Trials Working Group (PCWG-2) definition
[b]Radiographic PFS
[c]Biochemical PFS
[d]Radiographic PFS
[e]Withdrawal or reduction of level II or III analgesics according to WHO analgesics ladder
[f]Reduction of ≥30 % in the brief pain inventory-short form (BPI-SF) worst pain intensity score over the last 24 h observed at two consecutive evaluations 4 weeks apart without any increase in analgesic usage score; only patients experiencing a pain score ≥4 at baseline were included

protocols and the policy of post-AA treatment among different hospitals were the other weakness of the current study. Of note, unlike prospective study, regular imaging was not mandatory in our study and this could deprive some patients from other life-prolonging treatment earlier before any clinical or biochemical progression existed. Finally, the follow-up time for the chemo-naive group is comparatively inadequate and the inferior outcome in this group may not be the ultimate result. Our group will plan for another follow-up study in the future.

Conclusions

The present study reported the unanticipated short survival after AA in chemo-naïve patient outside clinical trial setting. The overall survival was particularly short in those with visceral diseases, and further clinical trial for AA in this subgroup of patients is warranted. In contrast, AA was well tolerated and efficacious in mCRPC patients with prior chemotherapy. AA resulted in comparable pain control in both groups of patients. PSA response, in particular present within the first 3 months after AA, could serve as a prognostic biomarker for survival outcome and may have a potential role in selecting patients for additional or alternative treatment earlier in future clinical trial.

Ethics approval and consent to participate

The study was approved by the institutional review board of the authors' institutions (Joint Chinese University of Hong Kong – New Territories East Cluster Clinical Research Ethics Committee/Ref no: CRE-2015.481). Informed consent has been exempted by the review board as most of the patients in this study were dead when the data was collected.

Abbreviations

AA: abiraterone acetate; ADT: androgen deprivation therapy; AR: androgen receptor; mCRPC: metastatic castration-resistant prostate cancer; PCWG-2: Prostate Cancer Clinical Trials Working Group; PSA: prostate-specific antigen; PSA-DT: PSA doubling time.

Competing interests

The authors declare that they have no competing interests.

Authors' contributions

DMP contributed to conception, analysis and interpretation of data. DMP was also involved in drafting and revising the manuscript. DMP, KC, SHL, TWC, HS, EKL, DL and MFC contributed to acquisition of data. DMP, KC, SHL, TWC, HS, EKL, DL and MFC read and approved the final manuscript.

Acknowledgement

The authors wish to thank Ms Lee-Wai Yee, Dr. Leung-Sing Fai and Dr. Michael Kam for their input and contributions to the study.

Funding

The authors declare that they have no funding resources for this particular study.

Author details

[1]Department of Clinical Oncology, State Key Laboratory in Oncology in South China, Sir YK Pao Centre for Cancer, Hong Kong Cancer Institute and Prince of Wales Hospital, The Chinese University of Hong Kong, Hong Kong, Hong Kong. [2]Department of Clinical Oncology, Pamela Youde Nethersole Eastern Hospital, Hong Kong, Hong Kong. [3]Department of Oncology, Princess Margaret Hospital, Hong Kong, Hong Kong. [4]Department of Clinical Oncology, Queen Elizabeth Hospital, Hong Kong, Hong Kong. [5]Department of Clinical Oncology, Queen Mary Hospital, Hong Kong, Hong Kong. [6]Department of Clinical Oncology, Tuen Mun Hospital, Hong Kong, Hong Kong. [7]Hong Kong Society of Uro-Oncology (HKSUO), Hong Kong, Hong Kong.

References

1. Schroder F, Crawford ED, Axcrona K, Payne H, Keane TE. Androgen deprivation therapy: past, present and future. BJU Int. 2012;109 Suppl 6:1–12.
2. Donkena KV, Yuan H, Young CY. Recent advances in understanding hormonal therapy resistant prostate cancer. Curr Cancer Drug Targets. 2010;10(4):402–10.
3. Tannock IF, de Wit R, Berry WR, Horti J, Pluzanska A, Chi KN, Oudard S, Theodore C, James ND, Turesson I, et al. Docetaxel plus prednisone or mitoxantrone plus prednisone for advanced prostate cancer. N Engl J Med. 2004;351(15):1502–12.
4. Petrylak DP, Tangen CM, Hussain MH, Lara Jr PN, Jones JA, Taplin ME, Burch PA, Berry D, Moinpour C, Kohli M, et al. Docetaxel and estramustine compared with mitoxantrone and prednisone for advanced refractory prostate cancer. N Engl J Med. 2004;351(15):1513–20.
5. Basch E, Loblaw DA, Oliver TK, Carducci M, Chen RC, Frame JN, Garrels K, Hotte S, Kattan MW, Raghavan D, et al. Systemic therapy in men with metastatic castration-resistant prostate cancer: American Society of Clinical Oncology and Cancer Care Ontario clinical practice guideline. J Clin Oncol. 2014;32(30):3436–48.
6. de Bono JS, Logothetis CJ, Molina A, Fizazi K, North S, Chu L, Chi KN, Jones RJ, Goodman OB, Jr., Saad F, et al. Abiraterone and increased survival in metastatic prostate cancer. N Engl J Med. 2011;364(21):1995–2005.
7. Ryan CJ, Smith MR, Fizazi K, Saad F, Mulders PF, Sternberg CN, Miller K, Logothetis CJ, Shore ND, Small EJ, et al. Abiraterone acetate plus prednisone versus placebo plus prednisone in chemotherapy-naive men with metastatic castration-resistant prostate cancer (COU-AA-302): final overall survival analysis of a randomised, double-blind, placebo-controlled phase 3 study. Lancet Oncol. 2015;16(2):152–60.
8. Templeton AJ, Vera-Badillo FE, Wang L, Attalla M, De Gouveia P, Leibowitz-Amit R, Knox JJ, Moore M, Sridhar SS, Joshua AM, et al. Translating clinical trials to clinical practice: outcomes of men with metastatic castration resistant prostate cancer treated with docetaxel and prednisone in and out of clinical trials. Ann Oncol. 2013;24(12):2972–7.
9. Poon D, Ng J, Kuen C. The importance of cycles of chemotherapy and post-docetaxel novel therapies in metastatic castration-resistant prostate cancer (mCRPC). Prostate Int. 2015;0(0):0.
10. Beer TM, Armstrong AJ, Rathkopf DE, Loriot Y, Sternberg CN, Higano CS, Iversen P, Bhattacharya S, Carles J, Chowdhury S, et al. Enzalutamide in metastatic prostate cancer before chemotherapy. N Engl J Med. 2014;371(5):424–33.
11. Scher HI, Halabi S, Tannock I, Morris M, Sternberg CN, Carducci MA, Eisenberger MA, Higano C, Bubley GJ, Dreicer R, et al. Design and end points of clinical trials for patients with progressive prostate cancer and castrate levels of testosterone: recommendations of the Prostate Cancer Clinical Trials Working Group. J Clin Oncol. 2008;26(7):1148–59.
12. Goodman Jr OB, Flaig TW, Molina A, Mulders PF, Fizazi K, Suttmann H, Li J, Kheoh T, de Bono JS, Scher HI. Exploratory analysis of the visceral disease subgroup in a phase III study of abiraterone acetate in metastatic castration-resistant prostate cancer. Prostate Cancer Prostatic Dis. 2014;17(1):34–9.

13. van Soest RJ, van Royen ME, de Morree ES, Moll JM, Teubel W, Wiemer EA, Mathijssen RH, de Wit R, van Weerden WM. Cross-resistance between taxanes and new hormonal agents abiraterone and enzalutamide may affect drug sequence choices in metastatic castration-resistant prostate cancer. Eur J Cancer. 2013;49(18):3821–30.

14. Berthold DR, Pond GR, Soban F, de Wit R, Eisenberger M, Tannock IF. Docetaxel plus prednisone or mitoxantrone plus prednisone for advanced prostate cancer: updated survival in the TAX 327 study. J Clin Oncol. 2008;26(2):242–5.

15. Xu XS, Ryan CJ, Stuyckens K, Smith MR, Saad F, Griffin TW, Choi Park Y, Yu MK, Vermeulen A, Poggesi I, et al. Correlation between prostate-specific antigen kinetics and overall survival in abiraterone acetate-treated castration-resistant prostate cancer patients. Clin Cancer Res. 2015;21(14):3170–7.

16. Caffo O, De Giorgi U, Fratino L, Lo Re G, Basso U, D'Angelo A, Donini M, Verderame F, Ratta R, Procopio G, et al. Safety and clinical outcomes of patients treated with abiraterone acetate after docetaxel: results of the Italian Named Patient Programme. BJU Int. 2015;115(5):764–71.

17. Loriot Y, Massard C, Albiges L. Personalizing treatment in patients with castrate-resistant prostate cancer: a study of predictive factors for secondary endocrine therapies activity. J Clin Oncol. 2012;30 (Suppl. 5).

18. Fitzpatrick JM, Bellmunt J, Fizazi K, Heidenreich A, Sternberg CN, Tombal B, Alcaraz A, Bahl A, Bracarda S, Di Lorenzo G, et al. Optimal management of metastatic castration-resistant prostate cancer: highlights from a European Expert Consensus Panel. Eur J Cancer. 2014;50(9):1617–27.

27

Reliability of radioisotope-guided sentinel lymph node biopsy in penile cancer: verification in consideration of the European guidelines

Tim Schubert[1], Jens Uphoff[1], Rolf-Peter Henke[2], Friedhelm Wawroschek[1] and Alexander Winter[1*]

Abstract

Background: Lymph node (LN) staging in penile cancer has strong prognostic implications. This contrasts with the high morbidity of extended inguinal LN dissection (LND) or over-treatment of many patients. Therefore, inguinal dynamic sentinel node biopsy (DSNB) or modified LND is recommended by the European Association of Urology (EAU) guidelines to evaluate the nodal status of patients with clinically node-negative penile cancer. This study analyzed the reliability and morbidity of radioguided DSNB in penile cancer under consideration of the current EAU recommendations in an experienced center with long-term follow-up.

Methods: Thirty-four patients who received primary surgery and had radioguided inguinal DSNB for penile cancer (≥T1G2) were included (July 2004 to July 2013). Preoperative sentinel LN (SLN) mapping was performed using lymphoscintigraphy after peritumoral injection of ^{99m}Technetium nanocolloid on the day of surgery. During surgery, SLNs were detected using a gamma probe. According to the EAU guidelines, a secondary ipsilateral radical inguinal LND was performed in patients who had positive SLNs. The false-negative and complication rates of DSNB were assessed.

Results: A total of 32 patients were analyzed. Two patients were lost to follow-up. A total of 166 SLNs (median, 5; range, 1–15) were removed and 216 LNs (SLNs + non-SLNs; median, 6; range, 2–19) were dissected. LN metastases were found in five of the 32 (15.6 %) patients and nine of the 166 (5.4 %) SLNs were found to contain metastases. None of the remaining 50 non-SLNs contained metastases. In only one of the five SLN-positive patients, a singular further metastasis was detected by secondary radical inguinal LND. During follow-up (median, 30.5; range, 5–95 months) no inguinal nodal recurrence was detected. DSNB-related complications occurred in 11.1 % of explored groins.

Discussion and Conclusions: Radioguided DSNB is a suitable procedure for LN staging in penile cancer considering the EAU recommendations and with the required experience. Under these circumstances, patients can be spared from higher morbidity without compromising the detection of LN metastases or therapeutic implications. Improvement of the methodology used to perform DSNB should be developed further to decrease the risk of missing LN metastases and to simplify the procedure.

Keywords: Penile cancer, Sentinel node biopsy, Inguinal lymph node dissection, Lymph node metastases

* Correspondence: winter.alexander@klinikum-oldenburg.de
[1]University Hospital for Urology, Klinikum Oldenburg, School of Medicine and Health Sciences, Carl von Ossietzky University Oldenburg, Rahel-Straus-Straße 10, 26133 Oldenburg, Germany
Full list of author information is available at the end of the article

Background

In penile cancer, lymph node (LN) metastasis is the main known prognostic factor affecting patients' survival [1]. A recent published analysis showed an overall 5-year cancer-specific survival of patients with primary invasive tumors of 81 %, but only 56 % of patients with LN metastases survived the first 5 years after diagnosis [2]. Inguinal LNs are the first nodal group affected in penile cancer. Early inguinal LN dissection (LND) or the resection of clinically occult LN metastases improves survival compared with removal when the metastases become clinically apparent [2–4]. Only one-third of penile cancer patients with regional recurrence are alive after 5 years [4].

Consequently, management of inguinal LN is crucial for prognosis in patients with penile cancer. Patients with palpable inguinal nodes are at high risk for LN metastases. In patients with nonpalpable inguinal nodes (cN0), the likelihood of the presence of metastasis is approximately 20–25 % [5]. However, current imaging techniques are not reliable for detecting micro-metastases [6]. Moreover, nomograms are also inappropriate for predicting LN metastases in penile cancer. The accuracy of currently available predictive models is below 80 % [6].

Therefore, in cases of palpable inguinal LNs, radical inguinal LND is required. Patients with normal inguinal nodes and an intermediate or high risk of lymphatic metastasis (≥T1G2) should also receive invasive LN staging [6]. Because only 20–25 % of patients with normal inguinal LNs experience regional lymphatic spread, performing a radical inguinal LND may be an overtreatment in approximately 80 % of these cases, resulting in considerable morbidity [7]. Complications, such as wound infection, skin necrosis, wound dehiscence, lymphedema, and lymphoceles, can occur [8].

To reduce the morbidity associated with radical inguinal LND, two invasive procedures are recommended by the European Association of Urology (EAU) guidelines for patients with nonpalpable nodes: modified inguinal LND and dynamic sentinel node biopsy (DSNB) [6]. If either modified LND or DSNB show LN metastases, an ipsilateral radical inguinal LND should be performed. Fine needle aspiration cytology (FNAC) has been advised in clinically node-negative patients by former guidelines [9], but it is no longer recommended by the EAU owing to low specificity [6]. Moreover, FNAC is not reliable for the detection of micro-metastases.

Modified inguinal LND includes a limitation of the dissection field and preservation of the saphenous vein. As a result, morbidity of the inguinal LND procedure can be reduced. However, limitation of the dissection area results in a higher probability of false-negative cases [8]. According to the current EAU guidelines, the false-negative rate of modified inguinal

LND is not known [6]. There are few data on this aspect of this disease.

DSNB in penile cancer was first described by Cabanas [10]. The modern sentinel concept in penile cancer using a radioactive tracer with or without blue dye was introduced around the turn of the millennium and was recently further developed [5, 11, 12]. The reliability and low morbidity of this technique have been reported by various research groups [7, 13–16].

This study aimed to analyze the reliability of radioisotope-guided DSNB in penile cancer in an experienced center under consideration of the current EAU recommendations and with a long-term follow-up.

Methods

Patient population and inclusion criteria for analysis

A total of 49 patients with penile cancer were operated on at our institute from July 2004 to July 2013 and documented in a consecutive data bank. In this retrospective study, 34 patients with ≥ T1G2 tumors who received radioisotope-guided inguinal DSNB were included. Of these, 32 could be analyzed. Two patients died a few months after surgery. Causes of death were not related to complications of the operation or penile cancer.

All of the patients were informed orally and in writing regarding inguinal DSNB and penile surgery, and they gave informed consent.

Surgical treatment

The DSNB was performed in accordance with the current EAU guidelines [6]. A FNAC, which is still recommended by others to reduce the false-negative rate, was not performed [9].

Surgical treatment of the primary tumor depended on the tumor stage, and included circumcision ($n = 5$), resection of the glans with or without circumcision ($n = 11$), or partial resection of the penis ($n = 16$). All included patients presented with a tumor stage ≥ T1G2 and received an inguinal DSNB. In 17 patients, the DSNB was performed in a one-step manner in the same operation. Fifteen cases received a secondary inguinal DSNB. Two patients additionally received stage-adapted modified or radical inguinal LND. In one of these patients, radical LND of the left groin and a DSNB of the right groin were performed. The radical LND was indicated because of an ipsilateral suspicious LN. The other patient had bilateral enlarged inguinal LNs.

According to the EAU guidelines, a secondary ipsilateral radical inguinal LND was performed in patients who had positive SLNs (pN1 stage). Secondary inguinal and pelvic LND was performed if histopathological evaluation of the inguinal LND specimen revealed two or more tumor-positive LNs (pN2 stage).

Sentinel tracer injection

The sentinel tracer (⁹⁹ᵐTechnetium nanocolloid, radio-activity ca. 30 MBq) was preoperatively injected peritumorally on the day of surgery approximately 4 hours before the operation ($n = 17$) (Fig. 1) or in a two-step procedure in the area of the resection ($n = 15$). Lymphoscintigraphy was then carried out. The SLNs were intraoperatively detected using two different gamma probes (C-Trak System, Care Wise, Morgan Hill, CA, USA; Crystal Probe SG04, Crystal Photonics GmbH, Berlin, Germany).

Intraoperative procedures and histopathology

LNs identified as SLNs by the gamma probe were dissected. For surgical reasons, LNs other than SLNs directly adjoining and adhering to SLNs were also removed, if in situ separation was not possible.

All LNs were initially cut in 3-mm transverse sections, routinely processed, and completely embedded in paraffin. Sections that were 4–5 μm thick were stained with hematoxylin–eosin.

Follow-up

All intra- and postoperative complications were recorded according to the Clavien–Dindo classification. Follow-up was performed on an outpatient basis by urologists in the community in accordance with our instructions. As recommended by the EAU guidelines [6], for patients with negative inguinal nodes after local treatment, follow-up visits included physical examination of the penis and the groin for detection of local and/or regional recurrence. On indication, ultrasound, computed tomography (CT), or magnetic resonance imaging (MRI) was used. In patients with positive LNs, CT or MRI scanning was carried out at 3-monthly intervals during the first 2 years for the detection of regional recurrence or systematic disease.

Analysis

We classified DSNB as a false-negative procedure only if non-SLNs were positive or regional nodal recurrence developed after a negative SLN procedure. The false-negative rate of DSNB was calculated according to the standard definition: false-negative procedures/true-positive procedures + false-negative procedures.

Ethical approval

The study was approved by the Ethics Committee of the Carl von Ossietzky University Oldenburg.

Results

A summary of the patient and tumor characteristics is shown in Table 1.

A total of 166 SLNs (median, 5; range, 1–15) were removed and 216 LNs (SLNs + non-SLNs; median, 6; range, 2–19) were dissected. LN metastases were found in five of the 32 (15.6 %) patients and nine of 166 (5.4 %) SLNs were found to contain metastases. None of the remaining 50 non-SLNs contained metastasis. Of the five patients with positive SLNs, three presented with pN1 stage. In secondary radical inguinal LND, a singular further metastasis was detected only in one of these patients, while the other two patients had pN2 stage disease. These two patients were also clinically node positive. One of these patients, who showed preoperative enlarged LNs bilaterally, was the only patient with LN

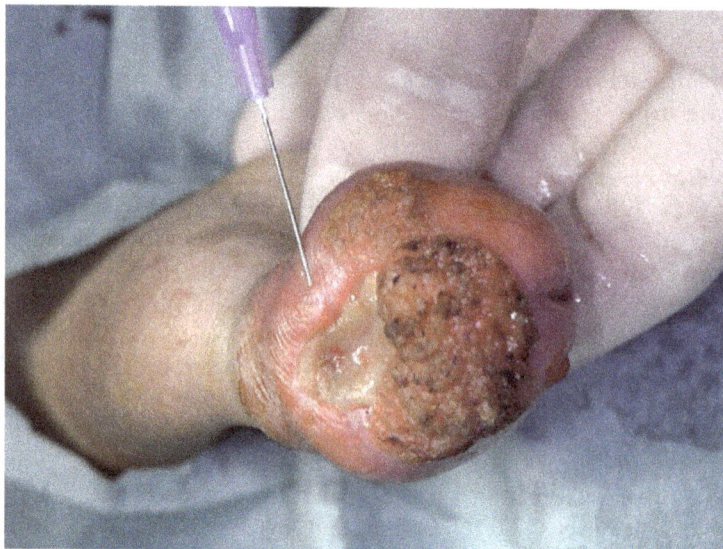

Fig. 1 Peritumoral injection of the sentinel tracer (⁹⁹ᵐTechnetium nanocolloid)

Table 1 Summary of patient and tumor characteristics

Characteristic	No. of patients
Total	32
Grade by T stage	
T1	20
G1	excluded from study
G2	18
G3	2
T2	10
G1	1
G2	9
G3	0
T3	2
G1	0
G2	0
G3	2
T4	0
Follow-up, month	
Median	30.5
Range	5–95
Age, years	
Median	67
Range	39–78

metastases in both groins. All other nodal positive patients presented with unilateral metastases. On secondary iliacal LND in one of the two cases, pelvic LN metastases were found (3 of 11 removed LNs were positive). In the other patient, all further LNs were free of metastases. The histopathological findings are shown in detail in Table 2. During follow-up, no inguinal nodal recurrence was detected. Accordingly, no patient had false-negative DSNB taking into account the EAU recommended procedure, including a secondary radical LN in the case of positive SLNs.

Recurrence of primary tumors was identified in two patients at 11 or 12 months after surgery by physical examination or by MRI. In one patient, a Merkel cell carcinoma of the right thigh was diagnosed simultaneously with penile cancer. During follow-up, diffuse metastasis of the Merkel cell carcinoma appeared.

Table 2 Nodal status related to histopathological tumor stage

Stage	pN0 (n = 26)	pN+ inguinal (n = 5)	pN+ pelvic (n = 1)
pT1 G2	16 (89 %)	2	0
pT1 G3	1 (50 %)	1	1
pT2 G1	1 (100 %)	0	0
pT2 G2	8 (89 %)	1	0
pT3 G3	1 (50 %)	1	0

Four patients died during the follow-up. The median follow-up for these patients was 44.5 months (range, 22–69 months). Reasons for death were pulmonary emphysema, advanced renal cell carcinoma, and systemic metastatic disease. In one patient, the cause of death remained unclear.

DSNB-related complications were assessed in a total of five patients, but intervention was only required in three patients (Clavien–Dindo grade III). One patient underwent a revision operation of both groins owing to wound infection. Wound healing was achieved by vacuum bandages and antibiotics after the revision operation (Clavien–Dindo grade IIIb). Two patients had unilateral inguinal lymphoceles. In these two patients, the lymphoceles were drained (Clavien–Dindo grade IIIa). Two other patients suffered from prolonged wound secretion of the groin and were treated with clinical surveillance without any re-intervention procedures (Clavien–Dindo grade I). Five patients had complications (Clavien–Dindo grade III) after radical LND of the groins. Two patients underwent a revision operation of one groin owing to wound infection (Clavien–Dindo grade IIIb). Wound healing was achieved either by vacuum bandages and antibiotics after the revision operation or secondary operation. Drainage of lymphoceles was performed in the other three patients (Clavien–Dindo grade IIIa). Therefore, the complication rate concerning DSNB alone was 11.1 % (per groin). Complications occurred in all patients with radical inguinal LND (100 %, per groin). In these patients, an intervention was always required.

Discussion

In this study, we performed a retrospective analysis of patients who underwent radioisotope-guided DSNB in a center with wide expertise in sentinel procedures related to urological malignancies. The reliability of this approach was investigated under consideration of the current EAU guidelines (2014) [6]. The median follow-up was 30.5 months in the present study. Because recurrence of tumors occurs typically within 2 years, a false-negative rate of DSNB should become clinically apparent at that time [17]. Accordingly, a median follow-up of 30.5 months is sufficient to address this issue. This is underlined by the fact that, in our study, no inguinal recurrence was detected if patients who were only followed up for at least 24 months (n = 19; median follow-up, 60 months; range, 24–95 months) were analyzed.

A DSNB or an EAU recommended procedure [6], including secondary LND in patients with positive SLNs, showed reliable results in the examined population. In only one patient with a tumor-positive SLN, a singular further LN metastasis was detected on secondary radical LND. None of the patients suffered recurrence of inguinal LN. Our results are in line with recent studies in which DSNBs showed high reliability. In a prospective study, Lam et al. analyzed a total of 264 patients with penile cancer undergoing DSNB [14]. The false-negative rate per patient was 6 %. Fuchs et al. found an inguinal nodal recurrence in only 3.7 % of their patients [18], while Leijte et al. investigated 323 patients and calculated a false-negative rate of 7 % per groin [19]. In a recent national multicenter study from Denmark, the overall false-negative rate was 13.3 % per patient [20]. However, caution is advised, because in our study, 56 % of the patients had a low stage (T1G2). At a median of 30 months, there are still many patients at risk for recurrence. For this reason, our results may not reflect the outcome of series with a different mixture of patients. In an initial DSNB series by Kirrander et al., the recurrence rate was 15 % [21]. However, in their study, 50 % of the patients had T2 or greater primary tumors.

Some more potential limitations of this study need to be discussed. The results from the present study are based on the data of one center and on a relatively small cohort. In this context, the low incidence of penile cancer in Germany has to be taken into account. However, this study represents the largest published German DSNB series in penile cancer to date.

Another limitation is the fact that the DSNB was performed either primarily or secondarily after resection of penile tumors in the present study. LN metastases were found in five patients. Three patients underwent primary DSNB, and two underwent a secondary procedure after resection of the primary tumor. However, a study by Graafland et al. suggested that the results of a primary DSNB were equal to those of a two-step procedure [22]. In their study, 40 patients who had undergone DSNB after previous resection of the primary penile tumor were analyzed, and no recurrences developed in the groins during a median follow-up of 28 months.

Whether a DSNB should be performed is still controversial, mostly because a false-negative result is associated with a significant risk of death. Therefore, some authors have stressed that a DSNB cannot be considered as a real gold standard for evaluation of patients with cN0 penile carcinoma [23, 24]. This is because initial results of DSNB in penile cancer show a high false-negative rate of 19.2–22 % [7, 25]. In a recent study, an experienced research group in Amsterdam showed that the 5-year cancer-specific survival for all patients with pN+ disease is better than that in series that prefer primary inguinal LND in all patients who are considered at risk for LN metastases [2]. After performing several modifications to the DSNB procedure, the false-negative rate dropped to 4.8 % [7]. As mentioned above, other studies have shown that DSNB is a reliable and safe method for inguinal LN staging in penile cancer [7, 13–16]. Moreover, excellent results concerning sensitivity, false-negative

rates, and complication rates for DSNB have been reported in several studies [14, 19, 26]. These findings show the importance of methodology in DSNB. However, the conclusion cannot be made that a lower false-negative rate is only caused by these modifications; experience in performing DSNB might also be a contributing factor.

Re-routing of the radioactive tracer due to tumor blockage of lymph vessels has been proposed as a mechanism for increasing the risk for false-negative SLN procedures [27]. One fundamental problem with the sentinel technique is that when LNs are fully metastasized or lymph pathways are blocked, the afferent lymph will be directed to other LNs/non-SLNs [28]. Therefore, Leijte et al. added preoperative ultrasound of the groins with FNAC of suspicious nodes to identify and cytologically examine possible blocked SLNs [7]. This procedure was advised in clinically node-negative patients in former guidelines [9], but it is no longer recommended by the EAU owing to the low specificity of FNAC [6]. The current EAU guidelines take the possibility of fully metastasized LNs or blocked lymphatic vessels into account by recommending a primary radical inguinal LND in patients with clinical enlarged LNs or a secondary radical LND in cases with tumor-positive SLNs, respectively.

Further investigations have been made to improve the reliability of DSNBs. Brouwer et al. recently showed indocyanine green-^{99m}Technetium-nanocolloid as a hybrid radioactive and fluorescent tracer for performing DSNB [12]. This tracer was successfully used for combined radio- and fluorescence-guided DSNB in penile carcinoma. A large improvement in optical SLN detection compared with blue dye has been achieved using this new approach.

The low risk of a false-negative rate in DSNB has to be weighed against the morbidity of conventional inguinal LND in penile cancer. Inguinal LND is a potential over-treatment in patients without regional LN involvement, which constitutes about 80 % of those with cN0 disease [29]. The rate of complications of DSNB in the present study was 11.1 % (per groin), which is in line with recent studies [21, 30]. We found no cancer in non-SLNs. This suggests that more extensive node sampling is unnecessary and may contribute to morbidity. Other authors have reported a lower rate of complications after DSNB [7, 14, 18, 24]. Leijte et al. were able to decrease the complication rate of inguinal DSNB from 10.2 to 5.7 % [7]. In a systemic review, Neto et al. reported a complication rate of 3.6 % when performing inguinal DSNB [31]. However, inguinal LND is a procedure with a considerably higher complication rate of 40–50 % [23, 31]. Protzel et al. pointed out that the potential advantage of reduced morbidity with DSNB appears to be less pronounced compared with modified inguinal LND [8]. However, there are only limited data regarding the false-negative rate of modified LND [6]. Therefore, further studies are needed to compare the false-negative rates of DSNB and modified LND.

Conclusions

Radioguided DSNB is a suitable procedure for LN staging in penile cancer patients under consideration of the EAU recommended procedure in experienced centers. Under these circumstances, patients can be spared from higher morbidity without compromising the detection of LN metastases or therapeutic implications in LN positive patients. Improvement of the methodology used to perform DSNB (e.g., new tracers) should be developed further to decrease the risk of missing LN metastases and to simplify the procedure.

Abbreviations
CT: Computed tomography; DSNB: Dynamic sentinel node biopsy; EAU: European Association of Urology; FNAC: Fine needle aspiration cytology; LN: Lymph node; LND: Lymph node dissection; MRI: Magnetic resonance imaging; SLN: Sentinel lymph node.

Competing interests
The authors declare that they have no competing interests.

Authors' contributions
TS performed the analysis, reviewed the literature, and drafted the manuscript. JU participated in the acquisition of data and analysis. RPH carried out histological examinations and was involved in critically revising the manuscript for important intellectual content. FW participated in the conception and design of the study and interpretation of data, and was involved in critically revising the manuscript for important intellectual content. AW participated in the conception of the study, acquisition and interpretation of data, and was involved in critically revising the manuscript for important intellectual content. All authors have read and approved the final manuscript.

Authors' information
TS: Resident, University Hospital for Urology, Klinikum Oldenburg, School of Medicine and Health Sciences, Carl von Ossietzky University Oldenburg, Oldenburg, Germany.
JU: Senior Physician, University Hospital for Urology, Klinikum Oldenburg, School of Medicine and Health Sciences, Carl von Ossietzky University Oldenburg, Oldenburg, Germany.
RPH: Director of the Oldenburg Institute of Pathology, Oldenburg, Germany; member of the International Society of Urological Pathologists.
FW: Medical Director, University Hospital for Urology, Klinikum Oldenburg, School of Medicine and Health Sciences, Carl von Ossietzky University Oldenburg, Oldenburg, Germany.
AW: Senior Physician, University Hospital for Urology, Klinikum Oldenburg, School of Medicine and Health Sciences, Carl von Ossietzky University Oldenburg, Oldenburg, Germany.

Acknowledgements
The authors have not received any source of funding.

Author details
¹University Hospital for Urology, Klinikum Oldenburg, School of Medicine and Health Sciences, Carl von Ossietzky University Oldenburg, Rahel-Straus-Straße 10, 26133 Oldenburg, Germany. ²Oldenburg Institute of Pathology, Taubenstraße 28, 26122 Oldenburg, Germany.

References
1. Horenblas S. Lymphadenectomy for squamous cell carcinoma of the penis. Part 2: the role and technique of lymph node dissection. BJU Int. 2001;88:473–83.
2. Djajadiningrat RS, Graafland NM, van Werkhoven E, Meinhardt W, Bex A, van der Poel HG, et al. Contemporary management of regional nodes in penile cancer-improvement of survival? J Urol. 2014;191:68–73.
3. Kroon BK, Horenblas S, Lont AP, Tanis PJ, Gallee MP, Nieweg OE. Patients with penile carcinoma benefit from immediate resection of clinically occult lymph node metastases. J Urol. 2005;173:816–9.
4. Leijte JA, Kirrander P, Antonini N, Windahl T, Horenblas S. Recurrence patterns of squamous cell carcinoma of the penis: recommendations for follow-up based on a two-centre analysis of 700 patients. Eur Urol. 2008;54:161–8.
5. Horenblas S, Jansen L, Meinhardt W, Hoefnagel CA, de Jong D, Nieweg OE. Detection of occult metastasis in squamous cell carcinoma of the penis using a dynamic sentinel node procedure. J Urol. 2000;163:100–4.
6. Hakenberg OW, Compérat EM, Minhas S, Necchi A, Protzel C, Watkin N. EAU Guidelines on Penile Cancer: 2014 Update. Eur Urol. 2015;67:142–50.
7. Leijte JA, Kroon BK, Valdés Olmos RA, Nieweg OE, Horenblas S. Reliability and safety of current dynamic sentinel node biopsy for penile carcinoma. Eur Urol. 2007;52:170–7.
8. Protzel C, Alcaraz A, Horenblas S, Pizzocaro G, Zlotta A, Hakenberg OW. Lymphadenectomy in the surgical management of penile cancer. Eur Urol. 2009;55:1075–88.
9. Pizzocaro G, Algaba F, Horenblas S, Solsona E, Tana S, Van Der Poel H, et al. EAU penile cancer guidelines 2009. Eur Urol. 2010;57:1002–12.
10. Cabanas RM. An approach for the treatment of penile carcinoma. Cancer. 1977;39:456–66.
11. Wawroschek F, Vogt H, Bachter D, Weckermann D, Hamm M, Harzmann R. First experience with gamma probe guided sentinel lymph node surgery in penile cancer. Urol Res. 2000;28:246–9.
12. Brouwer OR, van den Berg NS, Mathéron HM, van der Poel HG, van Rhijn BW, Bex A, et al. A hybrid radioactive and fluorescent tracer for sentinel node biopsy in penile carcinoma as a potential replacement for blue dye. Eur Urol. 2014;65:600–9.
13. Nicolai N. Has dynamic sentinel node biopsy achieved its top performance in penile cancer? What clinicians still need to manage lymph nodes in early stage penile cancer. Eur Urol. 2013;63:664–6.
14. Lam W, Alnajjar HM, La-Touche S, Perry M, Sharma D, Corbishley C, et al. Dynamic sentinel lymph node biopsy in patients with invasive squamous cell carcinoma of the penis: a prospective study of the long-term outcome of 500 inguinal basins assessed at a single institution. Eur Urol. 2013;63:657–63.
15. Hughes B, Leijte J, Shabbir M, Watkin N, Horenblas S. Non-invasive and minimally invasive staging of regional lymph nodes in penile cancer. World J Urol. 2009;27:197–203.
16. Horenblas S. Sentinel lymph node biopsy in penile carcinoma. Semin Diagn Pathol. 2012;29:90–5.
17. Lubke WL, Thompson IM. The case for inguinal lymph node dissection in the treatment of T2-T4, N0 penile cancer. Semin Urol. 1999;11:80–4.
18. Fuchs J, Hamann MF, Schulenburg F, Knüpfer S, Osmonov D, Lützen U, et al. Sentinel lymph node biopsy for penile carcinoma: Assessment of reliability. Urologe A. 2013;52:1447–50.
19. Leijte JA, Hughes B, Graafland NM, Kroon BK, Olmos RA, Nieweg OE, et al. Two-center evaluation of dynamic sentinel node biopsy for squamous cell carcinoma of the penis. J Clin Oncol. 2009;27:3325–9.
20. Jakobsen JK, Krarup KP, Sommer P, Nerstrøm H, Bakholdt V, Sørensen JA, et al. DaPeCa-1: Diagnostic Accuracy of Sentinel Node Biopsy in 222 Penile Cancer Patients at four Tertiary Referral Centres - a National Study from Denmark. BJU Int. 2015. doi:10.1111/bju.13127. Epub ahead of print.
21. Kirrander P, Andrén O, Windahl T. Dynamic sentinel node biopsy in penile cancer: initial experiences at a Swedish referral centre. BJU Int. 2013;111:E48–53.
22. Graafland NM, Valdés Olmos RA, Meinhardt W, Bex A, van der Poel HG, van Boven HH, et al. Nodal staging in penile carcinoma by dynamic sentinel node biopsy after previous therapeutic primary tumour resection. Eur Urol. 2010;58:748–51.
23. Ficarra V, Galfano A. Should the dynamic sentinel node biopsy (DSNB) be considered the gold standard in the evaluation of lymph node status in patients with penile carcinoma? Eur Urol. 2007;52:17–9.

24. Spiess PE, Izawa JI, Bassett R, Kedar D, Busby JE, Wong F, et al. Preoperative lymphoscintigraphy and dynamic sentinel node biopsy for staging penile cancer: results with pathological correlation. J Urol. 2007;177:2157–61.

25. Tanis PJ, Lont AP, Meinhardt W, Olmos RA, Nieweg OE, Horenblas S. Dynamic sentinel node biopsy for penile cancer: reliability of a staging technique. J Urol. 2002;168:76–80.

26. Jensen JB, Jensen KM, Ulhøi BP, Nielsen SS, Lundbeck F. Sentinel lymph-node biopsy in patients with squamous cell carcinoma of the penis. BJU Int. 2009;103:1199–203.

27. Kroon BK, Horenblas S, Estourgie SH, Lont AP, Valdés Olmos RA, Nieweg OE. How to avoid false-negative dynamic sentinel node procedures in penile carcinoma. J Urol. 2004;171:2191–4.

28. Morgan-Parkes JH. Metastases: mechanisms, pathways, and cascades. AJR Am J Roentgenol. 1995;164:1075–82.

29. Sadeghi R, Gholami H, Zakavi SR, Kakhki VR, Tabasi KT, Horenblas S. Accuracy of sentinel lymph node biopsy for inguinal lymph node staging of penile squamous cell carcinoma: systematic review and meta-analysis of the literature. J Urol. 2012;187:25–31.

30. Kroon BK, Horenblas S, Meinhardt W, van der Poel HG, Bex A, van Tinteren H, et al. Dynamic sentinel node biopsy in penile carcinoma: evaluation of 10 years experience. Eur Urol. 2005;47:601–6.

31. Neto AS, Tobias-Machado M, Ficarra V, Wroclawski ML, Amarante RD, Pompeo AC, et al. Dynamic sentinel node biopsy for inguinal lymph node staging in patients with penile cancer: a systematic review and cumulative analysis of the literature. Ann Surg Oncol. 2011;18:2026–34.

28

Cancer detection rate of prebiopsy MRI with subsequent systematic and targeted biopsy are superior to non-targeting systematic biopsy without MRI in biopsy naïve patients

Satoshi Washino[1,3*], Shigeru Kobayashi[2], Tomohisa Okochi[4], Tomohiro Kameda[1], Tsuzumi Konoshi[3], Tomoaki Miyagawa[3], Tatsuya Takayama[1] and Tatsuo Morita[1]

Abstract

Background: To determine whether prebiopsy multiparametric magnetic resonance imaging (mpMRI) with subsequent systematic plus targeted biopsies for suspicious lesions improve prostate cancer detection compared with standard non-targeting systematic biopsies without mpMRI in biopsy-naïve patients.

Methods: Patients who underwent their first prostate biopsy due to suspicion of prostate cancer were analyzed retrospectively to compare the biopsy outcomes between patients who received prebiopsy mpMRI (215 patients) and those who did not (281 patients). mpMRI was performed to determine pre-biopsy likelihood of the presence of prostate cancer using a three-point scale (1 = low level of suspicion, 2 = equivocal, and 3 = high level of suspicion). Systematic biopsies were performed in both groups. Targeted biopsies were added for a high level of suspicious lesions on mpMRI. All biopsies were performed by transperineal biopsy technique. After biopsy, Prostate Imaging Reporting and Data System ver. 2 (PIRADS-2) scoring was performed to describe the mpMRI findings and predictive value of PIRADS-2 was evaluated.

Results: The detection rate of total and clinically significant prostate cancer was significantly higher in patients who received prebiopsy mpMRI than in those who did not (55.3 and 46.0% vs. 42.0 and 35.2%, respectively; $p = 0.004$ and $p = 0.016$). The clinically insignificant prostate cancer detection rate was similar between the two groups (9.3% vs. 6.8%; $p = 0.32$). Of 86 patients who underwent systematic plus targeted biopsy in the MRI cohort and were diagnosed with prostate cancer, seven patients were detected by addition of targeted biopsy whereas 29 patients were missed by targeted biopsy but detected by systematic biopsy. There was a correlation between the PIRADS-2 and prostate cancer detection rate, and a receiver-operator curve analysis yielded an area under the curve of 0.801 ($p < 0.0001$).

Conclusions: Prebiopsy mpMRI with subsequent systematic plus targeted biopsies for suspicious lesions can yield a higher cancer detection rate than non-targeting systematic biopsies. PIRADS-2 scoring is useful for predicting the biopsy outcome.

Keywords: Magnetic resonance imaging, Biopsy, Target, Random, Prostate cancer

---

* Correspondence: suwajiisan@jichi.ac.jp
[1]Department of Urology, Jichi Medical University, 3311-1 Yakushiji, Shimotsuke, Tochigi 329-0498, Japan
[3]Department of Urology, Jichi Medical University Saitama Medical Center, 1-847, Amanuma-cho, Omiya-ku, Saitama 330-8503, Japan
Full list of author information is available at the end of the article

Background

Prostate cancer (PCa) is the most common male malignancy and the second most common cause of male cancer-related death [1]. It is usually diagnosed based on systematic transrectal ultrasound (TRUS)-guided random biopsies of the prostate gland. However, a significant number of transrectal biopsies are negative for cancer, yielding inaccurate results [2–4]. The cancer detection rate with a standard TRUS-guided prostate biopsy is only 20~40% [5]. Furthermore, TRUS-guided transrectal biopsies have a limited ability to sample the anterior prostate [6].

The ideal prostate biopsy goal would be to identify clinically significant PCa and minimize the detection of indolent disease. The growing availability of prostate multiparametric magnetic resonance imaging (mpMRI), novel functional imaging modalities, and increased standardization have created an opportunity for the detection, localization, and staging of PCa [7]. Screening patients using mpMRI may avoid the morbidity associated with a biopsy if no lesions are seen [8]. In addition, targeted biopsies should identify more clinically significant PCa than non-targeted TRUS-guided biopsies [9]. High PCa detection rates have been reported using magnetic resonance imaging (MRI)-targeted biopsies, both in patients with prior negative TRUS biopsies and in biopsy-naïve patients [9–13]. However, it is not clear whether prebiopsy MRI with a subsequent targeted biopsy is superior to the traditional systematic non-targeted TRUS biopsy in biopsy-naïve patients [14–16]. Therefore, this study examined whether prebiopsy mpMRI with the subsequent addition of targeted biopsies for suspicious lesions could improve the PCa detection rate in biopsy-naïve patients. These results were compared with those of a standard cohort of patients who underwent systematic non-targeted TRUS biopsies without MRI.

Methods

Patients

This retrospective observational study was approved by the local Institutional Review Board. The eligibility criteria were as follows: patients with a prostate-specific antigen (PSA) level < 15 ng/mL who underwent their first prostate biopsy for suspected PCa at Jichi Medical University or Jichi Medical University Saitama Medical Center between January 2010 and April 2014. Patients who underwent mpMRI before their prostate biopsy were assigned to the MRI cohort, whereas those who did not undergo MRI were assigned to the non-MRI cohort. Physicians decided who was to undergo MRI as their beliefs and patients' preferences after discussion with patients. A total of 557 patients were eligible: 383 at Jichi Medical University and 174 at Jichi Medical University Saitama Medical Center. Sixty-one patients were excluded based on the following criteria: interval from mpMRI to biopsy > 6 months (25 patients), < 12 biopsy cores (17 patients), MRI performed in another hospital (11 patients), the use of 5α-reductase inhibitors or anti-androgen therapy at the time of biopsy (6 patients), previous prostate surgical intervention (1 patient), and a blurred MRI scan (1 patient). Data from 496 patients were analyzed, and 215 and 281 patients were assigned to the MRI and non-MRI cohorts, respectively.

Imaging

All patients in the MRI cohort underwent mpMRI, which was performed using a 1.5-Tesla (Excelart Vantage, Toshiba Medical Systems, Otawara, Japan; MAGNETOM Symphony Advanced, Siemens, Munich, Germany; MAGNEOM Avanto, Siemens; or Achieva, Philips, Amsetrdam, Netherlands) or 3-Tesla (Vantage Titan 3 T, Toshiba Medical Systems; or MAGNETOM Skyra, Siemens) machine with a 16-channel phased-array body coil. The protocol included T2-weighted imaging, diffusion-weighted imaging, and dynamic contrast-enhanced imaging. Radiologists evaluated the mpMRI results and determined the locations of suspicious lesions. The likelihood of the presence of PCa was determined using a three-point scale (1 = low level of suspicion, 2 = equivocal, and 3 = high level of suspicion) because the standardized Prostate Imaging Reporting and Data System (PIRADS) criteria were not used to evaluate the images when the biopsies were performed. However, one very experienced genitourinary radiologist (T.O. or S.K.) at each institute blinded to the biopsy and the first MRI evaluation before biopsy reviewed and scored each suspicious lesion in the mpMRI image from 1 to 5 points according to the PIRADS criteria (ver. 2.0; PIRADS-2) [17, 18]. PI-RADS is both quantitative and qualitative, but only qualitative scoring was used in this study. The highest overall PIRADS-2 score of each mpMRI scan was used.

Biopsy protocol

All biopsies were performed using a transperineal approach with an 18-gauge needle biopsy gun under general or spinal anesthesia. In the non-MRI cohort, 12 to 14 cores were biopsied during non-targeted systematic TRUS-guided transperineal biopsies. In the MRI cohort, 12 to 14 cores were also biopsied during systematic TRUS-guided transperineal biopsies. However, in patients who had suspicious lesions on mpMRI, each lesion was targeted in one of the systematic biopsies and, typically, two cores of targeted biopsies were added for each lesion (Fig. 1). The targeted biopsies were performed using the cognitive registration technique described previously [19], with a minor modification: we used an ultrasound-guided freehand biopsy instead of a transperineal template.

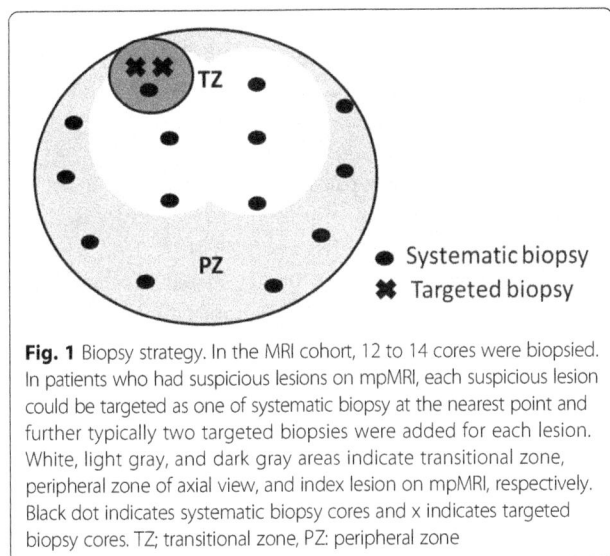

Fig. 1 Biopsy strategy. In the MRI cohort, 12 to 14 cores were biopsied. In patients who had suspicious lesions on mpMRI, each suspicious lesion could be targeted as one of systematic biopsy at the nearest point and further typically two targeted biopsies were added for each lesion. White, light gray, and dark gray areas indicate transitional zone, peripheral zone of axial view, and index lesion on mpMRI, respectively. Black dot indicates systematic biopsy cores and x indicates targeted biopsy cores. TZ; transitional zone, PZ: peripheral zone

Clinically significant cancer

Clinically significant PCa was defined as a Gleason score (GS) $\geq 3 + 4$ or a maximum cancer core length ≥ 4 mm; all other lesions were deemed as clinically insignificant PCa. This threshold has been validated to predict lesions with tumor volumes ≥ 2 mL [19].

Study endpoints

Patients' characteristics and cancer detection rate were compared between the MRI and non-MRI cohort. The endpoint of this study was the detection rate of all PCa and clinically significant PCa.

Statistical analysis

The data were analyzed using the Mann–Whitney U test or Fisher's exact test. Univariate and multivariate analyses were performed using logistic regression analysis to determine significant predictors of PCa. A p-value ≤ 0.05 was considered significant. The statistical analyses were performed using GraphPad Prism (ver. 5.0; GraphPad, La Jolla, CA, USA) and SPSS for Windows software (ver. 19.0; SPSS Inc., Chicago, IL, USA).

Results

Patient characteristics, MRI images, and biopsy strategy
There were no significant differences in patient characteristics between the two cohorts, except for prostate volume, which was significantly smaller in the MRI cohort than in the non-MRI cohort (median = 27.7 vs. 32.0 cm^3, $p = 0.0002$; Table 1). Examples of 1.5- and 3-Tesla MRI images are shown in Fig. 2. The 3-Tesla MRI seems to show the suspicious lesion clearly, compared to 1.5-Tesla MRI. Systematic biopsies were

Table 1 Patient characteristics and biopsy outcomes

	MRI (+) n = 215		MRI (−) n = 281		p Value
	Median	IQR	Median	IQR	
Age	68	(62–72)	68	(63–72)	0.21
PSA (ng/mL)	6.4	(5.2–8.8)	6.7	(5.5–9.4)	0.25
Prostate volume (cm^3)	27.7	(21.0–36.0)	32.0	(23.0–45.8)	0.0002
PSA density (ng/mL/cm^3)	0.22	(0.16–0.34)	0.23	(0.16–0.34)	0.79
DRE positive, n (%)	44	(20.5)	41	(14.6)	0.09
TRUS positive, n (%)	32	(14.9)	29	(10.3)	0.13
MRI type, n (%)					
1.5 Tesla	161	(74.9%)	(−)		
3 Tesla	54	(25.1%)	(−)		
Prostate cancer, n (%)	119	(55.3%)	118	(42.0%)	0.004
Gleason sum, n (%)					
3 + 3	34	(15.8%)	42	(14.9%)	0.80
3 + 4	43	(20.0%)	40	(14.5%)	0.08
4 + 3	16	(7.4%)	11	(3.9%)	0.11
8 or more	26	(12.1%)	25	(8.9%)	0.30
Clinical significance, n (%)					
Insignificant cancer	20	(9.3%)	19	(6.8%)	0.32
Significant cancer	99	(46.0%)	99	(35.2%)	0.016
Cancer positive cores	3	(1.25–5)	2	(1–4)	0.28

performed in all patients and the median number of cores collected was 12 [interquartile range (IQR) = 12–14] in both cohorts. Targeted biopsies for suspicious lesions on mpMRI were performed in 129 patients (60.0%) in the MRI cohort; 345 cores were targeted for 145 suspicious lesions; the median targeted core number per prostate was two (IQR = 2–4).

Cancer detection rate

The cancer detection rate was significantly higher in the MRI cohort than in the non-MRI cohort (55.3% vs. 42.0%, $p = 0.004$; Table 1). When cancer grade was compared between the two cohorts, there was no significant difference in the detection rate of low-grade cancer (GS 3 + 3; 15.8% in the MRI cohort vs. 14.9% in the non-MRI cohort, $p = 0.80$). However, detection of intermediate- or high-grade cancer (GS ≥ 3 + 4) was significantly higher in the MRI cohort compared with the non-MRI cohort (39.5% vs. 27.0%, respectively, $p = 0.004$). The clinically significant PCa detection rate was also higher in the MRI cohort than in the non-MRI cohort (46.0% vs. 35.2%, respectively, $p = 0.016$).

Systematic and targeted cores in each cohort

Table 2 summarizes the outcomes of the systematic and targeted cores in each cohort. The rate of cancer-positive cores and cores including a Gleason pattern of 4 or more was significantly higher in targeted biopsies than in systematic biopsies in the MRI and non-MRI cohorts, respectively (31.3 and 23.1% vs. 12.3 and 8.4%, and 10.0 and 5.9%, all $p < 0.0001$) (Table 2). The cancer-positive core rate for systematic biopsies in the MRI cohort was also significantly higher than that in the non-MRI cohort (12.3% vs. 10.0%, $p = 0.004$). The percentage of core length involved by cancer in

targeted cores was also significantly higher than that in systematic biopsies, in both the MRI and non-MRI cohorts [median (IQR) = 50% (20–70) vs. 30% (10–60) and 20% (10–50), $p = 0.0011$ and $p < 0.0001$].

Addition of targeted biopsies to systematic biopsies

Of the 129 patients who underwent systematic and targeted biopsies in the MRI cohort, 86 had PCa. We performed a subgroup analysis on these patients to assess the performance of the targeted biopsies (Fig. 3). Seven and four patients were diagnosed with PCa and upgraded to an intermediate and high grade, respectively, by the addition of targeted biopsies. The index lesions in seven patients missed by systematic biopsies but detected by targeted biopsies were in the anterior transitional zone ($n = 4$), anterior stroma ($n = 1$), anterior peripheral zone ($n = 1$), and posterolateral peripheral zone ($n = 1$). Twenty-nine patients were missed by targeted biopsies but detected by systematic biopsies.

Factors predicting prostate cancer detection

Univariate and multivariate analyses were performed to identify predictors of PCa detection (Table 3). Multivariate logistic regression analysis revealed that PSA level, prostate volume, performing prebiopsy mpMRI, and digital rectal examination findings were independent predictors of PCa detection.

Cancer detection rate according to PIRADS-2 score

The detection rate of all PCa and clinically significant PCa, stratified according to PIRADS-2 scores of 1, 2, 3, 4, and 5 in the MRI cohort, was 31.8 and 18.2%, 9.1 and 9.1%, 14.5 and 10.9%, 78.3 and 66.0%, and 83.3 and 80.0%, respectively (Table 4). The detection rate of clinically significant cancer was significantly higher in patients with

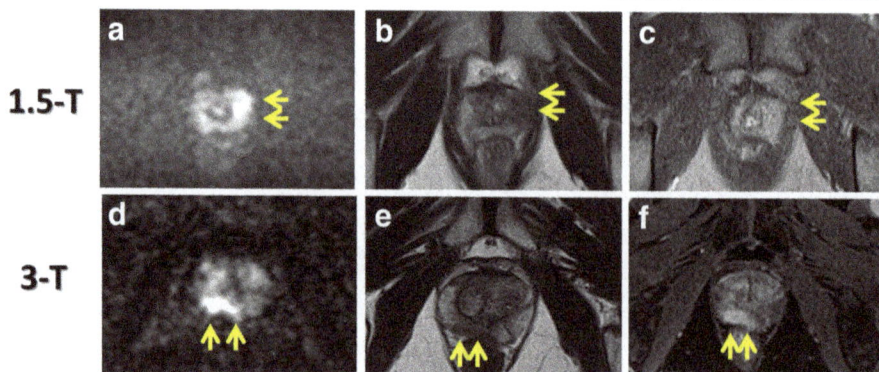

Fig. 2 MRI images. 1.5-Tesla MRI images obtained from a patient with a PSA level of 3.86 ng/mL (A – C). Diffusion weighted image (DWI) with a b-value 1500 s/mm^2 (A) showed a high intensity area in the left peripheral zone (Arrow). T2 weighted image (T2WI: B) and dynamic contrast enhancement image (DCEI: C) showed a low intensity area and an enhancement, respectively, in the same lesion, which was considered to be a high level of suspicious. 3-Tesla MRI images obtained from a patient with a PSA level of 3.57 ng/mL (D – F). DWI with a b-value 2000 s/mm^2 (D) showed a high intensity area in the right peripheral zone (Arrow). T2WI (E) and dynamic DCEI (F) showed a low intensity area and an enhancement, respectively, in the same lesion, which was considered to be a high level of suspicious

Table 2 Systematic and targeted cores in each cohort

	MRI (+)				MRI (−)		p Value		
	Systematic cores n = 2696 (A)		Targeted cores n = 345 (B)		Systematic cores n = 3542 (C)		A vs B	A vs C	B vs C
Cores of cancer, n (%)	333	(12.3)	108	(31.3)	355	(10.0)	< 0.0001	0.004	< 0.0001
Cores including GP 4 or more, n (%)	229	(8.4)	80	(23.1)	210	(5.9)	< 0.0001	0.0001	< 0.0001
Median percentage of core length involved by cancer (IQR)	30	(10–60)	50	(20–70)	20	(10–50)	0.0011	0.10	< 0.0001

a PIRADS-2 score of 4 or 5 compared with those with a PIRADS-2 score of 1–3 (69.3% vs. 12.5%; $p < 0.0001$). By contrast, there was no significant difference in the detection rate of clinically insignificant PCa between groups (10.2% vs. 5.7%; $p = 0.32$). When a PIRADS-2 score of 4 or 5 was considered positive, the sensitivity, specificity, positive predictive value (PPV), and negative predictive value (NPV) for PCa detection were 0.87 [95% confidence intervals (CI), 0.79–0.92], 0.75 (95% CI, 0.65–0.83), 0.81 (95% CI, 0.73–0.88), and 0.82 (95% CI, 0.72–0.89), respectively. Receiver operating characteristic (ROC) curve analysis for predicting PCa detection using the PIRADS-2 score revealed an area under the curve (AUC) of 0.801 (95% CI, 0.738–0.864), which was superior to AUC of 0.738 (95% CI, 0.670–0.806) in the three-point scale at the first radiological evaluation before biopsy.

Discussion

In this study, the detection rate of clinically significant PCa was significantly higher in the MRI cohort than the non-MRI cohort, whereas the clinically insignificant PCa detection rate was similar in both groups (Table 1). Performing MRI was an independent predictor of PCa detection (Table 3). These results suggest that prebiopsy MRI has the potential to improve biopsy outcomes in biopsy-naïve patients. We believe that a prebiopsy MRI has at least two advantages: patients can be selected more efficiently and a targeted biopsy of the index lesion can be added.

Traditionally, the decision regarding whether a prostate biopsy should be performed has been based mainly on the PSA, digital rectal examination findings, and age, which leads to inaccurate results. MRI can provide more precise information about the likelihood of the presence of PCa and prostate volume before biopsy. The prostate volume is negatively associated with the cancer detection rate, as shown in this (Table 3) and previous studies [20] and prostate volume was significantly smaller in the MRI cohort than the non-MRI cohort in this study (Table 1). These suggest that prostate biopsies might not be recommended in patients with a large prostate volume and/or normal MRI. Patient selection may partially explain the higher cancer detection rate in the MRI cohort. The combination of MRI findings and other biomarkers may better determine which patients should undergo prostate biopsy. Recently, we reported that the combination of PIRADS-2 score and PSA density was useful for decision-making before a prostate biopsy [21]. In that study, no patients with a PIRADS-2 score of ≤ 3 and PSA density of < 0.15 ng/mL/cm^3 were diagnosed with clinically significant PCa. In the present study, 27 patients had a PIRADS-2 score of ≤ 3 and PSA density of < 0.15 ng/mL/cm^3. Of these, no patients were diagnosed with clinically significant PCa (data not shown).

In this study, targeted biopsies based on MRI detected PCa more efficiently than systematic biopsies (Table 2). Furthermore, some patients in the MRI cohort were diagnosed with PCa or upgraded by the addition of targeted biopsies (Fig. 3). In particular, targeted biopsy

		Targeted				
		No cancer	GS 3+3	GS 7	GS 8 or more	Total
Systematic	No cancer	0	4	3	0	7
	GS 3+3	8	11	2	0	21
	GS 7	17	2	21	2	42
	GS 8 or more	4	0	1	11	16
	Total	29	17	27	13	86

Fig. 3 Cross-tabulation of histology (Gleason score) of targeted and systematic biopsy among patients who received both biopsies and had prostate cancer. Seven patients were diagnosed with prostate cancer by addition of targeted biopsies (dark gray box). Additionally, four patients were upgraded to intermediate or high grade by addition of targeted biopsies (light gray box). GS, Gleason score

Table 3 Univariate and multivariate analysis for prostate cancer detection in all patients

		N	Univariate analysis			Multivariate analysis		
			HR	95% CI	p-value	HR	95% CI	p-value
Age	≤ 65	189	–	–	–	(–)	(–)	0.101
	66–70	147	1.166	0.755–1.801	0.488			
	> 70	160	1.836	1.119–2.812	0.005			
PSA	≤ 5.0	89	–	–	–	–	–	–
	5.01–7.50	219	1.194	0.721–1.978	0.491	1.346	0.767–2.363	0.300
	7.51–10	97	1.949	1.085–3.499	0.026	2.620	1.342–5.115	0.005
	> 10.0	91	2.712	1.484–4.955	0.001	3.947	1.995–7.806	< 0.001
Prostate volume	≤ 25.0	176	–	–	–	–	–	–
	25.1–35.0	147	0.361	0.228–0.571	< 0.001	0.336	0.205–0.551	< 0.001
	> 35.0	173	0.135	0.084–0.217	< 0.001	0.112	0.073–0.204	< 0.001
MRI	No	281	–	–	–	–	–	–
	Yes	215	1.712	1.197–2.450	0.003	1.749	1.160–2.636	0.008
DRE	Negative	411	–	–	–	–	–	–
	Positive	85	4.193	2.467–7.126	< 0.001	3.068	1.704–5.526	< 0.001
TRUS	Negative	435	-	-	-	(–)	(–)	0.154
	Positive	61	2.500	1.418–4.407	0.002			

was beneficial for the diagnosis of anterior cancer because most of the tumors detected by targeted biopsies, but missed by systematic biopsies, were located in the anterior zone. Collectively, the addition of a targeted biopsy might improve the biopsy outcome. However, the effectiveness of targeted biopsy in this study may have been underestimated because the urologist was not blinded to the suspicious lesions on MRI, so that these could be targeted in systematic biopsies. This suggestion is supported by the fact that the cancer-positive core rate in systematic biopsies in the MRI cohort was significantly higher than that in the non-MRI cohort (Table 2). However, performing the study with the urologists blinded to the MRI during the systematic biopsies would be preferred to evaluate the effectiveness of systematic and targeted biopsies accurately. The cancer detection rate of 55.3% in the MRI cohort in this study was somewhat lower than that reported in previous series that performed targeted biopsies with or without systematic biopsies (56–64%) [10, 13, 22, 23]. Furthermore, one third of the tumors were missed by targeted biopsies, but detected by systematic biopsies (Fig. 3). Three

techniques have been reported for targeted biopsies: MRI-guided in-bore biopsy; MRI-TRUS fusion-guided biopsy; and cognitive registration. Although few direct comparisons have been performed, MRI-guided in-bore and MRI-TRUS fusion-guided biopsies likely yield a higher detection rate of clinically significant PCa compared with cognitive registration [13, 14, 22–24]. The cognitive registration technique was used in this study, which may have caused the somewhat low PCa detection rate. However, MRI-guided in-bore and MRI-TRUS fusion-guided biopsies have limited availability and are complex and costly to introduce and/or perform; therefore, they are not feasible for routine use so far. These suggest that targeted biopsies using cognitive registration are more practical and may improve the performance of prostate biopsy.

This study found a correlation between the PIRADS-2 score and PCa detection rate, especially in clinically significant PCa. ROC analysis revealed an AUC of 0.801 which was superior to that of 0.738 in the three-point scale; the sensitivity, specificity, PPV, and NPV were 0.87, 0.75, 0.81, and 0.82, respectively. A meta-analysis

Table 4 Cancer detection rate according to PI-RADS v2 score

	PI-RADS v2 score				
	1 n = 22	2 n = 11	3 n = 55	4 n = 97	5 n = 30
Insignificant PCa, n (%)	3 (13.6%)	0 (0%)	2 (3.6%)	12 (12.4%)	1 (3.3%)
Significant PCa, n (%)	4 (18.2%)	1 (9.1%)	6 (10.9%)	64 (66.0%)	24 (80.0%)
Total PCa, n (%)	7 (31.8%)	1 (9.1%)	8 (14.5%)	76 (78.3%)	25 (83.3%)

assessing the performance of mpMRI for detecting PCa found a specificity of 0.88 (95% CI, 0.82–0.92), sensitivity of 0.74 (95% CI, 0.66–0.81), and NPV of 0.64–0.94, which is consistent with our results. Recently, PIRADS was annotated, revised, and published as a second version, PIRADS-2, to define standards of high-quality clinical service for mpMRI, including image creation and reporting [17, 18]. Kuru et al. performed ROC analysis for PCa detection using the PIRADS score and found an excellent specificity of 0.90–0.98 [25]. Grey et al. [26] reported that a ROC analysis of clinically significant PCa yielded an AUC of 0.88–0.89 and sensitivity, specificity, PPV, and NPV of 0.95–0.97, 0.6, 0.58–0.61, and 0.97–0.98, respectively. The difference in the ability to predict biopsy outcome among studies may be due to differences in the MRI machines and protocols used, as well as to variations in the PIRADS scoring, biopsy protocols, and patient characteristics.

Two recent randomized controlled trials (RCTs) compared the outcomes between prebiopsy MRI with the addition of a targeted biopsy and a conventional TRUS-guided random biopsy [15, 16]. One used a MRI-TRUS fusion targeted biopsy, while the other used the cognitive registration technique, similar to our study. Both found that the PCa detection rate was similar between the MRI and control groups, which is not consistent with our results. Selection bias in our retrospective study could have been the major reason for the difference versus the two RCTs, and patient selection after MRI may have been one of the major causes of the higher cancer detection rate in our MRI cohort. There were also differences in the study protocols, sample sizes, and biopsy protocols among studies. Furthermore, the PCa detection rate of 54–57% for the conventional TRUS-guided biopsy of the two RCTs was higher than that in our study, and another reported study [5].

This study had some limitations. First, the analysis was retrospective and patient selection bias may have been present, as described above. However, it appears based on the statistics that the two cohorts were very similar other than prostate size. Second, PIRADS scoring was not performed at the same time as the biopsy. Third, some patients underwent 1.5-Tesla MRI, whereas others underwent 3-Tesla MRI, reflecting technological changes. However, the PCa detection rate did not differ significantly between 1.5-Tesla and 3-Tesla MRI (data not shown). Fourth, there is no widely accepted definition of clinically significant PCa. Fifth, the promise of targeted biopsies is to reduce the number of total biopsies. However, our study suggests that systematic biopsies should not be omitted when cognitive fusion transperineal

biopsies are performed because one third of the tumors were missed by targeted biopsies but detected by systematic biopsies (Fig. 3). Sixth, several radiologists were involved in reporting the MRIs and several urologists performed biopsies. However, this could be deemed an advantage, since clinical effectiveness of prebiopsy mpMRI was demonstrated despite this heterogeneity. Finally, only one radiologist was involved in the MRI review of the PIRADS-2 scoring in each institution; therefore, inter-observer reliability could not be assessed.

Conclusions
Prebiopsy mpMRI with subsequent systematic plus targeted biopsies could yield a more clinically significant PCa detection rate than a non-targeted TRUS-guided biopsy in biopsy-naïve patients. PIRADS-2 scoring is useful for predicting biopsy outcome. However, large prospective studies are needed to confirm our results.

Abbreviations
AUC: Area under the curve; CI: Confidence intervals; GS: Gleason score; IQR: Interquartile range; mpMRI: multiparametric magnetic resonance imaging; MRI: Magnetic resonance imaging; NPV: Negative predictive values; PCa: Prostate cancer; PIRADS: Prostate imaging reporting and data system; PIRADS-2: Prostate imaging reporting and data system version 2.0; PPV: Positive predictive values; ROC: Receiver operating characteristic; TRUS: Transrectal ultrasound

Funding
There was no financial or material support for this article.

Authors' contributions
SW contributed to the study design, data collection, interpretation and manuscript writing. SK, TO, T Kameda, and T Konishi contributed to data collection and interpretation. T Miyagawa, TT, and T Morita contributed to data analysis and manuscript writing. All authors read and approved the final manuscript.

Ethics approval and consent to participate
The study protocol was reviewed and approved by the Institutional Review Board at Jichi Medical University or Jichi Medical University Saitama Medical Center (Rin15–29 and RinA14–096) and obtaining additional informed consent from patients was not required by the ethics committee for this retrospective study.

Competing interests
The authors declare that they have no competing interests.

Author details
[1]Department of Urology, Jichi Medical University, 3311-1 Yakushiji, Shimotsuke, Tochigi 329-0498, Japan. [2]Department of Radiology, Jichi Medical University, 3311-1 Yakushiji, Shimotsuke, Tochigi 329-0498, Japan. [3]Department of Urology, Jichi Medical University Saitama Medical Center, 1-847, Amanuma-cho, Omiya-ku, Saitama 330-8503, Japan. [4]Department of Radiology, Jichi Medical University Saitama Medical Center, 1-847, Amanuma-cho, Omiya-ku, Saitama 330-8503, Japan.

References

1. Center MM, Jemal A, Lortet-Tieulent J, Ward E, Ferlay J, Brawley O, Bray F. International Variation in Prostate Cancer Incidence and Mortality Rates. European Urology. 2012;61(6):1079–92.

2. Sinnott M, Falzarano SM, Hernandez AV, Jones JS, Klein EA, Zhou M, Magi-Galluzzi C. Discrepancy in prostate cancer localization between biopsy and prostatectomy specimens in patients with unilateral positive biopsy: implications for focal therapy. Prostate. 2012;72(11):1179–86.

3. Han M, Chang D, Kim C, Lee BJ, Zuo Y, Kim H-J, Petrisor D, Trock B, Partin AW, Rodriguez R, et al. Geometric evaluation of systematic transrectal ultrasound guided prostate biopsy. J Urol. 2012;188(6):2404–9.

4. de Rooij M, Hamoen EHJ, Futterer JJ, Barentsz JO, Rovers MM. Accuracy of multiparametric MRI for prostate Cancer detection: a meta-analysis. Am J Roentgenol. 2014;202(2):343–51.

5. Trabulsi EJ, Halpern EJ, Gomella LG. Ultrasonography and biopsy of the prostate. In: Wein AJ, editor. Campbell-Walsh Urology. 10th ed; 2011. p. 2735.

6. Hossack T, Patel MI, Huo A, Brenner P, Yuen C, Spernat D, Mathews J, Haynes A-M, Sutherland R, Del Prado W, et al. Location and pathological characteristics of cancers in radical prostatectomy specimens identified by Transperineal biopsy compared to Transrectal biopsy. J Urol. 2012;188(3):781–5.

7. Mazaheri Y, Shukla-Dave A, Muellner A, Hricak H. MR imaging of the prostate in clinical practice. Magn Reson Mater Phys Biol Med. 2008;21(6):379–92.

8. Hamoen E, de Rooij M, Witjes J, Barentsz J, Rovers M. Use of the prostate imaging reporting and data system (PI-RADS) for prostate Cancer detection with multiparametric magnetic resonance imaging: a diagnostic meta-analysis. Eur Urol. 2015;67(6):1112–21.

9. Siddiqui MM, Rais-Bahrami S, Hong T, Stamatakis L, Vourganti S, Nix J, Hoang AN, Walton-Diaz A, Shuch B, Weintraub M, et al. Magnetic resonance imaging/ultrasound-fusion biopsy significantly upgrades prostate Cancer versus systematic 12-core Transrectal ultrasound biopsy. Eur Urol. 2013;64(5):713–9.

10. Overduin CG, Futterer JJ, Barentsz JO. MRI-guided biopsy for prostate Cancer detection: a systematic review of current clinical results. Curr Urol Rep. 2013;14(3):209–13.

11. Park BK, Park JW, Park SY, Kim CK, Lee HM, Jeon SS, Seo SI, Jeong BC, Choi HY. Prospective evaluation of 3-T MRI performed before initial Transrectal ultrasound-guided prostate biopsy in patients with high prostate-specific antigen and no previous biopsy. Am J Roentgenol. 2011;197(5):W876–81.

12. Haffner J, Lemaitre L, Puech P, Haber G-P, Leroy X, Jones JS, Villers A. Role of magnetic resonance imaging before initial biopsy: comparison of magnetic resonance imaging-targeted and systematic biopsy for significant prostate cancer detection. BJU Int. 2011;108(8B):E171–8.

13. Quentin M, Blondin D, Arsov C, Schimmoeller L, Hiester A, Godehardt E, Albers P, Antoch G, Rabenalt R. Prospective evaluation of magnetic resonance imaging guided in-bore prostate biopsy versus systematic Transrectal ultrasound guided prostate biopsy in biopsy naive men with elevated prostate specific antigen. J Urol. 2014;192(5):1374–9.

14. Delongchamps NB, Peyromaure M, Schull A, Beuvon F, Bouazza N, Flam T, Zerbib M, Muradyan N, Legman P, Cornud F. Prebiopsy magnetic resonance imaging and prostate Cancer detection: comparison of random and targeted biopsies. J Urol. 2013;189(2):493–9.

15. Tonttila PP, Lantto J, Paakko E, Piippo U, Kauppila S, Lammentausta E, Ohtonen P, Vaarala MH. Prebiopsy multiparametric magnetic resonance imaging for prostate cancer diagnosis in biopsy-naive men with suspected prostate cancer based on elevated prostate-specific antigen values: results from a randomized prospective blinded controlled trial. Eur Urol. 2016;69(3):419–25.

16. Baco E, Rud E, Eri LM, Moen G, Vlatkovic L, Svindland A, Eggesbo HB, Ukimura O. A randomized controlled trial to assess and compare the outcomes of two-core prostate biopsy guided by fused magnetic resonance and Transrectal ultrasound images and traditional 12-core systematic biopsy. Eur Urol. 2016;69(1):149–56.

17. Barentsz JO, Richenberg J, Clements R, Choyke P, Verma S, Villeirs G, Rouviere O, Logager V, Futterer JJ. ESUR prostate MR guidelines 2012. Eur Radiol. 2012;22(4):746–57.

18. Weinreb JC, Barentsz JO, Choyke PL, Cornud F, Haider MA, Macura KJ, Margolis D, Schnall MD, Shtern F, Tempany CM, et al. PI-RADS prostate imaging - reporting and data system: 2015, version 2. Eur Urol. 2016;69(1):16–40.

19. Kasivisvanathan V, Dufour R, Moore CM, Ahmed HU, Abd-Alazeez M, Charman SC, Freeman A, Allen C, Kirkham A, van der Meulen J, et al. Transperineal magnetic resonance image targeted prostate biopsy versus Transperineal template prostate biopsy in the detection of clinically significant prostate Cancer. J Urol. 2013;189(3):860–6.

20. Symons JL, Huo A, Yuen CL, Haynes A-M, Matthews J, Sutherland RL, Brenner P, Stricker PD. Outcomes of transperineal template-guided prostate biopsy in 409 patients. BJU Int. 2013;112(5):585–93.

21. Washino S, Okochi T, Saito K, Konishi T, Hirai M, Kobayashi Y, Miyagawa T. Combination of PI-RADS score and PSA density predicts biopsy outcome in biopsy naïve patients. BJU Int. 2017;119(2):225–33.

22. Miyagawa T, Ishikawa S, Kimura T, Suetomi T, Tsutsumi M, Irie T, Kondoh M, Mitake T. Real-time virtual sonography for navigation during targeted prostate biopsy using magnetic resonance imaging data. Int J Urol. 2010;17(10):855–60.

23. Pokorny MR, De Rooij M, Duncan E, Schroeder FH, Parkinson R, Barentsz JO, Thompson LC. Prospective study of diagnostic accuracy comparing prostate Cancer detection by Transrectal ultrasound-guided biopsy versus magnetic resonance (MR) imaging with subsequent MR-guided biopsy in men without previous prostate biopsies. Eur Urol. 2014;66(1):22–9.

24. Cool DW, Zhang X, Romagnoli C, Izawa JI, Romano WM, Fenster A. Evaluation of MRI-TRUS fusion versus cognitive registration accuracy for MRI-targeted, TRUS-guided prostate biopsy. Am J Roentgenol. 2015;204(1):83–91.

25. Kuru TH, Roethke MC, Rieker P, Roth W, Fenchel M, Hohenfellner M, Schlemmer H-P, Hadaschik BA. Histology core-specific evaluation of the European Society of Urogenital Radiology (ESUR) standardised scoring system of multiparametric magnetic resonance imaging (mpMRI) of the prostate. BJU Int. 2013;112(8):1080–7.

26. Grey ADR, Chana MS, Popert R, Wolfe K, Liyanage SH, Acher PL. Diagnostic accuracy of magnetic resonance imaging (MRI) prostate imaging reporting and data system (PI-RADS) scoring in a transperineal prostate biopsy setting. BJU Int. 2015;115(5):728–35.

Permissions

All chapters in this book were first published in UROLOGY, by BioMed Central; hereby published with permission under the Creative Commons Attribution License or equivalent. Every chapter published in this book has been scrutinized by our experts. Their significance has been extensively debated. The topics covered herein carry significant findings which will fuel the growth of the discipline. They may even be implemented as practical applications or may be referred to as a beginning point for another development.

The contributors of this book come from diverse backgrounds, making this book a truly international effort. This book will bring forth new frontiers with its revolutionizing research information and detailed analysis of the nascent developments around the world.

We would like to thank all the contributing authors for lending their expertise to make the book truly unique. They have played a crucial role in the development of this book. Without their invaluable contributions this book wouldn't have been possible. They have made vital efforts to compile up to date information on the varied aspects of this subject to make this book a valuable addition to the collection of many professionals and students.

This book was conceptualized with the vision of imparting up-to-date information and advanced data in this field. To ensure the same, a matchless editorial board was set up. Every individual on the board went through rigorous rounds of assessment to prove their worth. After which they invested a large part of their time researching and compiling the most relevant data for our readers.

The editorial board has been involved in producing this book since its inception. They have spent rigorous hours researching and exploring the diverse topics which have resulted in the successful publishing of this book. They have passed on their knowledge of decades through this book. To expedite this challenging task, the publisher supported the team at every step. A small team of assistant editors was also appointed to further simplify the editing procedure and attain best results for the readers.

Apart from the editorial board, the designing team has also invested a significant amount of their time in understanding the subject and creating the most relevant covers. They scrutinized every image to scout for the most suitable representation of the subject and create an appropriate cover for the book.

The publishing team has been an ardent support to the editorial, designing and production team. Their endless efforts to recruit the best for this project, has resulted in the accomplishment of this book. They are a veteran in the field of academics and their pool of knowledge is as vast as their experience in printing. Their expertise and guidance has proved useful at every step. Their uncompromising quality standards have made this book an exceptional effort. Their encouragement from time to time has been an inspiration for everyone.

The publisher and the editorial board hope that this book will prove to be a valuable piece of knowledge for researchers, students, practitioners and scholars across the globe.

List of Contributors

Pridvi Kandagatla
Department of Urology, Wayne State University School of Medicine, 9200 Scott Hall 540 E. Canfield Avenue, Detroit, MI 48201, USA

Sreenivasa R Chinni
Department of Urology, Wayne State University School of Medicine, 9200 Scott Hall 540 E. Canfield Avenue, Detroit, MI 48201, USA
Department of Pathology, Wayne State University School of Medicine, 9200 Scott Hall 540 E. Canfield Avenue, Detroit, MI 48201, USA
The Barbara Ann Karmanos Cancer Institute, Detroit, MI 48201, USA

Donald Wong and Walter Korz
British Canadian Bio Science Corporation, Vancouver, Canada

Klaus-Peter Dieckmann, Petra Anheuser and Raphael Ikogho
Albertinen-Krankenhaus, Department of Urology, Suentelstrasse 11a, D-22457 Hamburg, Germany

Ralf Gehrckens
Albertinen-Krankenhaus, Department of Diagnostic Radiology, Hamburg, Germany

Sven Philip Aries
Elbpneumologie, Mörkenstrasse 47, D-22767 Hamburg, Germany

Wiebke Hollburg
Hämatologisch-onkologische Praxis Altona (HOPA), Mörkenstrasse 47, D-22767 Hamburg, Germany
Joanna Kubicka-Wołkowska, Sylwia Dębska-Szmich, Maja Lisik-Habib and Piotr Potemski
Department of Chemotherapy, Medical University of Lodz, Paderewskiego 4, 93-509 Lodz, Poland

Marcin Noweta
Department of Dermatology, Paediatric Dermatology and Dermatological Oncology, Medical University of Lodz, Lodz, Poland

Karsten Günzel, Hannes Cash, John Buckendahl, Maximilian Königbauer, Jörg Neymeyer, Stefan Hinz, Kurt Miller and Carsten Kempkensteffen
Department of Urology, Charité — University Medicine Berlin, Hindenburgdamm 30, 12203 Berlin, Germany

Patrick Asbach and Matthias Haas
Departement of Radiology, Charité — University Medicine Berlin, Hindenburgdamm 30, 12203 Berlin, Germany

Evgenii Kim and Zephaniah Phillips V
School of Information and Communications, Gwangju Institute of Science and Technology, Gwangju 500-712, Korea

Songhyun Lee and Jae G Kim
Department of Medical System Engineering, Gwangju Institute of Science and Technology, Gwangju 500-712, Korea

Andrea Fuschi
Sapienza University of Rome, Department of Medical and Surgical Biotechnologies, Unit of Urology, ICOT, Via Franco Faggiana 1668, 04100 Latina, Italy

Giovanni Palleschi, Antonio Carbone and Antonio Luigi Pastore
Sapienza University of Rome, Department of Medical and Surgical Biotechnologies, Unit of Urology, ICOT, Via Franco Faggiana 1668, 04100 Latina, Italy
Uroresearch Association, non profit association, Via Franco Faggiana 1668, 04100 Latina, Italy

Vincenzo Petrozza, Natale Porta and Jessica Cacciotti
Department of Medical and Surgical Biotechnologies, Histopathology Unit, ICOT Latina, via Faggiana 1668, Latina, Italy

Giorgia Manfredonia
ICOT Hospital, CADI Centre, via Faggiana 1668, Latina, Italy

Cosimo de Nunzio
Sapienza University of Rome, Department of Urology, Sant'Andrea Hospital, Rome, Italy

Zhengbang Dong, Haijing Yang, Jingdong Zhang and Fei Wang
Department of Dermatology, Zhongda Hospital, Southeast University, Nanjing, Jiangsu 210009, China

Chao Qin, Qijie Zhang and Lei Zhang
Department of Urology, First Affiliated Hospital of Nanjing Medical University, Nanjing, Jiangsu 210029, China

Haifeng Huang, Wei Wang, Tingsheng Lin, Qing Zhang, Xiaozhi Zhao and Huibo Lian
Department of Urology, Affiliated Drum Tower Hospital, Medical School of Nanjing University, Nanjing 210008, China

Hongqian Guo
Department of Urology, Affiliated Drum Tower Hospital, Medical School of Nanjing University, Nanjing 210008, China
Institute of Urology, Nanjing University, Nanjing 210008, China

Franz Hamann, C. Hamann, A. Trettel, K P Jünemann and C M Naumann
Department of Urology and Pediatric Urology, University Hospital Schleswig Holstein, Campus Kiel, Arnold Heller Str. 3, 24105 Kiel, Germany

Tian-Fu Li, Qiu-Yue Wu, Cui Zhang, Wei-Wei Li, Qing Zhou, Wei-Jun Jiang, Ying-Xia Cui and Xin-Yi Xia
Department of Reproduction and Genetics, Institute of Laboratory Medicine, Jinling Hospital, Nanjing University School of Medicine, Nanjing 210002, PR China

Yi-Chao Shi
Center for Reproduction and Genetics, Suzhou Municipal Hospital, Nanjing Medical University Affiliated Suzhou Hospital, 26 Daoqian Street, Suzhou 215002, PR China

Richard Morgan, Angie Boxall, Guy R Simpson, Agnieszka Michael and Hardev S Pandha
Faculty of Health and Medical Sciences, University of Surrey, Guildford, UK

Kevin J Harrington
Targeted Therapy Team, Chester Beatty Laboratories, The Institute of Cancer Research, London, UK

Riina-Minna Väänänen, Natalia Tong Ochoa and Kim Pettersson
Department of Biotechnology, University of Turku, Turku, Finland

Peter J. Boström
Department of Urology, Turku University Hospital, Turku, Finland

Pekka Taimen
Department of Pathology, University of Turku and Turku University Hospital, Turku, Finland

Marrissa Martyn-St James, Katy Cooper, Eva Kaltenthaler, Kath Dickinson and Anna Cantrell
School for Health and Related Research (ScHARR), University of Sheffield, Regent Court, 30 Regent Street, Sheffield S1 4DA, UK

Kevan Wylie
Porterbrook Clinic, Sexual Medicine, Sheffield, UK

Leila Frodsham
Institute of Psychosexual Medicine, London, UK

Catherine Hood
St George's Hospital, London, UK

Eva Gupta and Winston Tan
Mayo Clinic, 4500 San Pablo Rd S, Jacksonville 32224, FL, USA

Troy Guthrie
Baptist Cancer Institute, Jacksonville, FL, USA

Isaura Danielli Borges de Sousa and Maria do Desterro Soares Brandão Nascimento
Tumors and DNA Bank of Maranhão, Federal University of Maranhão (UFMA), São Luís, Brazil

Flávia Castello Branco Vidal
Tumors and DNA Bank of Maranhão, Federal University of Maranhão (UFMA), São Luís, Brazil
Department of Morphology, Federal University of Maranhão (UFMA), São Luís, Brazil

Luciane Maria Oliveira Brito
Tumors and DNA Bank of Maranhão, Federal University of Maranhão (UFMA), São Luís, Brazil
Department of Medicine III, Federal University of Maranhão (UFMA), São Luís, Brazil

João Paulo Castello Branco Vidal
José Alencar Gomes da Silva National Cancer Institute, Department of Genetics, Rio de Janeiro, Brazil

George Castro Figueira de Mello
Maranhão State Institute of Oncology Aldenora Bello (IMOAB), São Luis, MA, Brazil

Yasushi Nakai, Satoshi Anai, Masaomi Kuwada, Makito Miyake, Yoshitomo Chihara, Nobumichi Tanaka, Akihide Hirayama, Katsunori Yoshida, Yoshihiko Hirao and Kiyohide Fujimoto
Department of Urology, Nara Medical University, 840 Shijo-cho, Kashihara-shi, Nara 634-8522, Japan

Jae Young Joung, Jeong Eun Kim, Sung Han Kim, Ho Kyung Seo, Jinsoo Chung and Kang Hyun Lee
Center for Prostate Cancer, National Cancer Center, Goyang, South Korea

Weon Seo Park and Eun Kyung Hong
Department of Pathology, National Cancer Center, Goyang, South Korea

Paulo Príncipe
Department of Urology, Porto Hospital Centre – St. António Hospital, Largo Prof. Abel Salazar, 4000-001 Porto, Portugal
Center for Urological Research, Department of Urology, Porto Hospital Centre – St. António Hospital, Porto, Portugal

Avelino Fraga
Department of Urology, Porto Hospital Centre – St. António Hospital, Largo Prof. Abel Salazar, 4000-001 Porto, Portugal
Center for Urological Research, Department of Urology, Porto Hospital Centre – St. António Hospital, Porto, Portugal

Ricardo Ribeiro
Center for Urological Research, Department of Urology, Porto Hospital Centre – St. António Hospital, Porto, Portugal
Molecular Oncology Group - CI, Portuguese Institute of Oncology, Porto, Portugal
Genetics Laboratory, Faculty of Medicine, University of Lisbon, Lisbon, Portugal

Carlos Lopes
ICBAS, Abel Salazar Biomedical Sciences Institute, University of Porto, Porto, Portugal

Rui Medeiros
ICBAS, Abel Salazar Biomedical Sciences Institute, University of Porto, Porto, Portugal
Molecular Oncology Group - CI, Portuguese Institute of Oncology, Porto, Portugal

André Coelho and José Ramon Vizcaíno
Department of Pathology, Porto Hospital Centre – St. António Hospital, Porto, Portugal

Helena Coutinho
Department of Pathology and Oncology, Faculty of Medicine, University of Porto, Porto, Portugal

José Manuel Lopes
Department of Pathology and Oncology, Faculty of Medicine, University of Porto, Porto, Portugal
Institute of Pathology and Molecular Immunology of University of Porto (IPATIMUP), Porto, Portugal

Carlos Lobato
Department of Urology, Porto Military Hospital, Porto, Portugal

Steffen Rausch, Joerg Hennenlotter, Josef Wiesenreiter, Andrea Hohneder, Julian Heinkele, Christian Schwentner and Arnulf Stenzl
Department of Urology, Eberhard-Karls-University Tuebingen, Hoppe-Seyler-Str. 3, 72076 Tuebingen, Germany

Tilman Todenhöfer
Department of Urology, Eberhard-Karls-University Tuebingen, Hoppe-Seyler-Str. 3, 72076 Tuebingen, Germany
Vancouver Prostate Centre, University of British Columbia, 2660 Oak Street, Vancouver V6H 3Z6, Canada

Divya Shenoy
University of Mississippi Medical School, Jackson, MS, USA

Satyaseelan Packianathan
University of Mississippi Medical Center, 2500 North State Street, 39216-4505 Jackson, MS, USA

Srinivasan Vijayakumar
University of Mississippi Medical Center, 2500 North State Street, 39216-4505 Jackson, MS, USA
UMMC Cancer Institute, Department of Radiation Oncology, 2500 North State Street, 39216-4505 Jackson, MS, USA

Allen M. Chen
University of California, Los Angeles-David Geffen School of Medicine, Los Angeles, California, USA

Catherine Coyle
Public Health Agency, Belfast, Northern Ireland

Eileen Morgan and Anna Gavin
Northern Ireland Cancer Registry, Queen's University, Belfast, Northern Ireland

Frances J. Drummond
National Cancer Registry Ireland, Cork, Ireland
Department of Epidemiology and Public Health, University College Cork, Cork, Ireland

Linda Sharp
National Cancer Registry Ireland, Cork, Ireland
Institute of Health & Society, Newcastle University, Newcastle, UK

Götz Geiges
Arztpraxis für Urologie (Partnerpraxis der Charité), Berlin, Germany

Thomas Harms
Gemeinschaftspraxis Urologikum, Köln, Germany

Gerald Rodemer
Praxisgemeinschaft für Onkologie und Urologie, Wilhelmshaven, Germany

Ralf Eckert
Urologische Arztpraxis, Lutherstadt Eisleben, Germany

Frank König and Jörg Schroder
ATURO – Praxis für Urologie, Berlin, Germany

Rolf Eichenauer
Urologikum Hamburg, Hamburg, Germany

Seiji Hoshi, Yuichi Sato, Junya Hata, Hidenori Akaihata, Soichiro Ogawa, Nobuhiro Haga and Yoshiyuki Kojima
Department of Urology, Fukushima Medical University School of Medicine, 1, Hikarigaoka, Fukushima 960-1295, Japan

Jannicke Frugård
Department of Urology, Haukeland University Hospital, N-5021 Bergen, Norway

Karsten Gravdal
Department of Pathology, Haukeland University Hospital, N-5021 Bergen, Norway

Yngve Nygård, Svein A. Haukaas and Christian Beisland
Department of Urology, Haukeland University Hospital, N-5021 Bergen, Norway
Department of Clinical Medicine, University of Bergen, Bergen, Norway

Ole J. Halvorsen and Lars A. Akslen
Department of Pathology, Haukeland University Hospital, N-5021 Bergen, Norway
Center for Cancer Biomarkers CCBIO, Department of Clinical Medicine, University of Bergen, Bergen, Norway

M. Raghavendran
Department Of Urology, Apollo BGS Hospitals, Adichunchunagiri Road, Kuvempunagar, Mysore, Karnataka 570009, India

A. Venugopal
Apollo BGS Hospitals, Mysore, Karnataka, India

G. Kiran Kumar
Department Of Urology, Apollo Hospitals, Mysore, Karnataka, India

Darren M. C. Poon and Daisy Lam
Department of Clinical Oncology, State Key Laboratory in Oncology in South China, Sir YK Pao Centre for Cancer, Hong Kong Cancer Institute and Prince of Wales Hospital, The Chinese University of Hong Kong, Hong Kong, Hong Kong
Hong Kong Society of Uro-Oncology (HKSUO), Hong Kong, Hong Kong

Kuen Chan
Department of Clinical Oncology, Pamela Youde Nethersole Eastern Hospital, Hong Kong, Hong Kong
Hong Kong Society of Uro-Oncology (HKSUO), Hong Kong, Hong Kong

S. H. Lee
Department of Oncology, Princess Margaret Hospital, Hong Kong, Hong Kong
Hong Kong Society of Uro-Oncology (HKSUO), Hong Kong, Hong Kong T. W. Chan
Department of Clinical Oncology, Queen Elizabeth Hospital, Hong Kong, Hong Kong
Hong Kong Society of Uro-Oncology (HKSUO), Hong Kong, Hong Kong

Henry Sze and Michelle F. T. Chan
Department of Clinical Oncology, Queen Mary Hospital, Hong Kong, Hong Kong

Hong Kong Society of Uro-Oncology (HKSUO), Hong Kong, Hong Kong

Eric K. C. Lee
Department of Clinical Oncology, Tuen Mun Hospital, Hong Kong, Hong Kong
Hong Kong Society of Uro-Oncology (HKSUO), Hong Kong, Hong Kong

Tim Schubert, Jens Uphoff, Friedhelm Wawroschek and Alexander Winter
University Hospital for Urology, Klinikum Oldenburg, School of Medicine and Health Sciences, Carl von Ossietzky University Oldenburg, Rahel-Straus-Straße 10, 26133 Oldenburg, Germany

Rolf-Peter Henke
Oldenburg Institute of Pathology, Taubenstraße 28, 26122 Oldenburg, Germany

Tomohiro Kameda, Tatsuya Takayama and Tatsuo Morita
Department of Urology, Jichi Medical University, 3311-1 Yakushiji, Shimotsuke, Tochigi 329-0498, Japan

Satoshi Washino
Department of Urology, Jichi Medical University, 3311-1 Yakushiji, Shimotsuke, Tochigi 329-0498, Japan
Department of Urology, Jichi Medical University Saitama Medical Center, 1-847, Amanuma-cho, Omiya-ku, Saitama 330-8503, Japan

Shigeru Kobayashi
Department of Radiology, Jichi Medical University, 3311-1 Yakushiji, Shimotsuke, Tochigi 329-0498, Japan

Tsuzumi Konoshi and Tomoaki Miyagawa
Department of Urology, Jichi Medical University Saitama Medical Center, 1-847, Amanuma-cho, Omiya-ku, Saitama 330-8503, Japan

Tomohisa Okochi
Department of Radiology, Jichi Medical University Saitama Medical Center, 1-847, Amanuma-cho, Omiya-ku, Saitama 330-8503, Japan

Index